MULTIPLE MYELOMA – AN OVERVIEW

Edited by **Ajay Gupta**

Multiple Myeloma – An Overview
Edited by Ajay Gupta

Published by InTech
Janeza Trdine 9, 51000 Rijeka, Croatia

Publishing Process Manager Oliver Kurelic

Technical Editor Teodora Smiljanic

Cover Designer InTech Design Team

Additional hard copies can be obtained from orders@intechopen.com

Multiple Myeloma – An Overview, Edited by Ajay Gupta
p. cm.
ISBN 978-953-307-768-0

Meet the editor

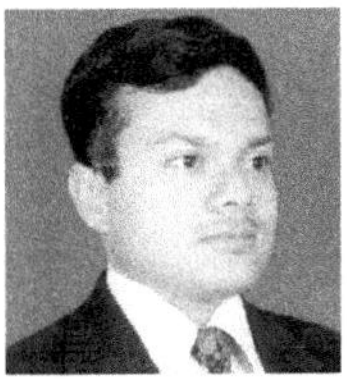

Dr. Ajay Gupta MD, is a Senior Consultant in Medical Oncology at Max Cancer Center in New Delhi. He received the 2008 American Society of Clinical Oncology (ASCO) Foundation Brigid Leventhal Award for Pediatric Oncology (for the best work in pediatric cancer research) for his work entitled 'Randomized control trial comparing efficacy of oral amoxicillin-clavulanate and ofloxacin with intravenous ceftriaxone and amikacin as outpatient therapy in pediatric low-risk febrile neutropenia'. His professional interests include hematology and bone marrow transplants. He received his medical oncology fellowship from the All India Institute of Medical Sciences in New Delhi. Dr Gupta also trained in cardiology and internal medicine and has received the Certificate of Completion of Specialist Training (CCST) from the Specialist Training Authority of Medical Royal Colleges in General Internal Medicine in the UK.

Contents

Preface

Multiple myeloma is a malignant disorder characterized by the proliferation of plasma cells. It accounts for 10% of hematological cancers and 1% of all cancers. The disease is uniformly fatal with a median survival of approximately three years with conventional chemotherapy, although the outlook has improved with the integration of newer therapies including high-dose therapy followed by autologous stem cell transplantation.

Much insight has been gained into the molecular pathways that lead to myeloma and indeed much more remains to be done. The understanding of these pathways is closely linked to their therapeutic implications and is stressed upon in the initial chapters.

The role of multiple pro-inflammatory pathways, hypoxia inducing factor, tumor necrosis factor, proteasomes , sumoylation pathways and their therapeutic importance is examined as is the role of experimental therapies like dendritic cell therapy.

Recently, the introduction of newer agents such as bortezomib, lenalidomide, thalidomide, liposomal doxorubicin, etc. has led to a flurry of trials aimed at testing various combinations in order to improve survival. Higher response rates observed with these agents have led to their integration into induction therapies. It has raised questions in terms of redefining the inclusion criteria/timing and expected benefits of stem cell transplantation.

The role of various new therapies vis a vis transplantation has also been examined. Recent advances in the management of plasmacytomas , renal dysfunction, dentistry as well as mobilization of stem cells in the context of myeloma have also found exclusive mention. These areas are clinically very relevant and are often neglected in text books on multiple myeloma. A complete book on the topic would be too exhaustive: as such, since brevity is the soul of wit our attempt has been to present before the reader a comprehensive yet brief text on this important subject.

Ajay Gupta
MD, DM, CCST (UK), Senior Consultant,
Medical Oncology, Max Cancer Centre, Saket, New Delhi,
India

Part 1

Multiple Myeloma: Disease Biology and It's Therapeutic Applications

1

Proteasome Inhibitors in the Treatment of Multiple Myeloma

Lisa J. Crawford and Alexandra E. Irvine
Centre for Cancer Research and Cell Biology, Queen's University Belfast
Northern Ireland

1. Introduction

The ubiquitin proteasome system is responsible for the degradation of proteins involved in a wide range of cellular processes such as the cell cycle, apoptosis, transcription, cell signalling, immune response and antigen presentation. Protein homeostasis is essential for normal cell growth and inhibition of proteasome function has emerged as a viable strategy for anti-cancer treatment. The first proteasome inhibitor to enter clinical practice, bortezomib, was approved by the Food and Drug Administration as a single agent to treat relapsed/refractory Multiple Myeloma in 2003 and expanded to first-line treatment in combination with melphalan and prednisone in 2008. It is now a routine component of Multiple Myeloma therapy and has had a major impact on expanding treatment options in the last few years. Bortezomib exhibits novel action against Multiple Myeloma by targeting both intracellular mechanisms and interactions within the bone marrow environment. Although it demonstrates significant anti-Myeloma activity when used alone, it has been shown to have even greater benefits when used in combination with conventional and novel chemotherapeutic agents. There are currently over 200 clinical trials ongoing or recently completed examining bortezomib alone and in combination in various stages of disease and treatment. The clinical success of bortezomib has prompted the development of a number of second generation proteasome inhibitors with improved pharmacological properties. In this chapter, we review the development of bortezomib as a novel therapeutic agent in Multiple Myeloma and summarize the key observations from recently completed and ongoing studies on the effect of bortezomib both as a single agent and in combination therapies in the setting of newly diagnosed Multiple Myeloma and for relapsed disease. We also discuss the progress of next generation proteasome inhibitors in the clinic.

2. The ubiquitin proteasome system

The ubiquitin proteasome pathway represents the major pathway for intracellular protein degradation. It is responsible for the degradation of approximately 80% of cellular proteins, including misfolded and mutated proteins as well as those involved in the regulation of development, differentiation, cell proliferation, signal transduction, apoptosis and antigen presentation. Proteins are degraded by the ubiquitin proteasome pathway via two distinct and successive steps: the covalent attachment of multiple monomers of ubiquitin molecules to a protein substrate and degradation of the tagged protein by the 26S proteasome. Tagging of a protein by ubiquitin requires the action of three classes of enzymes - ubiquitin activating enzyme (E1), ubiquitin conjugating enzyme (E2) and ubiquitin ligase (E3). A single E1 enzyme activates ubiquitin by forming a thiol ester bond between E1 and ubiquitin in an ATP-dependent step. Following activation, ubiquitin is then transferred to an active site residue within an E2 enzyme which shuttles ubiquitin either directly or in concert with an E3 enzyme to a lysine residue in the target protein. There are more than 30 different E2 and over 500 E3 enzymes, which work in cooperation to confer exquisite substrate specificity to the ubiquitin proteasome pathway. The successive conjugation of ubiquitin moieties generates a polyubiquitin chain that acts as a signal to target the protein for degradation by the 26S proteasome (Figure 1a).

The 26S or constitutive proteasome is found in the nucleus and cytoplasm of all eukaryotic cells. It is composed of a core 20S particle capped with a 19S structure at each end. The 20S catalytic core is made up of 28 subunits arranged into four stacked rings, creating a central chamber where proteolysis occurs. The two outer rings are composed of 7 different α subunits, which are predominantly structural and the two inner rings are composed of 7 different β subunits, at least three of which contain catalytic sites (Groll et al., 1997). Catalytic activities of the proteasome are classified into three major categories, based upon preference to cleave a peptide bond after a particular amino acid residue. These activities are referred to as chymotrypsin-like, trypsin-like and caspase-like and are associated with β5, β2 and β1 subunits respectively. The chymotrypsin-like activity cleaves after hydrophobic residues, the trypsin-like activity cleaves after basic residues and the caspase-like activity cleaves after acidic residues (Groll et al., 1999; Heinemeyer et al., 1997). Substrates gain access to the proteolytic chamber by binding to the 19S regulatory particle at either end of the 20S proteasome. Polyubiquitin-tagged proteins are recognised by the 19S particle, where ubiquitin is cleaved off and recycled and the target protein is unfolded and fed into the 20S catalytic chamber (Groll et al., 2000; Navon & Goldberg, 2001). An alternative proteasome isoform known as the immunoproteasome can be formed in response to cytokine signalling. Interferon-γ and tumour necrosis factor - α induce the expression of a different set of catalytic β-subunits and regulatory cap to form the immunoproteasome. Subunits β1i (LMP2), β2i (MECL1) and β5i (LMP7) replace constitutive subunits β1, β2 and β5 and the 19S regulatory cap is replaced with an 11S regulatory structure (Figure 1b). These modifications allow the immunoproteasome to generate antigenic peptides for presentation by the major histocompatability (MHC) class 1 mediated immune response (Rock & Goldberg, 1999). The expression of the immunoproteasome appears to be tissue specific and is particularly abundant in immune-related cells. Immunoproteasomes are highly expressed in haemopoietic tumours such as Multiple Myeloma.

3. Proteasome inhibitors as drug candidates

As the ubiquitin proteasome pathway plays a critical role in regulating many cellular processes, it is not surprising that defects within this pathway have been associated with a number of pathologies, including neurodegenerative diseases and cancer. Proteasome inhibitors were initially synthesized as *in vitro* probes to investigate the function of the proteasome's catalytic activity. However, as the essential role of the proteasome in cell function was established, the proteasome emerged as an attractive target for cancer therapy. Early studies showed that proteasome inhibitors induced apoptosis in leukaemic cell lines

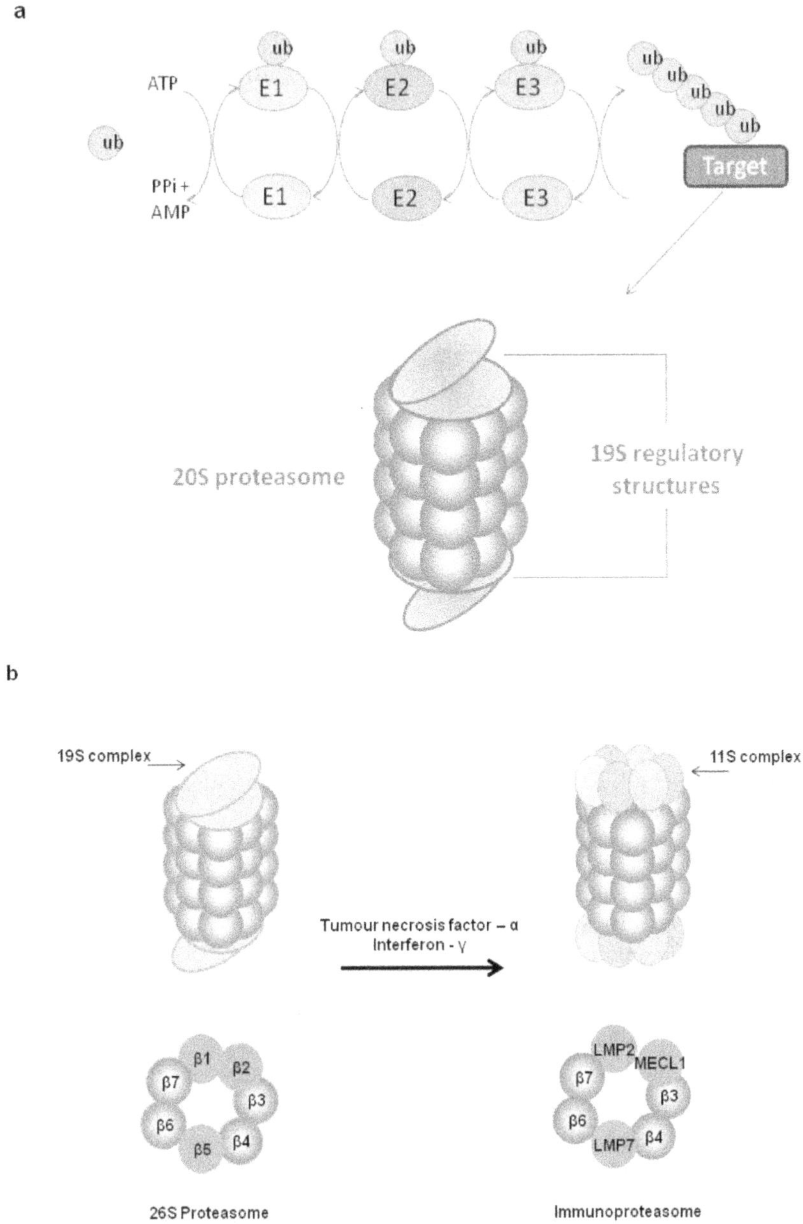

Fig. 1. a. Ubiquitin proteasome pathway mediated degradation. b. Proteasome composition.

(Imajoh-Ohmi et al., 1995; Shinohara et al., 1996; Drexler, 1997) and were active in an *in vivo* model of Burkitt's lymphoma (Orlowski et al., 1998). Further *in vitro* investigations demonstrated that proteasome inhibitors displayed a broad spectrum anti-proliferative and pro-apoptotic activity against haematological and solid tumours. While these studies established the potential of proteasome inhibitors as anti-cancer agents, many of the compounds available were limited to laboratory studies due to a relative lack of potency, specificity or stability. This led to the development of a series of dipeptide boronic acids, which were more potent and selective than many previously available inhibitors. These inhibitors were screened *in vitro* against the National Cancer Institute's panel of cancer cell lines and on the basis of its cytotoxicity, the compound bortezomib (PS-341, Velcade®) was brought forward for further testing.

4. Mechanisms of action of bortezomib in multiple myeloma

Bortezomib is a reversible proteasome inhibitor, primarily of the chymotrypsin-like activity of both the constitutive (β5) and immunoproteasome (LMP7) (Lightcap et al., 2000; Crawford et al., 2006). Initial *in vitro* evaluation of bortezomib demonstrated that it induced an accumulation of intracellular proteins, leading to G2-M arrest and then apoptosis through dual activation of caspase - 8 and caspase - 9 (Adams et al., 1999, Mitsiades et al., 2002). Importantly, bortezomib was also demonstrated to be significantly more toxic to Multiple Myeloma tumour cells than to normal counterparts. Hideshima et al. (2001) demonstrated that Multiple Myeloma cell lines and primary patient cells were 20-40 times more sensitive to bortezomib-induced apoptosis than bone marrow or peripheral blood mononuclear cells from healthy donors. Another novel aspect for bortezomib in Multiple Myeloma was that it was found to act not only on the Multiple Myeloma cells themselves but also on the protective bone marrow microenvironment. In addition, inhibition of proteasome function was found to both sensitize tumour cells to conventional chemotherapy and to overcome chemotherapy resistance. Finally, studies in murine xenograft models demonstrated that bortezomib significantly inhibited Multiple Myeloma cell growth and angiogenesis and prolonged survival (Leblanc et al., 2002). The main mechanisms attributed to bortezomib-induced apoptosis in Multiple Myeloma are outlined below.

4.1 NFκB

One of the first mechanisms of action attributed to bortezomib in Multiple Myeloma was inhibition of the inflammation associated transcription factor NFκB. NFκB, is constitutively activated in Multiple Myeloma and plays an important role in cell survival, proliferation and resistance to cytotoxic agents. NFκB is bound to its inhibitor IκB in the cytoplasm and is activated by proteasomal degradation of IκB. When activated, this transcription factor induces the expression of cell adhesion molecules (e.g. vascular cell adhesion molecule) and anti-apoptotic proteins (e.g. Bcl-2 and XIAP) and increases interleukin-6 production in bone marrow stromal cells. There are two pathways which activate NFκB, known as the canonical (or classical) pathway and the alternative non-canonical pathway (Gilmore, 2006). Inhibition of proteasome activity was demonstrated to prevent degradation of IκB and subsequent activation and translocation of NFκB to the nucleus to activate downstream pathways (Hideshima et al., 2001; Russo et al., 2001; Sunwoo et al., 2001). However, recent studies are challenging the concept that proteasome inhibitors inhibit NFκB activation and suggest that bortezomib may actually activate upstream NFκB activating kinases via the canonical pathway and increase NFκB activity (Markovina et al., 2008; Hideshima et al., 2009). In contrast, Chauhan et al. (2011) recently assessed the action of the second generation proteasome inhibitor MLN2238 on NFκB and report that this compound inhibits both the canonical and non-canonical pathways of activation. As MLN2238 is structurally distinct from bortezomib, this suggests that different proteasome inhibitors may exert differential effects on the NFκB pathway by blocking either one or both pathways of activation.

4.2 Apoptosis

Apoptosis is regulated by the opposing activities of pro-apoptotic and anti-apoptotic molecules. Cancer cells often have disregulated apoptotic signalling pathways with increased levels of anti-apoptotic proteins which provide a survival advantage and confer resistance to chemotherapeutic agents. Inhibition of proteasome activity by bortezomib is associated with an upregulation of pro-apoptotic factors such as p53, Bik, BIM and NOXA and a related decrease in anti-apoptotic proteins such as Bcl-$_{XL}$ and Bcl-2. Induction of NOXA has been reported to be a key mechanism in bortezomib-mediated apoptosis which is independent of p53 status but dependent on c-Myc (Qin et al., 2005; Gomez-Bougie et al., 2007; Nikiforov et al., 2007; Fennell et al., 2008). Bortezomib-mediated apoptosis is accompanied by induction of c-Jun-NH2 terminal kinase, generation of reactive oxygen species, release of cytochrome c, second mitochondria-derived activator of caspases and apoptosis-inducing factor and activation of the intrinsic caspase-8 pathway and extrinsic caspase-9 pathway.

4.3 Unfolded protein response

The endoplasmic reticulum plays a central role in protein homeostasis. Proteins are processed and folded in the lumen of the endoplasmic reticulum and misfolded proteins are returned to the cytosol and degraded in the proteasome. Multiple Myeloma cells have a high rate of protein synthesis and this is inherently associated with a high level of misfolded proteins. Accumulation of misfolded proteins in the endoplasmic reticulum triggers the Unfolded Protein Response. This process is mediated through three endoplasmic reticulum transmembrane receptors: ATF6, IRE1 and PERK. In resting cells the endoplasmic reticulum chaperone BiP (GRP 78) maintains these receptors in a resting state; BiP becomes dissociated from the endoplasmic reticulum receptors when unfolded proteins accumulate and triggers the Unfolded Protein Response.

It has been recognised for some time that bortezomib can induce the Unfolded Protein Response in Multiple Myeloma cells and that this contributes to its pro-apoptotic activity (Obeng et al., 2006; Meister et al., 2007). Numerous studies have now shown that treatment of Multiple Myeloma cell lines *in vitro* with bortezomib triggers activation of ATF6, IRE 1 and PERK (Davenport et al., 2007; Gu et al., 2008; Dong et al., 2009). Caspase 2 is believed to act upstream of mitochondrial signalling in this bortezomib ER stress- induced apoptosis (Gu et al., 2008). Similar mechanisms have been implicated in mantle cell lymphoma cell lines (Rao et al., 2010; Roue et al., 2011). It is clear that a greater understanding of the Unfolded Protein Response is fundamental to allow the rational development of combination therapies (Kawaguchi et al., 2011).

4.4 Bone marrow microenvironment

Interactions between Multiple Myeloma cells and bone marrow stroma regulate the growth and survival of Myeloma cells and play a critical role in angiogenesis, bone disease and drug resistance. The success of bortezomib in Multiple Myeloma has been attributed not only to direct effects on Myeloma cells but also its effect on the bone marrow microenvironment. Vascular cell adhesion molecule-1 is a major ligand on bone marrow stromal cells that mediates binding of Multiple Myeloma cells via the cell surface molecule very late antigen-4. Early studies on proteasome inhibitors demonstrated that they downregulate cytokine-induced expression of vascular cell adhesion molecule-1 (Read et al., 1995). Hideshima et al., (2001) subsequently reported that treatment with bortezomib decreased binding of Myeloma cells to bone marrow stromal cells by 50% and consequently inhibited the related upregulation of interleukin-6 secretion and paracrine tumour growth.

Bortezomib has also been demonstrated to have both direct and indirect effects on angiogenesis. Initial studies found that bortezomib treatment decreased the secretion of vascular endothelial growth factor from Myeloma cells, thereby decreasing vasculogenesis and angiogenesis (Nawrocki et al., 2002). More recent studies using functional assays including chemotaxis, adhesion to fibronectin and capillary formation demonstrated that bortezomib has direct anti-proliferative effects on vascular endothelial cells. Tamura et al. (2010) demonstrated that bortezomib potently inhibits cell growth of vascular endothelial cells by suppressing the G2/M transition of the cell cycle and increasing permeability, thus acting as a vascular targeting drug.

A critical role of the bone marrow microenvironment in the efficacy of bortezomib in Multiple Myeloma was further established by Edwards et al. (2009). *In vivo* studies demonstrated that bortezomib had a greater effect on tumour burden when Myeloma cells were grown in the bone marrow of mice than when they were grown at sub-cutaneous sites.

4.5 Bortezomib and bone formation

Osteolytic lesions characterised with activated osteoclast activity accompanied with a reduction in osteoblast activity are a major feature of Multiple Myeloma. Bortezomib exhibits important effects on the development and progression of Myeloma-associated bone disease by reducing osteoclast activity and increasing osteoblast function, therefore reducing bone resorption and stimulating new bone formation. Both preclinical and clinical analysis have demonstrated that bortezomib exerts these effects in part by inhibiting dickkopf-1 and receptor activator of nuclear factor-kappa B ligand and increasing levels of alkaline phosphatase and osteocalcin (Terpos et al., 2006; Heider et al., 2006; Giuliani et al., 2007). However, a recent study by Lund and colleagues (2010) found that the combination of a glucocorticoid such as dexamethasone with bortezomib could inhibit the positive effects of bortezomib on osteoblast proliferation and differentiation, suggesting that bortezomib may result in better healing of osteolytic lesions when used without a glucocorticoid.

4.6 Gene expression studies

While a number of mechanisms of action of bortezomib have been outlined above, the full mechanism of bortezomib-induced cytotoxicity remains to be elucidated. Gene expression studies have been employed to try and increase our understanding of the cytotoxic action of this compound in Multiple Myeloma. Mitsiades et al., (2002) performed gene expression profiling in a Multiple Myeloma cell line and demonstrated that bortezomib resulted in a downregulation of growth and survival signalling pathways and upregulation of molecules implicated in pro-apoptotic cascades, as well as upregulation of heat shock proteins and ubiquitin proteasome pathway members. Chen et al. (2010) performed a genome-wide siRNA screen in malignant cell lines to evaluate the genetic determinants that confer sensitivity to bortezomib. They found that bortezomib promotes apoptosis primarily by disregulating Myc and polyamines, interfering with protein translation and disrupting DNA damage repair pathways. More recently, Takeda and colleagues (2011) investigated genes affecting the toxicity of bortezomib in the fission yeast *S. pombe* and identified factors involved in the ubiquitin proteasome pathway, chromatin silencing, nuclear/cytoplasmic transportation, amino acid metabolism and vesicular trafficking. Gene expression profiling of Multiple Myeloma patients found that treatment with bortezomib resulted in an upregulation of proteasome genes and that high levels of the proteasome subunit PSMD4 was associated with an inferior prognosis (Shaughnessy et al., 2011). Further investigation into fully understanding the mechanism of action of bortezomib will help to identify therapeutic strategies to overcome resistance to bortezomib and to identify agents to enhance its efficacy.

5. Clinical use of bortezomib in Multiple Myeloma

5.1 Bortezomib therapy for relapsed or refractory Multiple Myeloma

Following encouraging preclinical results bortezomib was introduced into clinical trials to test for safety and efficacy in relapsed and refractory Multiple Myeloma. These studies established that bortezomib was effective and well-tolerated in Multiple Myeloma and led to approval of bortezomib in patients that had undergone at least two prior therapies. The incorporation of bortezomib into the treatment options for Myeloma represented a significant milestone as being the first proteasome inhibitor to be implemented into clinical use and also as the first novel therapy for Multiple Myeloma in over a decade. The main findings of the trials are outlined below.

Phase 1

Orlowski et al. (2002) conducted a Phase 1 trial evaluating the pharmacodynamics of bortezomib, along with toxicity and clinical responses in 27 patients with advanced refractory haematological malignancies. This study demonstrated that bortezomib could be safely administered, with a tolerable side-effect profile. There was significant evidence of anti-tumour activity in patients with Multiple Myeloma, with all 9 evaluable Multiple Myeloma patients showing some evidence of clinical benefit, including one complete response. Taken together with preclinical data this provided the rationale for Phase 2 clinical trials with bortezomib for the treatment of relapsed, refractory Myeloma.

Phase 2

The activity of bortezomib in relapsed and refractory Multiple Myeloma was confirmed with two Phase 2 trials, SUMMIT and CREST. SUMMIT (Study of Uncontrolled Multiple Myeloma managed with proteasome Inhibition Therapy) was a large multi-centre trial that enrolled 202 heavily pre-treated patients (Richardson et al., 2003). An overall response rate of 35% was achieved, including 10% of patients who achieved a complete or near complete response. Median time to progression was 7 months compared with 3 months on previous therapy. Grade 3 toxicities included cyclical thrombocytopenia, fatigue, peripheral neuropathy and neutropenia. Of these, the most clinically significant was peripheral neuropathy. The CREST (Clinical Response and Efficacy Study of PS-341 in the Treatment of relapsing Multiple Myeloma) trial was a smaller multicentre study that enrolled 54 patients with only one prior treatment (Jagannath et al., 2004). Patients were randomized to receive 1.0 or 1.3 mg/m^2 bortezomib. The overall response rates were 30% for patients receiving 1.0 mg/m^2 and 38% for patients receiving 1.3 mg/m^2. Adverse effects were similar to those seen in SUMMIT, however, less peripheral neuropathy was seen with reduced dose used in CREST. These findings led to the approval of bortezomib by the Food and Drug Administration and European Medicines Agency for relapsed/refractory Multiple Myeloma patients that had at least 2 prior therapies (Kane et al., 2006). Bortezomib was the first new therapy approved for Multiple Myeloma for over a decade.

Phase 3

APEX (Assessment of Proteasome inhibition for EXtending remissions) was a Phase 3 study of 668 patients with relapsed and refractory Multiple Myeloma after one to three prior treatments, who were randomized to receive either bortezomib or high-dose dexamethasone (Richardson et al., 2005). Bortezomib induced a better overall response rate than dexamethasone (38% vs. 18%), including a 13% vs. 2% complete or near complete response. Median time to progression for bortezomib was 6.22 months vs. 3.49 months for dexamethasone and overall survival was 29.3 months vs. 23.7 months. The adverse events were similar to those observed previously, however the rates of adverse events were higher for bortezomib.

5.2 Bortezomib-based combination therapy in relapsed or refractory Multiple Myeloma

Early preclinical work demonstrated that bortezomib sensitized Myeloma cells to other chemotherapeutic agents and this prompted clinical investigation of bortezomib-based combination therapies in relapsed or refractory Multiple Myeloma. Dexamethasone was the first agent to be combined with bortezomib in the clinic and is the most common agent to be used in bortezomib-based combinations. Both preclinical data and clinical trials showed that the combination increased anti-Myeloma activity. Data from the SUMMIT and CREST trials demonstrated additional responses in 18% and 33% of patients who received both drugs, including patients who had previously been refractory to dexamethasone. Bortezomib has since been demonstrated to enhance the activity of many chemotherapeutic agents in Multiple Myeloma, demonstrating promising response rates in early clinical trials (summarized in Table 1). Larger Phase 3 trials will be required to confirm response and survival to these combinations.

5.3 Bortezomib–based combinations with novel therapies

The increased understanding of intracellular pathways that are involved in the proliferation and survival of Myeloma cells has led to the identification of novel targets for therapeutic intervention. Numerous small molecule inhibitors have been developed in recent years, targeted against key cellular proteins or signalling pathways that may enhance the anti-tumour effect of bortezomib, or overcome resistance to bortezomib. These novel small molecule compounds include heat shock protein 90 inhibitors, histone deacetylase inhibitors, farnesyltransferase inhibitors, Bcl-2 inhibitors, monoclonal antibodies and a number of different kinase inhibitors. Many of these novel agents have demonstrated

Combination	Study	Overall Response	Reference
Bortezomib & alvocidib	Phase 1	44%	Holkova et al., 2011
Bortezomib & tanespimycin	Phase 1	27%	Richardson et al., 2011
Bortezomib, doxorubicin & intermediate dose dexamethasone	Phase 1		Takamatsu et al., 2010
Bortezomib, cyclophosphamide, thalidomide & dexamethasone	Phase 1	88%	Kim et al., 2010
Bortezomib & vorinostat	Phase 1	42%	Badros et al., 2009
Bortezomib & samarium lexidronam	Phase 1	21%	Berenson et al., 2009a
Bortezomib & temsirolimus	Phase 1/2	33%	Ghobrial et al., 2011
Bortezomib, low dose melphalan & dexamethasone	Phase 1/2	76%	Popat et al., 2009
Bortezomib, arsenic trioxide & ascorbic acid	Phase 1/2	27%	Berenson et al., 2007
Bortezomib, melphalan, prednisone & thalidomide	Phase 1/2	67%	Palumbo et al., 2007
Bortezomib & melphalan	Phase 1/2	68%	Berenson et al., 2006
Bortezomib, pegylated liposomal doxorubicin & thalidomide	Phase 2	55%	Chanan-Khan et al., 2009
Bortezomib, thalidomide & dexamethasone	Phase 2		Pineda-Roman et al., 2008
Bortezomib, melphalan, dexamethasone & intermittent thalidomide	Phase 2	66%	Terpos et al., 2008
Bortezomib, dexamethasone & cyclophosphamide	Phase 2	90%	Kropff et al., 2007

Table 1. Bortezomib-based combination therapy for relapsed/refractory Multiple Myeloma.

synergistic activity with bortezomib in preclinical studies and are under evaluation in early clinical trials in combination with bortezomib.

5.3.1 Heat shock protein 90 inhibitors

Heat shock protein 90 is a chaperone that stabilizes numerous proteins that contribute to tumour cell survival and proliferation. Inhibition of heat shock protein 90 in Myeloma cells results in decreased expression of insulin-like growth factor-1 and interleukin-6 receptors, with a related decrease in the PI3K/Akt signalling pathway. Preclinical studies with the heat shock protein 90 inhibitor tanespimycin in combination with bortezomib demonstrated a synergistic effect and resulted in enhanced accumulation of ubiquitinated proteins (Mitsiades et al., 2006). A Phase 1 clinical trial of bortezomib in combination with tanespimycin demonstrated significant and durable responses (Richardson et al., 2011) and a study of bortezomib in combination with KW-2478 is underway (NCT01063907).

5.3.2 Histone deactylase inhibitors

Ubiquitinated and misfolded proteins are degraded not only by proteasomes but also by aggresomes. Aggresome formation, which is dependent on the histone deacetylase HDAC6, is increased in response to inhibition of proteasome function. Histone deacetylase inhibitors are a class of compounds that regulate gene expression by interfering with the function of histone deacetylases. Preclinical studies demonstrated that the combination of bortezomib with a HDAC inhibitor resulted in significant cytotoxicity and show a marked accumulation of polyubiquitinated proteins (Catley et al., 2006; Nawrocki et al., 2008). A Phase 1 trial of bortezomib and vorinostat in relapsed/refractory myeloma demonstrated encouraging results, with an overall response rate of 42%, including 3 responses among 9 bortezomib refractory patients (Badros et al., 2009). Further trials of bortezomib along with HDAC inhibitors vorinostat and panobinostat are currently being investigated.

5.3.3 Farnesyltransferase inhibitors

Farnesyltransferase inhibitors block activation of the Ras dependent MAPK signalling pathway to regulate signal transduction and proliferation. Combination of the farnesyltranserase inhibitors lonafarnib and tipifarnib with bortezomib induced synergistic cell death and overcame cell adhesion-mediated drug resistance in Multiple Myeloma cell lines and primary cells (David et al., 2005; Yanamandra et al., 2006). David and colleagues (2005) observed that this combination resulted in a down-regulation of Akt signalling, an effect which was absent when either drug was used alone. Early phase clinical trials evaluating bortezomib and tipifarnib combination therapy are ongoing (NCT00243035; NCT00972712).

5.3.4 Bcl-2 inhibitors

Bcl-2 family members play a critical role in mediating tumour cell survival and chemoresistance in Multiple Myeloma. There are a number of small molecule inhibitors available that interfere with the function of Bcl-2 proteins and induce apoptosis in Multiple Myeloma cells. In preclinical studies, three Bcl-2 inhibitors obatoclax, ABT-737 and ABT-263 have shown synergistic activity with bortezomib (Chauhan et al., 2007; Trudel et al., 2007; Ackler et al., 2010). The combination of bortezomib with a Bcl-2 inhibitor resulted in enhanced NOXA-mediated activation of Bak and increased activation of the mitochondrial apoptotic pathways. Obatoclax is being investigated in combination with bortezomib in early clinical trials (NCT00719901).

5.3.5 Monoclonal antibodies

Monoclonal antibody therapy can selectively target specific molecules, proteins or receptors involved in disease processes. There are a number of antigens currently under investigation as potential targets in Multiple Myeloma in combination with bortezomib. Bevacizumab is a monoclonal antibody that is targeted towards vascular endothelial growth factor to disrupt angiogenensis (Brekken et al., 2000). The combination of bevacizumab and bortezomib is being evaluated in Phase 2 studies for relapsed Myeloma (NCT00464178). Interleukin-6, a key intermediate in Multiple Myeloma signalling pathways, is targeted by the chimeric antibody siltuximab. Preclinical evaluation of siltuximab and bortezomib demonstrated enhanced cytotoxicity of bortezomib in Myeloma cell lines and primary cells in the presence of bone marrow stromal cells (Voorhees et al., 2007). A Phase 2 trial is evaluating this combination in relapsed Myeloma (NCT00401843). Elotuzumab is directed towards CS1, a cell surface glycoprotein expressed at high levels on Multiple Myeloma cells. This anti-CS1 antibody demonstrated significantly enhanced anti-tumour activity in combination with bortezomib in *in vitro* and *in vivo* models of Myeloma (van Rhee et al., 2009) and Phase 1/2 trials are underway (NCT00726869). AVE1642 is an anti-insulin-like growth factor 1 antibody that demonstrated synergistic apoptosis in combination with bortezomib in preclinical studies (Descamps et al., 2009), however, response rates from a Phase 1 study were insufficient to warrant further investigation (Moreau et al., 2011). Early phase clinical trials combining bortezomib with anti-chemokine receptor 4 and anti-CD40 antibodies are also underway (NCT01359657 and NCT00664898).

5.3.6 Mammalian target of rapamycin inhibitor

Mammalian target of rapamycin (mTOR) inhibitors inhibit the mTOR kinase and related signalling pathways resulting in decreased expression of cyclins and c-Myc, increased expression of p27 and G_1 arrest. *In vitro* studies have demonstrated synergistic action of the mTOR inhibitors NVP-BEZ235 and pp242 with bortezomib (Baumann et al., 2009; Hoang et al., 2010). A Phase 1/2 study of bortezomib in combination with mTOR inhibitor temsirolimus demonstrated a partial response rate of 33% in heavily pre-treated refractory Myeloma (Ghobrial et al., 2011).

5.3.7 Cyclin-dependent kinase inhibitors

Cyclin-dependent kinase inhibitors are small molecule inhibitors that induce cell cycle arrest. Cyclin dependent kinase inhibitors (seliciclib and alvocidib) were shown to be synergistic with proteasome inhibitors in leukaemic cell lines (Dai et al., 2003, 2004). A subsequent study demonstrated that the cyclin dependent kinase inhibitor PD0332991 sensitizes an *in vivo* Multiple Myeloma model to bortezomib through enhanced induction of mitochondrial depolarization (Menu et al., 2008). A combination of bortezomib along with the cyclin dependent kinase inhibitor alvocidib (flavopiridol) was recently assessed in a Phase 1 trial for refractory B-cell malignancies and demonstrated an overall response rate of 44% with manageable toxicities (Holkova et al., 2011).

5.3.8 Akt inhibitors

Perifosine is an alkylphospholipid that inhibits Akt activation and associated growth and drug resistance in Multiple Myeloma. As a single agent, perifosine demonstrated significant toxicity both *in vivo* and *in vitro* and it has also been shown to inhibit bortezomib-induced upregulation of survivin resulting in enhanced bortezomib cytotoxicity (Hideshima et al., 2007). Perifosine is currently being evaluated in a Phase 1/2 study in combination with bortezomib with or without dexamethasone in relapsed Myeloma (NCT00401011) and a Phase 3 study of perifosine in combination with bortezomib and dexamethasone is currently recruiting (NCT01002248).

5.3.9 Multi-kinase inhibitors

Sorafenib and dasatinib are multi-kinase inhibitors that have been shown to enhance anti-Myeloma activity with bortezomib. Sorafenib inhibits RAF kinase, VEGF receptors, platelet-derived growth factor β, Flt-3, c-Kit and RET receptor tyrosine kinases. The combination of sorafenib and bortezomib produced synergistic apoptosis in a number of malignant cell lines and was dependent on Akt inhibition (Yu et al., 2006). This combination is currently being investigated in a Phase 1/2 trial in relapsed Myeloma (NCT00536575). Dasatinib is an inhibitor of c-abl, src family proteins, EphA2 and btk. The triple combination of dasatinib along with bortezomib and dexamethasone produced greater synergistic effects compared to single agents or double combinations in Multiple Myeloma cell line models and primary cells (de Queiroz Crusoe et al., 2011). A Phase 1 study combining all three agents in relapsed or refractory Myeloma has recently been completed (NCT00560352).

5.3.10 Other combinations

The combination of bortezomib with second generation immunomodulatory drug pomalidomide (NCT01212952), telomerase inhibitor GRN163L (NCT00718601), aurora A kinase inhibitor MLN8237 (Gorgun et al., 2010; NCT01034553), p38 mitogen-activated kinase inhibitor SCIO-469 (Navas et al., 2006; NCT00095680) and protease inhibitor nelfinavir mesylate (NCT01164709) are all being evaluated in early clinical trials. In addition there are numerous more novel targeted therapies under preclinical assessment in combination with proteasome inhibitors.

5.4 Bortezomib in front-line therapy

For over 40 years melphalan and prednisone was the standard therapy for patients with newly diagnosed Multiple Myeloma that were ineligible for high-dose therapy and autologous stem cell transplantation. Following encouraging activity of bortezomib combined with melphalan in patients with relapsed or refractory Myeloma, bortezomib plus melphalan and prednisone was evaluated in a Phase 1/2 trial for newly diagnosed Myeloma patients who were at least 65 years of age. The combination gave a response rate of 89% and a median time to progression of 27 months. This led to the Phase 3 trial VISTA (Velcade as Initial Standard Therapy in Multiple Myeloma), which compared bortezomib, melphalan and prednisone with melphalan and prednisone in newly diagnosed Myeloma patients who were ineligible for high-dose therapy. Results of this trial demonstrated that when bortezomib was included in the regimen the overall response rate increased from 30% to 71% and the time to progression was 24 months compared with 16.6 months (San Miguel et al., 2008). There was also fewer bone disease events, improvement in bone remodelling and evidence of bone healing. These results suggested a benefit for bortezomib at earlier use and provided the framework for approval of bortezomib for use as front-line therapy.

In newly diagnosed patients who were candidates for high-dose therapy with autologous stem cell transplantation, the combination of vincristine, doxorubicin and dexamethasone was the standard induction therapy. Four randomized trials evaluated the role of bortezomib-based combinations for induction therapy in transplant candidates. Bortezomib was combined with dexamethasone (Harousseau et al., 2010), with adriamycin and dexamethasone (Popat et al., 2008), with thalidomide and dexamethasone (Cavo et al., 2010) and with thalidomide, dexamethasone and chemotherapy (Barlogie et al., 2007). The bortezomib-based combinations all demonstrated superior response rates than the regimens without bortezomib. A number of other combinations incorporating bortezomib for both transplant eligible and ineligible patients are in clinical trials and are achieving overall response rates of up to 100% (Table 2).

Combination	Study Phase	Overall Response	Reference
Bortezomib, thalidomide & chemotherapy	Phase 1	83%	Badros et al., 2006
Bortezomib, dexamethasone, cyclophosphamide & lenalidomide	Phase 1	96%	Kumar et al., 2010
Bortezomib, doxorubicin & dexamethasone	Phase 1/2	89/95%	Popat et al., 2008
Bortezomib, lenalidomide & dexamethasone	Phase 1/2	100%	Richardson et al., 2010
Bortezomib, melphalan & prednisone	Phase 1/2	95%	Gasparetto et al., 2010
Bortezomib & melphelan	Phase 1/2	87%	Lonial et al., 2010
Bortezomib, lenanlidomide, pegylated liposomal doxorubicin & dexamethasone	Phase 1/2	96%	Jakubowiak et al., 2011
Bortezomib & dexamethasone	Phase 2	66%	Harousseau et al., 2006
Alternating bortezomib & dexamethasone	Phase 2	68%	Rosinol et al., 2007
Bortezomib, cyclophosphamide & dexamethasone	Phase 2	88%	Reeder et al., 2009
Bortezomib, ascorbic acid & melphalan	Phase 2	74%	Berenson et al., 2009b
Bortezomib, pegylated liposomal doxorubicin & dexamethasone	Phase 2	85%	Jakubowaik et al., 2009
Bortezomib & high dose melphalan	Phase 2	70%	Roussel et al., 2010
Bortezomib, cyclophosphamide & dexamethasone	Phase 2	95%	Besinger et al., 2010
Bortezomib & dexamethasone	Phase 2	86%	Corso et al., 2010
Vincristine, adriamycin & dexamethasone followed by bortezomib, thalidomide & dexamethasone	Phase 2	75%	Kim et al., 2011
Bortezomib & thalidomide	Phase 2	82%	Ghosh et al., 2011
Bortezomib, pegylated liposomal doxorubicin & thalidomide	Phase 2	78%	Sher et al., 2011
Bortezomib, thalidomide & dexamethasone	Phase 3	31%	Cavo et al., 2010
Bortezomib & dexamethasone	Phase 3	79%	Harousseau et al., 2010

Table 2. Bortezomib-based combinations for induction and front-line therapy.

6. Resistance to bortezomib

Despite the clinical success of bortezomib, many patients with Multiple Myeloma are unresponsive and drug resistance can also develop (Dispenzieri et al., 2010). The mechanisms underlying this drug resistance, both intrinsic and acquired, are as yet poorly understood.

Resistance to proteasome inhibitors may occur either at the level of the proteasome complex or in the downstream signalling pathways. Several researchers have approached this problem by growing cell lines in increasing concentration of bortezomib. Ri et al. (2010) found a unique point mutation in the proteasome β5 subunit (PSMB5) in bortezomib resistant Multiple Myeloma cell lines. Using overexpression studies they demonstrated that the mutation may act by interfering with the Unfolded Protein Response pathway. Shaughnessy and colleagues have recently applied gene expression studies to a group of 142 Multiple Myeloma patients and identified PSMD4 as associated with adverse response to bortezomib; PSMD4 is one of the non-ATPase subunits of the proteasome 19S regulator (Shaughnessy et al., 2011).

The anti-tumour effects of bortezomib have been mainly attributed to its' actions on the NFκB and Bcl-2 regulatory protein pathways. It is not therefore surprising that polymorphisms of the NFκB family genes have been associated with treatment outcome in Multiple Myeloma patients. Studies with lymphoid cell lines have recently shown Noxa/Bcl-2 interactions contribute to bortezomib resistance (Smith et al., 2011) and there have been similar reports in Mantle Cell Lymphoma cell lines (Weniger et al., 2011); there is no supporting clinical evidence as yet. Overexpression of apoptosis regulators REDD1 and survivin have also been associated with bortezomib resistance in cell line models (Decaux et al., 2010; Ling et al., 2010).

In cases where drug resistance is directly associated with the proteasome enzymatic complex it may be possible to overcome resistance by using second generation inhibitors which act through a different mechanism to bortezomib (Ruschak et al., 2011; Arastu-Kapur et al., 2011; Chauhan et al., 2011). Knowledge of the resistance mechanism may also allow rational design of future combination therapies.

7. Second generation inhibitors

The success of bortezomib in the clinic prompted the development of a new generation of structurally distinct proteasome inhibitors. In addition to bortezomib, there are currently five proteasome inhibitors in clinical development, representing three different structural classes - peptide boronic acids, peptide epoxyketones and β-lactones (Figure 2). These inhibitors bind either reversibly or irreversibly to catalytic sites within the proteasome.

7.1 Carfilzomib

Epoxomicin, a member of the epoxyketone family of natural peptide proteasome inhibitors, inhibits proteasome activity through a unique mechanism, by binding to both the hydroxyl and amino groups of the catalytic site threonine residue (Groll & Huber, 2004). Carfilzomib (formerly PR-171) is an epoxomicin-based proteasome inhibitor, with improved pharmaceutical properties. Unlike bortezomib, carfilzomib binds irreversibly to the chymotrypsin-like (β5 and LMP7) subunit, leading to more sustained proteasome inhibition. In preclinical studies carfilzomib was shown to exhibit equal potency but greater selectivity than bortezomib for the chymotrypsin-like activity. *In vitro* and *in vivo* studies demonstrated anti-tumour activity, tolerability and dosing flexibility in several xenograft models (Kuhn et al., 2007; Demo et al., 2007). Carfilzomib has also been shown to act synergistically with histone deacetylase inhibitors *in vitro* in lymphoma and leukaemia (Fuchs et al., 2009; Dasmahapatra et al., 2010; 2011). Results from Phase 1 studies in patients with haematological malignancies demonstrated that carfilzomib was well tolerated and may exhibit less peripheral neuropathy than bortezomib (O'Connor et al., 2009). Phase 2 trials of carfilzomib as a single agent in relapsed and refractory Multiple Myeloma demonstrated an overall response rate of 35.5% including patients with bortezomib-refractory disease. (Zangari et al., 2011) The main toxicities were fatigue and nausea, with limited peripheral neuropathy seen in less than 10% of patients. Carfilzomib is currently progressing in a number of trials for relapsed and newly diagnosed Multiple Myeloma and as both a single agent and in combination.

7.2 Marizomib (NPI-0052)

Marizomib, also known as Salinosporamide A, is a β-lactone compound derived from the marine bacterium *Salinospora tropica* (Macherla et al., 2005) and is structurally related to the lactacystin-derived proteasome inhibitor Omuralide. In contrast to bortezomib which is a slowly reversible inhibitor of chymotrypsin-like activity, marizomib binds irreversibly to all three catalytic activities of the proteasome. While bortezomib is administered intravenously, marizomib has the advantage of being orally bioactive. Initial *in vitro* studies established the effectiveness of this compound in Multiple Myeloma cell lines, including those that were resistant to bortezomib (Chauhan et al., 2005). Animal tumour model studies demonstrated reduced tumour growth without significant toxicity (Chauhan et al., 2005; Singh et al., 2010). Preclinical studies demonstrated synergistic results when marizomib was combined with bortezomib or lenalidomide (Chauhan et al., 2008; 2010a). Phase 1 trials of marizomib in Myeloma are currently ongoing. Marizomib displays a broader, faster acting and more durable proteasome inhibition than bortezomib and treatment does not appear to induce the limiting toxicities associated with bortezomib, such as peripheral neuropathy and thrombocytopenia.

7.3 MLN9708/MLN2238

MLN9708 like bortezomib is also a boron containing peptide proteasome inhibitor and was selected from a panel of inhibitors based on having a biochemical profile distinct from that of bortezomib. MLN9708 hydrolyses immediately in plasma to its biologically active form MLN2238. MLN2238 displays similar potency and selectivity for the chymotrypsin-like proteasome subunit, however, it has a substantially shorter half-life than bortezomib which may improve tissue distribution. Cell viability studies revealed a strong anti-proliferative effect on a variety of tumour cell lines and *in vivo* studies have demonstrated efficacy in human prostate xenograft, colon cancer and lymphoma models where both intravenous and oral dosing were effective (Kupperman et al., 2010). MLN2238 has been demonstrated to induce apoptosis in cells resistant to both conventional therapies and to bortezomib. Synergistic activity is seen by combining this compound with lenelidomide, HDAC inhibitors and dexamethasone *in vitro*. It is well tolerated in plasmacytoma xenograft mouse models and demonstrates significantly longer survival time than mice treated with bortezomib (Chauhan et al., 2011). This compound is currently being evaluated in Phase 1 studies in patients with lymphoma and non-haematological malignancies and in Phase 1/2 trials for Multiple Myeloma.

7.4 CEP-18770

CEP-18770 is a next-generation boronic acid-based proteasome inhibitor and in common with bortezomib it is a reversible inhibitor, primarily of the chymotrypsin-like activity. CEP-18770 was demonstrated to induce apoptosis in Multiple Myeloma cell lines and primary Myeloma cells, while displaying a favourable cytotoxicity profile towards normal cells (Piva et al., 2008; Dorsey et al., 2008). Its anti-tumour activity was demonstrated in several animal tumour models and it has been shown to demonstrate marked anti-Myeloma effects in combination with bortezomib and melphalan (Sanchez et al., 2010). CEP-18770 has completed early Phase 1 trials for solid tumours and non-Hodgkin's lymphoma and is currently being evaluated in Phase 1/2 trials for Multiple Myeloma.

7.5 ONX0912

ONX0912 (formerly PR-047) is a novel orally available analogue of the proteasome inhibitor carfilzomib. Carfilzomib, in common with bortezomib, is administered intravenously, however, proteasome inhibitor therapy requires twice weekly dosing and therefore an orally available inhibitor would be more advantageous. ONX0912 has demonstrated similar anti-tumour activity to carfilzomib *in vitro* in cell lines and primary cells and enhanced the anti-Myeloma activity of bortezomib, lenolidomide and histone deacetylase inhibitors; animal models of Multiple Myeloma, non-Hodgkin's lymphoma and colorectal cancer demonstrated reduced tumour progression and prolonged survival (Zhou et al., 2009; Roccaro et al., 2010; Chauhan et al., 2010b). A Phase 1 trial of ONX0912 in advanced solid tumours is currently recruiting.

7.6 Immunoproteasome Inhibitors

A novel approach that is looking promising is the use of proteasome inhibitors that specifically inhibit catalytic activities of the immunoproteasome. Immunoproteasomes are constitutively expressed in immune tissues and expressed at a much lower level in other cell types. Thus targeting immunoproteasomes confers a certain amount of specificity and provides an opportunity to overcome toxicities associated with proteasome inhibition, such as peripheral neuropathy and gastrointestinal effects. A number of immunoproteasome specific inhibitors have recently been described and exhibit encouraging preclinical activity in haematological malignancies. PR-924 is a tripeptide epoxyketone related to carfilzomib. It exhibits 100-fold greater selectivity for the LMP7 subunit than carfilzomib and was demonstrated to inhibit the growth of Multiple Myeloma cell lines and primary tumour cells and inhibited tumour growth in animal models without significant toxicity (Singh et al., 2010). The immunoproteasome inhibitor IPSI-101 is a peptide aldehyde which preferentially inhibits the LMP2 subunit. IPSI-101 induced accumulation of polyubiquitinated proteins and pro-apoptotic protein and inhibited proliferation in *in vitro* models of haematological malignancies (Kuhn et al., 2009). At the time of writing this review there were no clinical trials of immunoproteasome inhibitors in progress, however, it is likely that the encouraging preclinical data on PR-924 and ISPS-101 will form the basis for future clinical evaluation of these compounds.

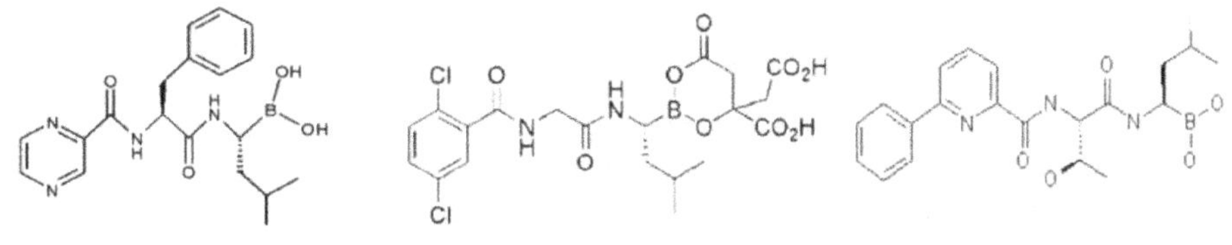

Bortezomib (Peptide Boronate) MLN9708 (Peptide Boronate) CEP-18770 (Peptide Boronate)

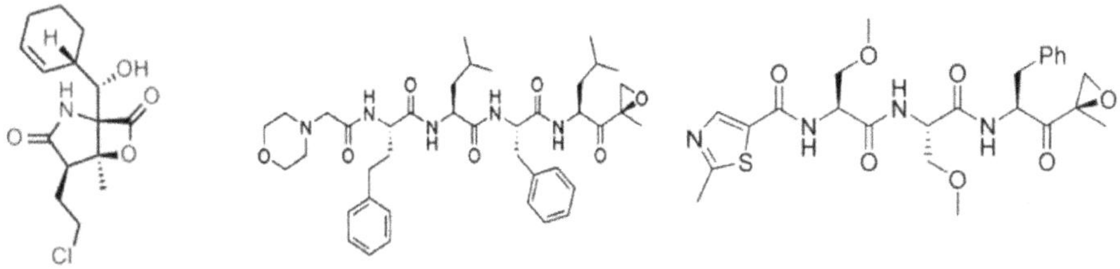

Marizomib (Salinosporamide A) Carfilzomib (Epoxykeytone) ONX 0912 (Epoxyketone)

Fig. 2. Structure and class of proteasome inhibitors in clinical trials.

8. Conclusion

Proteasome Inhibitors have provided a major new therapeutic strategy for the treatment of Multiple Myeloma. Bortezomib, the first-in-class of these inhibitors, has shown remarkable success since its introduction almost ten years ago. Second generation compounds are already demonstrating increased selectivity with a more acceptable therapeutic window. Researchers are turning to other parts of the Ubiquitin Proteasome Pathway to look for potential druggable targets which would confer greater specificity. The E3 ligases play a key role in substrate selection and the Pharma already have agents in their pipeline which show promise in modifying their action. Modulation of the Ubiquitin Proteasome Pathway with novel inhibitors offers a powerful approach to Myeloma therapy.

9. References

Ackler, S., M. J. Mitten, K. Foster, A. Oleksijew, M. Refici, S. K. Tahir, Y. Xiao, et al. 2010. The bcl-2 inhibitor ABT-263 enhances the response of multiple chemotherapeutic regimens in hematologic tumors in vivo. *Cancer Chemotherapy and Pharmacology* 66 (5) (Oct): 869-80.

Adams, J., V. J. Palombella, E. A. Sausville, J. Johnson, A. Destree, D. D. Lazarus, J. Maas, C. S. Pien, S. Prakash, and P. J. Elliott. 1999. Proteasome inhibitors: A novel class of potent and effective antitumor agents. *Cancer Research* 59 (11) (Jun 1): 2615-22.

Arastu-Kapur, S., J. L. Anderl, M. Kraus, F. Parlati, K. D. Shenk, S. J. Lee, T. Muchamuel, et al. 2011. Nonproteasomal targets of the proteasome inhibitors bortezomib and carfilzomib: A link to clinical adverse events. *Clinical Cancer Research* 17 (9) (May 1): 2734-43.

Badros, A., A. M. Burger, S. Philip, R. Niesvizky, S. S. Kolla, O. Goloubeva, C. Harris, et al. 2009. Phase I study of vorinostat in combination with bortezomib for relapsed and refractory multiple myeloma. *Clinical Cancer Research* 15 (16) (Aug 15): 5250-7.

Badros, A., O. Goloubeva, R. Fenton, A. P. Rapoport, G. Akpek, C. Harris, K. Ruehle, S. Westphal, and B. Meisenberg. 2006. Phase I trial of first-line bortezomib/thalidomide plus chemotherapy for induction and stem cell mobilization in patients with multiple myeloma. *Clinical Lymphoma & Myeloma* 7 (3) (Nov): 210-6.

Barlogie, B., E. Anaissie, F. van Rhee, J. Haessler, K. Hollmig, M. Pineda-Roman, M. Cottler-Fox, et al. 2007. Incorporating bortezomib into upfront treatment for multiple myeloma: Early results of total therapy 3. *British Journal of Haematology* 138 (2) (Jul): 176-85.

Baumann, P., S. Mandl-Weber, F. Oduncu, and R. Schmidmaier. 2009. The novel orally bioavailable inhibitor of phosphoinositol-3-kinase and mammalian target of rapamycin, NVP-BEZ235, inhibits growth and proliferation in multiple myeloma. *Experimental Cell Research* 315 (3) (Feb 1): 485-97.

Bensinger, W. I., S. Jagannath, R. Vescio, E. Camacho, J. Wolf, D. Irwin, G. Capo, et al. 2010. Phase 2 study of two sequential three-drug combinations containing bortezomib, cyclophosphamide and dexamethasone, followed by bortezomib, thalidomide and dexamethasone as frontline therapy for multiple myeloma. *British Journal of Haematology* 148 (4) (Feb): 562-8.

Berenson, J. R., J. Matous, R. A. Swift, R. Mapes, B. Morrison, and H. S. Yeh. 2007. A phase I/II study of arsenic trioxide/bortezomib/ascorbic acid combination therapy for the treatment of relapsed or refractory multiple myeloma. *Clinical Cancer Research* 13 (6) (Mar 15): 1762-8.

Berenson, J. R., H. H. Yang, K. Sadler, S. G. Jarutirasarn, R. A. Vescio, R. Mapes, M. Purner, et al. 2006. Phase I/II trial assessing bortezomib and melphalan combination therapy for the treatment of patients with relapsed or refractory multiple myeloma. *Journal of Clinical Oncology* 24 (6) (Feb 20): 937-44.

Berenson, J. R., O. Yellin, R. Patel, H. Duvivier, Y. Nassir, R. Mapes, C. D. Abaya, and R. A. Swift. 2009a. A phase I study of samarium lexidronam/bortezomib combination therapy for the treatment of relapsed or refractory multiple myeloma. *Clinical Cancer Research* 15 (3) (Feb 1): 1069-75.

Berenson, J. R., O. Yellin, D. Woytowitz, M. S. Flam, A. Cartmell, R. Patel, H. Duvivier, et al. 2009b. Bortezomib, ascorbic acid and melphalan (BAM) therapy for patients with newly diagnosed multiple myeloma: An effective and well-tolerated frontline regimen. *European Journal of Haematology* 82 (6) (Jun): 433-9.

Brekken, R. A., J. P. Overholser, V. A. Stastny, J. Waltenberger, J. D. Minna, and P. E. Thorpe. 2000. Selective inhibition of vascular endothelial growth factor (VEGF) receptor 2 (KDR/Flk-1) activity by a monoclonal anti-VEGF antibody blocks tumor growth in mice. *Cancer Research* 60 (18) (Sep 15): 5117-24.

Catley, L., E. Weisberg, T. Kiziltepe, Y. T. Tai, T. Hideshima, P. Neri, P. Tassone, et al. 2006. Aggresome induction by proteasome inhibitor bortezomib and alpha-tubulin hyperacetylation by tubulin deacetylase (TDAC) inhibitor LBH589 are synergistic in myeloma cells. *Blood* 108 (10) (Nov 15): 3441-9.

Cavo, M., P. Tacchetti, F. Patriarca, M. T. Petrucci, L. Pantani, M. Galli, F. Di Raimondo, et al. 2010. Bortezomib with thalidomide plus dexamethasone compared with thalidomide plus dexamethasone as induction therapy before, and consolidation therapy after, double autologous stem-cell transplantation in newly diagnosed multiple myeloma: A randomised phase 3 study. *Lancet* 376 (9758) (Dec 18): 2075-85.

Chanan-Khan, A., K. C. Miller, L. Musial, S. Padmanabhan, J. Yu, S. Ailawadhi, T. Sher, et al. 2009. Bortezomib in combination with pegylated liposomal doxorubicin and thalidomide is an effective steroid independent salvage regimen for patients with relapsed or refractory multiple myeloma: Results of a phase II clinical trial. *Leukemia & Lymphoma* 50 (7) (Jul): 1096-101.

Chauhan, D., L. Catley, G. Li, K. Podar, T. Hideshima, M. Velankar, C. Mitsiades, et al. 2005. A novel orally active proteasome inhibitor induces apoptosis in multiple myeloma cells with mechanisms distinct from bortezomib. *Cancer Cell* 8 (5) (Nov): 407-19.

Chauhan, D., A. Singh, M. Brahmandam, K. Podar, T. Hideshima, P. Richardson, N. Munshi, M. A. Palladino, and K. C. Anderson. 2008. Combination of proteasome inhibitors bortezomib and NPI-0052 trigger in vivo synergistic cytotoxicity in multiple myeloma. *Blood* 111 (3) (Feb 1): 1654-64.

Chauhan, D., A. V. Singh, B. Ciccarelli, P. G. Richardson, M. A. Palladino, and K. C. Anderson. 2010a. Combination of novel proteasome inhibitor NPI-0052 and lenalidomide trigger in vitro and in vivo synergistic cytotoxicity in multiple myeloma. *Blood* 115 (4) (Jan 28): 834-45.

Chauhan, D., A. V. Singh, M. Aujay, C. J. Kirk, M. Bandi, B. Ciccarelli, N. Raje, P. Richardson, and K. C. Anderson. 2010b. A novel orally active proteasome inhibitor ONX 0912 triggers in vitro and in vivo cytotoxicity in multiple myeloma. *Blood* 116 (23) (Dec 2): 4906-15.

Chauhan, D., Z. Tian, B. Zhou, D. J. Kuhn, R. Z. Orlowski, N. S. Raje, P. G. Richardson, and K. C. Anderson. 2011. In vitro and in vivo selective antitumor activity of a novel orally bioavailable proteasome inhibitor MLN9708 against multiple myeloma cells. *Clinical Cancer Research* 17 (16) (Aug 15): 5311-21.

Chauhan, D., M. Velankar, M. Brahmandam, T. Hideshima, K. Podar, P. Richardson, R. Schlossman, et al. 2007. A novel bcl-2/Bcl-X(L)/Bcl-w inhibitor ABT-737 as therapy in multiple myeloma. *Oncogene* 26 (16) (Apr 5): 2374-80.

Chen, S., J. L. Blank, T. Peters, X. J. Liu, D. M. Rappoli, M. D. Pickard, S. Menon, et al. 2010. Genome-wide siRNA screen for modulators of cell death induced by proteasome inhibitor bortezomib. *Cancer Research* 70 (11) (Jun 1): 4318-26.

Corso, A., L. Barbarano, S. Mangiacavalli, M. Spriano, E. P. Alessandrino, A. M. Cafro, C. Pascutto, et al. 2010. Bortezomib plus dexamethasone can improve stem cell collection and overcome the need for additional chemotherapy before autologous transplant in patients with myeloma. *Leukemia & Lymphoma* 51 (2) (Feb): 236-42.

Crawford, L. J., B. Walker, H. Ovaa, D. Chauhan, K. C. Anderson, T. C. Morris, and A. E. Irvine. 2006. Comparative selectivity and specificity of the proteasome inhibitors BzLLLCOCHO, PS-341, and MG-132. *Cancer Research* 66 (12) (Jun 15): 6379-86.

Dai, Y., M. Rahmani, and S. Grant. 2003. Proteasome inhibitors potentiate leukemic cell apoptosis induced by the cyclin-dependent kinase inhibitor flavopiridol through a SAPK/JNK- and NF-kappaB-dependent process. *Oncogene* 22 (46) (Oct 16): 7108-22.

Dai, Y., M. Rahmani, X. Y. Pei, P. Dent, and S. Grant. 2004. Bortezomib and flavopiridol interact synergistically to induce apoptosis in chronic myeloid leukemia cells resistant to imatinib mesylate through both Bcr/Abl-dependent and -independent mechanisms. *Blood* 104 (2) (Jul 15): 509-18.

Dasmahapatra, G., D. Lembersky, L. Kramer, R. I. Fisher, J. Friedberg, P. Dent, and S. Grant. 2010. The pan-HDAC inhibitor vorinostat potentiates the activity of the proteasome inhibitor carfilzomib in human DLBCL cells in vitro and in vivo. *Blood* 115 (22) (Jun 3): 4478-87.

Dasmahapatra, G., D. Lembersky, M. P. Son, E. Attkisson, P. Dent, R. I. Fisher, J. W. Friedberg, and S. Grant. 2011. Carfilzomib interacts synergistically with histone deacetylase inhibitors in mantle cell lymphoma cells in vitro and in vivo. *Molecular Cancer Therapeutics* 10 (9) (Sept): 1686-97.

Davenport, E. L., H. E. Moore, A. S. Dunlop, S. Y. Sharp, P. Workman, G. J. Morgan, and F. E. Davies. 2007. Heat shock protein inhibition is associated with activation of the unfolded protein response pathway in myeloma plasma cells. *Blood* 110 (7) (Oct 1): 2641-9.

David, E., S. Y. Sun, E. K. Waller, J. Chen, F. R. Khuri, and S. Lonial. 2005. The combination of the farnesyl transferase inhibitor lonafarnib and the proteasome inhibitor bortezomib induces synergistic apoptosis in human myeloma cells that is associated with down-regulation of p-AKT. *Blood* 106 (13) (Dec 15): 4322-9.

de Queiroz Crusoe, E., P. Maiso, D. Fernandez-Lazaro, L. San-Segundo, M. Garayoa, A. Garcia-Gomez, N. C. Gutierrez, et al. 2011. Transcriptomic rationale for the synergy observed with dasatinib + bortezomib + dexamethasone in multiple myeloma. *Annals of Hematology* (Jul 1) epub ahead of print.

Decaux, O., M. Clement, F. Magrangeas, W. Gouraud, C. Charbonnel, L. Campion, H. A. Loiseau, and S. Minvielle. 2010. Inhibition of mTORC1 activity by REDD1 induction in myeloma cells resistant to bortezomib cytotoxicity. *Cancer Science* 101 (4) (Apr): 889-97.

Demo, S. D., C. J. Kirk, M. A. Aujay, T. J. Buchholz, M. Dajee, M. N. Ho, J. Jiang, et al. 2007. Antitumor activity of PR-171, a novel irreversible inhibitor of the proteasome. *Cancer Research* 67 (13) (Jul 1): 6383-91.

Descamps, G., P. Gomez-Bougie, C. Venot, P. Moreau, R. Bataille, and M. Amiot. 2009. A humanised anti-IGF-1R monoclonal antibody (AVE1642) enhances bortezomib-induced apoptosis in myeloma cells lacking CD45. *British Journal of Cancer* 100 (2) (Jan 27): 366-9.

Dispenzieri, A., S. Jacobus, D. H. Vesole, N. Callandar, R. Fonseca, and P. R. Greipp. 2010. Primary therapy with single agent bortezomib as induction, maintenance and re-induction in patients with high-risk myeloma: Results of the ECOG E2A02 trial. *Leukemia, U.K* 24 (8) (Aug): 1406-11.

Dong, H., L. Chen, X. Chen, H. Gu, G. Gao, Y. Gao, and B. Dong. 2009. Dysregulation of unfolded protein response partially underlies proapoptotic activity of bortezomib in multiple myeloma cells. *Leukemia & Lymphoma* 50 (6) (Jun): 974-84.

Dorsey, B. D., M. Iqbal, S. Chatterjee, E. Menta, R. Bernardini, A. Bernareggi, P. G. Cassara, et al. 2008. Discovery of a potent, selective, and orally active proteasome inhibitor for the treatment of cancer. *Journal of Medicinal Chemistry* 51 (4) (Feb 28): 1068-72.

Drexler, H. C. 1997. Activation of the cell death program by inhibition of proteasome function. *Proceedings of the National Academy of Sciences of the United States of America* 94 (3) (Feb 4): 855-60.

Edwards, C. M., S. T. Lwin, J. A. Fowler, B. O. Oyajobi, J. Zhuang, A. L. Bates, and G. R. Mundy. 2009. Myeloma cells exhibit an increase in proteasome activity and an enhanced response to proteasome inhibition in the bone marrow microenvironment in vivo. *American Journal of Hematology* 84 (5) (May): 268-72.

Fennell, D. A., A. Chacko, and L. Mutti. 2008. BCL-2 family regulation by the 20S proteasome inhibitor bortezomib. *Oncogene* 27 (9) (Feb 21): 1189-97.

Fuchs, O., D. Provaznikova, I. Marinov, K. Kuzelova, and I. Spicka. 2009. Antiproliferative and proapoptotic effects of proteasome inhibitors and their combination with histone deacetylase inhibitors on leukemia cells. *Cardiovascular & Hematological Disorders Drug Targets* 9 (1) (Mar): 62-77.

Gasparetto, C., J. P. Gockerman, L. F. Diehl, C. M. de Castro, J. O. Moore, G. D. Long, M. E. Horwitz, et al. 2010. "Short course" bortezomib plus melphalan and prednisone as induction prior to transplant or as frontline therapy for nontransplant candidates in patients with previously untreated multiple myeloma. *Biology of Blood and Marrow Transplantation* 16 (1) (Jan): 70-7.

Ghobrial, I. M., E. Weller, R. Vij, N. C. Munshi, R. Banwait, M. Bagshaw, R. Schlossman, et al. 2011. Weekly bortezomib in combination with temsirolimus in relapsed or relapsed and refractory multiple myeloma: A multicentre, phase 1/2, open-label, dose-escalation study. *The Lancet Oncology* 12 (3) (Mar): 263-72.

Ghosh, N., X. Ye, A. Ferguson, C. A. Huff, and I. Borrello. 2011. Bortezomib and thalidomide, a steroid free regimen in newly diagnosed patients with multiple myeloma. *British Journal of Haematology* 152 (5) (Mar): 593-9.

Gilmore, T. D. 2006. Introduction to NF-kappaB: Players, pathways, perspectives. *Oncogene* 25 (51) (Oct 30): 6680-4.

Giuliani, N., F. Morandi, S. Tagliaferri, M. Lazzaretti, S. Bonomini, M. Crugnola, C. Mancini, et al. 2007. The proteasome inhibitor bortezomib affects osteoblast differentiation in vitro and in vivo in multiple myeloma patients. *Blood* 110 (1) (Jul 1): 334-8.

Gomez-Bougie, P., S. Wuilleme-Toumi, E. Menoret, V. Trichet, N. Robillard, M. Philippe, R. Bataille, and M. Amiot. 2007. Noxa up-regulation and mcl-1 cleavage are associated to apoptosis induction by bortezomib in multiple myeloma. *Cancer Research* 67 (11) (Jun 1): 5418-24.

Gorgun, G., E. Calabrese, T. Hideshima, J. Ecsedy, G. Perrone, M. Mani, H. Ikeda, et al. 2010. A novel aurora-A kinase inhibitor MLN8237 induces cytotoxicity and cell-cycle arrest in multiple myeloma. *Blood* 115 (25) (Jun 24): 5202-13.

Groll, M., M. Bajorek, A. Kohler, L. Moroder, D. M. Rubin, R. Huber, M. H. Glickman, and D. Finley. 2000. A gated channel into the proteasome core particle. *Nature Structural Biology* 7 (11) (Nov): 1062-7.

Groll, M., L. Ditzel, J. Lowe, D. Stock, M. Bochtler, H. D. Bartunik, and R. Huber. 1997. Structure of 20S proteasome from yeast at 2.4 A resolution. *Nature* 386 (6624) (Apr 3): 463-71.

Groll, M., W. Heinemeyer, S. Jager, T. Ullrich, M. Bochtler, D. H. Wolf, and R. Huber. 1999. The catalytic sites of 20S proteasomes and their role in subunit maturation: A mutational and crystallographic study. *Proceedings of the National Academy of Sciences of the United States of America* 96 (20) (Sep 28): 10976-83.

Groll, M., and R. Huber. 2004. Inhibitors of the eukaryotic 20S proteasome core particle: A structural approach. *Biochimica Et Biophysica Acta* 1695 (1-3) (Nov 29): 33-44.

Gu, H., X. Chen, G. Gao, and H. Dong. 2008. Caspase-2 functions upstream of mitochondria in endoplasmic reticulum stress-induced apoptosis by bortezomib in human myeloma cells. *Molecular Cancer Therapeutics* 7 (8) (Aug): 2298-307.

Harousseau, J. L., M. Attal, H. Avet-Loiseau, G. Marit, D. Caillot, M. Mohty, P. Lenain, et al. 2010. Bortezomib plus dexamethasone is superior to vincristine plus doxorubicin plus dexamethasone as induction treatment prior to autologous stem-cell transplantation in newly diagnosed multiple myeloma: Results of the IFM 2005-01 phase III trial. *Journal of Clinical Oncology* 28 (30) (Oct 20): 4621-9.

Harousseau, J. L., M. Attal, X. Leleu, J. Troncy, B. Pegourie, A. M. Stoppa, C. Hulin, et al. 2006. Bortezomib plus dexamethasone as induction treatment prior to autologous stem cell transplantation in patients with newly diagnosed multiple myeloma: Results of an IFM phase II study. *Haematologica* 91 (11) (Nov): 1498-505.

Heider, U., M. Kaiser, C. Muller, C. Jakob, I. Zavrski, C. O. Schulz, C. Fleissner, M. Hecht, and O. Sezer. 2006. Bortezomib increases osteoblast activity in myeloma patients irrespective of response to treatment. *European Journal of Haematology* 77 (3) (Sep): 233-8.

Heinemeyer, W., M. Fischer, T. Krimmer, U. Stachon, and D. H. Wolf. 1997. The active sites of the eukaryotic 20 S proteasome and their involvement in subunit precursor processing. *The Journal of Biological Chemistry* 272 (40) (Oct 3): 25200-9.

Hideshima, T., L. Catley, N. Raje, D. Chauhan, K. Podar, C. Mitsiades, Y. T. Tai, et al. 2007. Inhibition of akt induces significant downregulation of survivin and cytotoxicity in human multiple myeloma cells. *British Journal of Haematology* 138 (6) (Sep): 783-91.

Hideshima, T., H. Ikeda, D. Chauhan, Y. Okawa, N. Raje, K. Podar, C. Mitsiades, et al. 2009. Bortezomib induces canonical nuclear factor-kappaB activation in multiple myeloma cells. *Blood* 114 (5) (Jul 30): 1046-52.

Hideshima, T., P. Richardson, D. Chauhan, V. J. Palombella, P. J. Elliott, J. Adams, and K. C. Anderson. 2001. The proteasome inhibitor PS-341 inhibits growth, induces apoptosis, and overcomes drug resistance in human multiple myeloma cells. *Cancer Research* 61 (7) (Apr 1): 3071-6.

Hoang, B., P. Frost, Y. Shi, E. Belanger, A. Benavides, G. Pezeshkpour, S. Cappia, T. Guglielmelli, J. Gera, and A. Lichtenstein. 2010. Targeting TORC2 in multiple myeloma with a new mTOR kinase inhibitor. *Blood* 116 (22) (Nov 25): 4560-8.

Holkova, B., E. B. Perkins, V. Ramakrishnan, M. B. Tombes, E. Shrader, N. Talreja, M. D. Wellons, et al. 2011. Phase I trial of bortezomib (PS-341; NSC 681239) and alvocidib (flavopiridol; NSC 649890) in patients with recurrent or refractory B-cell neoplasms. *Clinical Cancer Research* 17 (10) (May 15): 3388-97.

Imajoh-Ohmi, S., T. Kawaguchi, S. Sugiyama, K. Tanaka, S. Omura, and H. Kikuchi. 1995. Lactacystin, a specific inhibitor of the proteasome, induces apoptosis in human monoblast U937 cells. *Biochemical and Biophysical Research Communications* 217 (3) (Dec 26): 1070-7.

Jagannath, S., B. Barlogie, J. Berenson, D. Siegel, D. Irwin, P. G. Richardson, R. Niesvizky, et al. 2004. A phase 2 study of two doses of bortezomib in relapsed or refractory myeloma. *British Journal of Haematology* 127 (2) (Oct): 165-72.

Jakubowiak, A. J., K. A. Griffith, D. E. Reece, C. C. Hofmeister, S. Lonial, T. M. Zimmerman, E. L. Campagnaro, et al. 2011. Lenalidomide, bortezomib, pegylated liposomal doxorubicin, and dexamethasone in newly diagnosed multiple myeloma: A phase 1/2 multiple myeloma research consortium trial. *Blood* 118 (3) (Jul 21): 535-43.

Jakubowiak, A. J., T. Kendall, A. Al-Zoubi, Y. Khaled, S. Mineishi, A. Ahmed, E. Campagnaro, et al. 2009. Phase II trial of combination therapy with bortezomib, pegylated liposomal doxorubicin, and dexamethasone in patients with newly diagnosed myeloma. *Journal of Clinical Oncology* 27 (30) (Oct 20): 5015-22.

Kane, R. C., A. T. Farrell, R. Sridhara, and R. Pazdur. 2006. United States food and drug administration approval summary: Bortezomib for the treatment of progressive multiple myeloma after one prior therapy. *Clinical Cancer Research* 12 (10) (May 15): 2955-60.

Kawaguchi, T., K. Miyazawa, S. Moriya, T. Ohtomo, X. F. Che, M. Naito, M. Itoh, and A. Tomoda. 2011. Combined treatment with bortezomib plus bafilomycin A1 enhances the cytocidal effect and induces endoplasmic reticulum stress in U266 myeloma cells: Crosstalk among proteasome, autophagy-lysosome and ER stress. *International Journal of Oncology* 38 (3) (Mar): 643-54.

Kim, H. J., S. S. Yoon, D. S. Lee, S. K. Sohn, H. S. Eom, J. L. Lee, J. S. Chung, et al. 2011. Sequential vincristine, adriamycin, dexamethasone (VAD) followed by bortezomib, thalidomide, dexamethasone (VTD) as induction, followed by high-dose therapy with autologous stem cell transplant and consolidation therapy with bortezomib for newly diagnosed multiple myeloma: Results of a phase II trial. *Annals of Hematology* (Jul 26) epub ahead of print.

Kim, Y. K., S. K. Sohn, J. H. Lee, D. H. Yang, J. H. Moon, J. S. Ahn, H. J. Kim, J. J. Lee, and Korean Multiple Myeloma Working Party (KMMWP). 2010. Clinical efficacy of a bortezomib, cyclophosphamide, thalidomide, and dexamethasone (vel-CTD) regimen in patients with relapsed or refractory multiple myeloma: A phase II study. *Annals of Hematology* 89 (5) (May): 475-82.

Kropff, M., G. Bisping, E. Schuck, P. Liebisch, N. Lang, M. Hentrich, T. Dechow, et al. 2007. Bortezomib in combination with intermediate-dose dexamethasone and continuous low-dose oral cyclophosphamide for relapsed multiple myeloma. *British Journal of Haematology* 138 (3) (Aug): 330-7.

Kuhn, D. J., Q. Chen, P. M. Voorhees, J. S. Strader, K. D. Shenk, C. M. Sun, S. D. Demo, et al. 2007. Potent activity of carfilzomib, a novel, irreversible inhibitor of the ubiquitin-proteasome pathway, against preclinical models of multiple myeloma. *Blood* 110 (9) (Nov 1): 3281-90.

Kuhn, D. J., S. A. Hunsucker, Q. Chen, P. M. Voorhees, M. Orlowski, and R. Z. Orlowski. 2009. Targeted inhibition of the immunoproteasome is a potent strategy against models of multiple myeloma that overcomes resistance to conventional drugs and nonspecific proteasome inhibitors. *Blood* 113 (19) (May 7): 4667-76.

Kumar, S. K., I. Flinn, S. J. Noga, P. Hari, R. Rifkin, N. Callander, M. Bhandari, et al. 2010. Bortezomib, dexamethasone, cyclophosphamide and lenalidomide combination for newly diagnosed multiple myeloma: Phase 1 results from the multicenter EVOLUTION study. *Leukemia, U.K* 24 (7) (Jul): 1350-6.

Kupperman, E., E. C. Lee, Y. Cao, B. Bannerman, M. Fitzgerald, A. Berger, J. Yu, et al. 2010. Evaluation of the proteasome inhibitor MLN9708 in preclinical models of human cancer. *Cancer Research* 70 (5) (Mar 1): 1970-80.

LeBlanc, R., L. P. Catley, T. Hideshima, S. Lentzsch, C. S. Mitsiades, N. Mitsiades, D. Neuberg, et al. 2002. Proteasome inhibitor PS-341 inhibits human myeloma cell growth in vivo and prolongs survival in a murine model. *Cancer Research* 62 (17) (Sep 1): 4996-5000.

Lightcap, E. S., T. A. McCormack, C. S. Pien, V. Chau, J. Adams, and P. J. Elliott. 2000. Proteasome inhibition measurements: Clinical application. *Clinical Chemistry* 46 (5) (May): 673-83.

Ling, X., D. Calinski, A. A. Chanan-Khan, M. Zhou, and F. Li. 2010. Cancer cell sensitivity to bortezomib is associated with survivin expression and p53 status but not cancer cell types. *Journal of Experimental & Clinical Cancer Research : CR* 29 (Jan 22): 8.

Lonial, S., J. Kaufman, M. Tighiouart, A. Nooka, A. A. Langston, L. T. Heffner, C. Torre, et al. 2010. A phase I/II trial combining high-dose melphalan and autologous transplant with bortezomib for multiple myeloma: A dose- and schedule-finding study. *Clinical Cancer Research* 16 (20) (Oct 15): 5079-86.

Lund, T., K. Soe, N. Abildgaard, P. Garnero, P. T. Pedersen, T. Ormstrup, J. M. Delaisse, and T. Plesner. 2010. First-line treatment with bortezomib rapidly stimulates both osteoblast activity and bone matrix deposition in patients with multiple myeloma, and stimulates osteoblast proliferation and differentiation in vitro. *European Journal of Haematology* 85 (4) (Oct): 290-9.

Macherla, V. R., S. S. Mitchell, R. R. Manam, K. A. Reed, T. H. Chao, B. Nicholson, G. Deyanat-Yazdi, et al. 2005. Structure-activity relationship studies of salinosporamide A (NPI-0052), a novel marine derived proteasome inhibitor. *Journal of Medicinal Chemistry* 48 (11) (Jun 2): 3684-7.

Markovina, S., N. S. Callander, S. L. O'Connor, J. Kim, J. E. Werndli, M. Raschko, C. P. Leith, B. S. Kahl, K. Kim, and S. Miyamoto. 2008. Bortezomib-resistant nuclear factor-kappaB activity in multiple myeloma cells. *Molecular Cancer Research : MCR* 6 (8) (Aug): 1356-64.

Meister, S., U. Schubert, K. Neubert, K. Herrmann, R. Burger, M. Gramatzki, S. Hahn, et al. 2007. Extensive immunoglobulin production sensitizes myeloma cells for proteasome inhibition. *Cancer Research* 67 (4) (Feb 15): 1783-92.

Menu, E., J. Garcia, X. Huang, M. Di Liberto, P. L. Toogood, I. Chen, K. Vanderkerken, and S. Chen-Kiang. 2008. A novel therapeutic combination using PD 0332991 and bortezomib: Study in the 5T33MM myeloma model. *Cancer Research* 68 (14) (Jul 15): 5519-23.

Mitsiades, C. S., N. S. Mitsiades, C. J. McMullan, V. Poulaki, A. L. Kung, F. E. Davies, G. Morgan, et al. 2006. Antimyeloma activity of heat shock protein-90 inhibition. *Blood* 107 (3) (Feb 1): 1092-100.

Mitsiades, N., C. S. Mitsiades, V. Poulaki, D. Chauhan, G. Fanourakis, X. Gu, C. Bailey, et al. 2002. Molecular sequelae of proteasome inhibition in human multiple myeloma cells. *Proceedings of the National Academy of Sciences of the United States of America* 99 (22) (Oct 29): 14374-9.

Moreau, P., F. Cavallo, X. Leleu, C. Hulin, M. Amiot, G. Descamps, T. Facon, M. Boccadoro, D. Mignard, and J. L. Harousseau. 2011. Phase I study of the anti insulin-like growth factor 1 receptor (IGF-1R) monoclonal antibody, AVE1642, as single agent and in combination with bortezomib in patients with relapsed multiple myeloma. *Leukemia* 25 (5) (May): 872-4.

Navas, T. A., A. N. Nguyen, T. Hideshima, M. Reddy, J. Y. Ma, E. Haghnazari, M. Henson, et al. 2006. Inhibition of p38alpha MAPK enhances proteasome inhibitor-induced apoptosis of myeloma cells by modulating Hsp27, bcl-X(L), mcl-1 and p53 levels in vitro and inhibits tumor growth in vivo. *Leukemia* 20 (6) (Jun): 1017-27.

Navon, A., and A. L. Goldberg. 2001. Proteins are unfolded on the surface of the ATPase ring before transport into the proteasome. *Molecular Cell* 8 (6) (Dec): 1339-49.

Nawrocki, S. T., C. J. Bruns, M. T. Harbison, R. J. Bold, B. S. Gotsch, J. L. Abbruzzese, P. Elliott, J. Adams, and D. J. McConkey. 2002. Effects of the proteasome inhibitor PS-341 on apoptosis and angiogenesis in orthotopic human pancreatic tumor xenografts. *Molecular Cancer Therapeutics* 1 (14) (Dec): 1243-53.

Nawrocki, S. T., J. S. Carew, K. H. Maclean, J. F. Courage, P. Huang, J. A. Houghton, J. L. Cleveland, F. J. Giles, and D. J. McConkey. 2008. Myc regulates aggresome formation, the induction of noxa, and apoptosis in response to the combination of bortezomib and SAHA. *Blood* 112 (7) (Oct 1): 2917-26.

Nikiforov, M. A., M. Riblett, W. H. Tang, V. Gratchouck, D. Zhuang, Y. Fernandez, M. Verhaegen, et al. 2007. Tumor cell-selective regulation of NOXA by c-MYC in response to proteasome inhibition. *Proceedings of the National Academy of Sciences of the United States of America* 104 (49) (Dec 4): 19488-93.

Oakervee, H. E., R. Popat, N. Curry, P. Smith, C. Morris, M. Drake, S. Agrawal, et al. 2005. PAD combination therapy (PS-341/bortezomib, doxorubicin and dexamethasone) for previously untreated patients with multiple myeloma. *British Journal of Haematology* 129 (6) (Jun): 755-62.

Obaidat, A., J. Weiss, B. Wahlgren, R. R. Manam, V. R. Macherla, K. McArthur, T. H. Chao, et al. 2011. Proteasome regulator marizomib (NPI-0052) exhibits prolonged inhibition, attenuated efflux, and greater cytotoxicity than its reversible analogs. *The Journal of Pharmacology and Experimental Therapeutics* 337 (2) (May): 479-86.

Obeng, E. A., L. M. Carlson, D. M. Gutman, W. J. Harrington Jr, K. P. Lee, and L. H. Boise. 2006. Proteasome inhibitors induce a terminal unfolded protein response in multiple myeloma cells. *Blood* 107 (12) (Jun 15): 4907-16.

O'Connor, O. A., A. K. Stewart, M. Vallone, C. J. Molineaux, L. A. Kunkel, J. F. Gerecitano, and R. Z. Orlowski. 2009. A phase 1 dose escalation study of the safety and pharmacokinetics of the novel proteasome inhibitor carfilzomib (PR-171) in patients with hematologic malignancies. *Clinical Cancer Research* 15 (22) (Nov 15): 7085-91.

Orlowski, R. Z., J. R. Eswara, A. Lafond-Walker, M. R. Grever, M. Orlowski, and C. V. Dang. 1998. Tumor growth inhibition induced in a murine model of human burkitt's lymphoma by a proteasome inhibitor. *Cancer Research* 58 (19) (Oct 1): 4342-8.

Orlowski, R. Z., T. E. Stinchcombe, B. S. Mitchell, T. C. Shea, A. S. Baldwin, S. Stahl, J. Adams, et al. 2002. Phase I trial of the proteasome inhibitor PS-341 in patients with refractory hematologic malignancies. *Journal of Clinical Oncology* 20 (22) (Nov 15): 4420-7.

Palumbo, A., M. T. Ambrosini, G. Benevolo, P. Pregno, N. Pescosta, V. Callea, C. Cangialosi, et al. 2007. Bortezomib, melphalan, prednisone, and thalidomide for relapsed multiple myeloma. *Blood* 109 (7) (Apr 1): 2767-72.

Pineda-Roman, M., M. Zangari, F. van Rhee, E. Anaissie, J. Szymonifka, A. Hoering, N. Petty, et al. 2008. VTD combination therapy with bortezomib-thalidomide-dexamethasone is highly effective in advanced and refractory multiple myeloma. *Leukemia* 22 (7) (Jul): 1419-27.

Piva, R., B. Ruggeri, M. Williams, G. Costa, I. Tamagno, D. Ferrero, V. Giai, et al. 2008. CEP-18770: A novel, orally active proteasome inhibitor with a tumor-selective pharmacologic profile competitive with bortezomib. *Blood* 111 (5) (Mar 1): 2765-75.

Popat, R., H. Oakervee, C. Williams, M. Cook, C. Craddock, S. Basu, C. Singer, et al. 2009. Bortezomib, low-dose intravenous melphalan, and dexamethasone for patients with relapsed multiple myeloma. *British Journal of Haematology* 144 (6) (Mar): 887-94.

Popat, R., H. E. Oakervee, S. Hallam, N. Curry, L. Odeh, N. Foot, D. L. Esseltine, M. Drake, C. Morris, and J. D. Cavenagh. 2008. Bortezomib, doxorubicin and dexamethasone (PAD) front-line treatment of multiple myeloma: Updated results after long-term follow-up. *British Journal of Haematology* 141 (4) (May): 512-6.

Qin, J. Z., J. Ziffra, L. Stennett, B. Bodner, B. K. Bonish, V. Chaturvedi, F. Bennett, et al. 2005. Proteasome inhibitors trigger NOXA-mediated apoptosis in melanoma and myeloma cells. *Cancer Research* 65 (14) (Jul 15): 6282-93.

Rao, R., S. Nalluri, W. Fiskus, A. Savoie, K. M. Buckley, K. Ha, R. Balusu, et al. 2010. Role of CAAT/enhancer binding protein homologous protein in panobinostat-mediated potentiation of bortezomib-induced lethal endoplasmic reticulum stress in mantle cell lymphoma cells. *Clinical Cancer Research* 16 (19) (Oct 1): 4742-54.

Read, M. A., A. S. Neish, F. W. Luscinskas, V. J. Palombella, T. Maniatis, and T. Collins. 1995. The proteasome pathway is required for cytokine-induced endothelial-leukocyte adhesion molecule expression. *Immunity* 2 (5) (May): 493-506.

Reeder, C. B., D. E. Reece, V. Kukreti, C. Chen, S. Trudel, J. Hentz, B. Noble, et al. 2009. Cyclophosphamide, bortezomib and dexamethasone induction for newly diagnosed multiple myeloma: High response rates in a phase II clinical trial. *Leukemia* 23 (7) (Jul): 1337-41.

Ri, M., S. Iida, T. Nakashima, H. Miyazaki, F. Mori, A. Ito, A. Inagaki, et al. 2010. Bortezomib-resistant myeloma cell lines: A role for mutated PSMB5 in preventing the accumulation of unfolded proteins and fatal ER stress. *Leukemia* 24 (8) (Aug): 1506-12.

Richardson, P. G., B. Barlogie, J. Berenson, S. Singhal, S. Jagannath, D. Irwin, S. V. Rajkumar, et al. 2003. A phase 2 study of bortezomib in relapsed, refractory myeloma. *The New England Journal of Medicine* 348 (26) (Jun 26): 2609-17.

Richardson, P. G., A. A. Chanan-Khan, S. Lonial, A. Y. Krishnan, M. P. Carroll, M. Alsina, M. Albitar, D. Berman, M. Messina, and K. C. Anderson. 2011. Tanespimycin and bortezomib combination treatment in patients with relapsed or relapsed and refractory multiple myeloma: Results of a phase 1/2 study. *British Journal of Haematology* 153 (6) (Jun): 729-40.

Richardson, P. G., P. Sonneveld, M. W. Schuster, D. Irwin, E. A. Stadtmauer, T. Facon, J. L. Harousseau, et al. 2005. Bortezomib or high-dose dexamethasone for relapsed multiple myeloma. *The New England Journal of Medicine* 352 (24) (Jun 16): 2487-98.

Richardson, P. G., E. Weller, S. Lonial, A. J. Jakubowiak, S. Jagannath, N. S. Raje, D. E. Avigan, et al. 2010. Lenalidomide, bortezomib, and dexamethasone combination therapy in patients with newly diagnosed multiple myeloma. *Blood* 116 (5) (Aug 5): 679-86.

Roccaro, A. M., A. Sacco, M. Aujay, H. T. Ngo, A. K. Azab, F. Azab, P. Quang, et al. 2010. Selective inhibition of chymotrypsin-like activity of the immunoproteasome and constitutive proteasome in waldenstrom macroglobulinemia. *Blood* 115 (20) (May 20): 4051-60.

Rock, K. L., and A. L. Goldberg. 1999. Degradation of cell proteins and the generation of MHC class I-presented peptides. *Annual Review of Immunology* 17 : 739-79.

Rosinol, L., A. Oriol, M. V. Mateos, A. Sureda, P. Garcia-Sanchez, N. Gutierrez, A. Alegre, et al. 2007. Phase II PETHEMA trial of alternating bortezomib and dexamethasone as induction regimen before autologous stem-cell transplantation in younger patients with multiple myeloma: Efficacy and clinical implications of tumor response kinetics. *Journal of Clinical Oncology* 25 (28) (Oct 1): 4452-8.

Roue, G., P. Perez-Galan, A. Mozos, M. Lopez-Guerra, S. Xargay-Torrent, L. Rosich, I. Saborit-Villarroya, E. Normant, E. Campo, and D. Colomer. 2011. The Hsp90 inhibitor IPI-504 overcomes bortezomib resistance in mantle cell lymphoma in vitro and in vivo by down-regulation of the prosurvival ER chaperone BiP/Grp78. *Blood* 117 (4) (Jan 27): 1270-9.

Roussel, M., P. Moreau, A. Huynh, J. Y. Mary, C. Danho, D. Caillot, C. Hulin, et al. 2010. Bortezomib and high-dose melphalan as conditioning regimen before autologous stem cell transplantation in patients with de novo multiple myeloma: A phase 2 study of the intergroupe francophone du myelome (IFM). *Blood* 115 (1) (Jan 7): 32-7.

Ruschak, A. M., M. Slassi, L. E. Kay, and A. D. Schimmer. 2011. Novel proteasome inhibitors to overcome bortezomib resistance. *Journal of the National Cancer Institute* 103 (13) (Jul 6): 1007-17.

Russo, S. M., J. E. Tepper, A. S. Baldwin Jr, R. Liu, J. Adams, P. Elliott, and J. C. Cusack Jr. 2001. Enhancement of radiosensitivity by proteasome inhibition: Implications for a role of NF-kappaB. *International Journal of Radiation Oncology, Biology, Physics* 50 (1) (May 1): 183-93.

San Miguel, J. F., R. Schlag, N. K. Khuageva, M. A. Dimopoulos, O. Shpilberg, M. Kropff, I. Spicka, et al. 2008. Bortezomib plus melphalan and prednisone for initial treatment of multiple myeloma. *The New England Journal of Medicine* 359 (9) (Aug 28): 906-17.

Sanchez, E., M. Li, J. A. Steinberg, C. Wang, J. Shen, B. Bonavida, Z. W. Li, H. Chen, and J. R. Berenson. 2010. The proteasome inhibitor CEP-18770 enhances the anti-myeloma activity of bortezomib and melphalan. *British Journal of Haematology* 148 (4) (Feb): 569-81.

Shaughnessy, J. D.,Jr, P. Qu, S. Usmani, C. J. Heuck, Q. Zhang, Y. Zhou, E. Tian, et al. 2011. Pharmacogenomics of bortezomib test-dosing identifies hyperexpression of proteasome genes, especially PSMD4, as novel high-risk feature in myeloma treated with total therapy 3. *Blood* 118 (13) (Sept 29): 3512-24.

Sher, T., S. Ailawadhi, K. C. Miller, D. Manfredi, M. Wood, W. Tan, G. Wilding, et al. 2011. A steroid-independent regimen of bortezomib, liposomal doxorubicin and thalidomide demonstrate high response rates in newly diagnosed multiple myeloma patients. *British Journal of Haematology* 154 (1) (Jul): 104-10.

Shinohara, K., M. Tomioka, H. Nakano, S. Tone, H. Ito, and S. Kawashima. 1996. Apoptosis induction resulting from proteasome inhibition. *The Biochemical Journal* 317 (Pt 2) (Pt 2) (Jul 15): 385-8.

Singh, A. V., M. Bandi, M. A. Aujay, C. J. Kirk, D. E. Hark, N. Raje, D. Chauhan, and K. C. Anderson. 2011. PR-924, a selective inhibitor of the immunoproteasome subunit LMP-7, blocks multiple myeloma cell growth both in vitro and in vivo. *British Journal of Haematology* 152 (2) (Jan): 155-63.

Singh, A. V., M. A. Palladino, G. K. Lloyd, B. C. Potts, D. Chauhan, and K. C. Anderson. 2010. Pharmacodynamic and efficacy studies of the novel proteasome inhibitor NPI-0052 (marizomib) in a human plasmacytoma xenograft murine model. *British Journal of Haematology* 149 (4) (May): 550-9.

Smith, A. J., H. Dai, C. Correia, R. Takahashi, S. H. Lee, I. Schmitz, and S. H. Kaufmann. 2011. Noxa/Bcl-2 protein interactions contribute to bortezomib resistance in human lymphoid cells. *The Journal of Biological Chemistry* 286 (20) (May 20): 17682-92.

Sunwoo, J. B., Z. Chen, G. Dong, N. Yeh, C. Crowl Bancroft, E. Sausville, J. Adams, P. Elliott, and C. Van Waes. 2001. Novel proteasome inhibitor PS-341 inhibits activation of nuclear factor-kappa B, cell survival, tumor growth, and angiogenesis in squamous cell carcinoma. *Clinical Cancer Research* 7 (5) (May): 1419-28.

Takamatsu, Y., K. Sunami, H. Hata, K. Nagafuji, I. Choi, M. Higuchi, K. Uozumi, Y. Masaki, K. Tamura, and Kyushu Hematology Organization for Treatment Study Group (K-

HOT). 2010. A phase I study of bortezomib in combination with doxorubicin and intermediate-dose dexamethasone (iPAD therapy) for relapsed or refractory multiple myeloma. *International Journal of Hematology* 92 (3) (Oct): 503-9.

Takeda, K., A. Mori, and M. Yanagida. 2011. Identification of genes affecting the toxicity of anti-cancer drug bortezomib by genome-wide screening in S. pombe. *PloS One* 6 (7): e22021.

Tamura, D., T. Arao, K. Tanaka, H. Kaneda, K. Matsumoto, K. Kudo, K. Aomatsu, et al. 2010. Bortezomib potentially inhibits cellular growth of vascular endothelial cells through suppression of G2/M transition. *Cancer Science* 101 (6) (Jun): 1403-8.

Terpos, E., D. J. Heath, A. Rahemtulla, K. Zervas, A. Chantry, A. Anagnostopoulos, A. Pouli, et al. 2006. Bortezomib reduces serum dickkopf-1 and receptor activator of nuclear factor-kappaB ligand concentrations and normalises indices of bone remodelling in patients with relapsed multiple myeloma. *British Journal of Haematology* 135 (5) (Dec): 688-92.

Terpos, E., E. Kastritis, M. Roussou, D. Heath, D. Christoulas, N. Anagnostopoulos, E. Eleftherakis-Papaiakovou, K. Tsionos, P. Croucher, and M. A. Dimopoulos. 2008. The combination of bortezomib, melphalan, dexamethasone and intermittent thalidomide is an effective regimen for relapsed/refractory myeloma and is associated with improvement of abnormal bone metabolism and angiogenesis. *Leukemia* 22 (12) (Dec): 2247-56.

Trudel, S., Z. H. Li, J. Rauw, R. E. Tiedemann, X. Y. Wen, and A. K. Stewart. 2007. Preclinical studies of the pan-bcl inhibitor obatoclax (GX015-070) in multiple myeloma. *Blood* 109 (12) (Jun 15): 5430-8.

Uy, G. L., S. D. Goyal, N. M. Fisher, A. Y. Oza, M. H. Tomasson, K. Stockerl-Goldstein, J. F. DiPersio, and R. Vij. 2009. Bortezomib administered pre-auto-SCT and as maintenance therapy post transplant for multiple myeloma: A single institution phase II study. *Bone Marrow Transplantation* 43 (10) (May): 793-800.

van Rhee, F., S. M. Szmania, M. Dillon, A. M. van Abbema, X. Li, M. K. Stone, T. K. Garg, et al. 2009. Combinatorial efficacy of anti-CS1 monoclonal antibody elotuzumab (HuLuc63) and bortezomib against multiple myeloma. *Molecular Cancer Therapeutics* 8 (9) (Sep): 2616-24.

Voorhees, P. M., Q. Chen, D. J. Kuhn, G. W. Small, S. A. Hunsucker, J. S. Strader, R. E. Corringham, M. H. Zaki, J. A. Nemeth, and R. Z. Orlowski. 2007. Inhibition of interleukin-6 signaling with CNTO 328 enhances the activity of bortezomib in preclinical models of multiple myeloma. *Clinical Cancer Research* 13 (21) (Nov 1): 6469-78.

Weniger, M. A., E. G. Rizzatti, P. Perez-Galan, D. Liu, Q. Wang, P. J. Munson, N. Raghavachari, et al. 2011. Treatment-induced oxidative stress and cellular antioxidant capacity determine response to bortezomib in mantle cell lymphoma. *Clinical Cancer Research* 17 (15) (Aug 1): 5101-12.

Yanamandra, N., N. M. Colaco, N. A. Parquet, R. W. Buzzeo, D. Boulware, G. Wright, L. E. Perez, W. S. Dalton, and D. M. Beaupre. 2006. Tipifarnib and bortezomib are synergistic and overcome cell adhesion-mediated drug resistance in multiple myeloma and acute myeloid leukemia. *Clinical Cancer Research* 12 (2) (Jan 15): 591-9.

Yu, C., B. B. Friday, J. P. Lai, L. Yang, J. Sarkaria, N. E. Kay, C. A. Carter, L. R. Roberts, S. H. Kaufmann, and A. A. Adjei. 2006. Cytotoxic synergy between the multikinase inhibitor sorafenib and the proteasome inhibitor bortezomib in vitro: Induction of apoptosis through akt and c-jun NH2-terminal kinase pathways. *Molecular Cancer Therapeutics* 5 (9) (Sep): 2378-87.

Zangari, M., M. Aujay, F. Zhan, K. L. Hetherington, T. Berno, R. Vij, S. Jagannath, et al. 2011. Alkaline phosphatase variation during carfilzomib treatment is associated with best response in multiple myeloma patients. *European Journal of Haematology* 86 (6) (Jun): 484-7.

Zhou, H. J., M. A. Aujay, M. K. Bennett, M. Dajee, S. D. Demo, Y. Fang, M. N. Ho, et al. 2009. Design and synthesis of an orally bioavailable and selective peptide epoxyketone proteasome inhibitor (PR-047). *Journal of Medicinal Chemistry* 52 (9) (May 14): 3028-38.

2

Regulatory Cells and Multiple Myeloma

Karthick Raja Muthu Raja[1,2] and Roman Hajek[1,2,3]
[1]*Babak Myeloma Group, Department of Pathological Physiology, Faculty of Medicine, Masaryk University, Brno,*
[2]*Department of Molecular and Cellular Biology, Faculty of Science, Masaryk University, Brno,*
[3]*Department of Internal Medicine- Hematooncology, Faculty Hospital, Brno,*
Czech Republic

1. Introduction

The concept of immune surveillance posits innate and adaptive immune cell mediated recognition and elimination of tumor cells, which express either tumor specific antigens or molecules by cellular stress. Both innate and adaptive immunity are important to inhibit tumor formation and rejection of transplanted tumors (Dunn et al., 2004; Pardoll, 2003). Despite immune surveillance, tumors do progress. Therefore, new concept immunoediting provides complete explanation of immune system in cancers. Immunoediting has three phases against tumors including elimination, equilibrium and escape (Swann & Smyth, 2007). Elimination phase is similar to immune surveillance, where the immune system detects tumor cells and kills them. In the equilibrium phase, tumor cells become dormant, and the immune system selectively destroys susceptible tumor clones and prevents tumor progression. In the escape phase, immune responses fail to suppress the tumor growth which leads to development of tumor variants that are resistant to anti-tumor responses. The major immune cells involved in targeting the tumor mass are CD8 T cells (MHC I dependent) and NK cells (MHC I independent/deficient) (Pardoll, 2003; Smyth et al., 2000, 2001). Perforin and Fas/FasL pathways constitute for contact-mediated cytotoxicity represented by NK and CD8 T cells (Lieberman, 2003; Russell & Ley, 2002). Also, other pathways play an important role in tumor elimination, such as IFN-γ and IFN-α/β. Regulatory T cells have been initially described in studies by Sakaguchi et al who proved the role of (CD4+CD25+) regulatory T (Treg) cells in maintaining the tolerance against self-antigens (Sakaguchi et al., 1995, 2004, 2008). Treg cells have been shown to contain distinct populations (Table 1) which are able to actively suppress the function of other immune cells, including CD4+CD25- T cells, CD8 T cells, dendritic cells, macrophages, B cells, NK cells and NKT cells (Azuma et al., 2003; Chen, 2006; Lim et al., 2005; Murakami et al., 2002; Romagnani et al., 2005; Trzonkowski et al., 2004). Several studies recently proved that Treg cells could induce tolerance against tumors (Nagai et al., 2004; von Boehmer, 2005; Yamaguchi & Sakaguchi, 2006). Also, studies addressed the expansion of Treg cells in various non-hematological and hematological malignancies (Beyer & Schultze, 2006b). Treg cells were also proved to inversely correlate with outcome of various cancers, including gastric malignancies, ovarian and breast cancers (Curiel et al., 2004; Merlo et al., 2009; Sasada et al., 2003). However, it appears that in certain diseases, such as follicular lymphoma and Hodgkin's lymphoma, higher number of FoxP3+ cells correlate with better survival (Alvaro et al., 2005; Carreras et al., 2006).

Multiple myeloma is a plasma cell proliferative disorder and the second most common hematological malignancy standing next to lymphoma (Kyle & Rajkumar, 2008). Multiple myeloma is clinically characterized by ≥ 10% of plasma cell infiltration in the bone marrow, ≥ 30g/L of monoclonal protein and presence of CRAB symptoms (hypercalcemia, renal insufficiency, anemia and bone lytic lesions) (Raja et al., 2010). It has been proved that B and T lymphocyte populations in multiple myeloma significantly associate with survival (Kay et al., 2001). Multiple myeloma patients commonly present with defects in numbers and function of various immune cells including dendritic cells, B cells, T cells and NK cells (Pratt et al., 2007). Concept of immunoediting also fits in multiple myeloma because of its several stages, starting from premalignant stage known as monoclonal gammopathy of undetermined significance to symptomatic stage (Swann & Smyth, 2007). Elimination phase of immunoediting has been explained in premalignant stage of myeloma, where strong T cell response was observed against the tumor clone compared to malignant stage (Dhodapkar, 2005). Followed by surveillance, T cells patrol the premalignant clone (equilibrium) and finally lose responses against malignant clones which lead to symptomatic myeloma (escape) (Dhodapkar et al., 2003). Recently, in multiple myeloma several studies showed elevated level of Treg cells; these cells were functionally active in suppressing the function of naïve T cells. In this chapter, we focus on describing general aspects of Treg cells, including subtypes, functions, migration and induction of tolerance at tumor microenvironment. Then, we discuss the role of CD4 Treg cells in multiple myeloma and their association with stages and survival, and influence of immunomodulatory drugs on multiple myeloma patient's Treg cells. Additionally, we discuss the role of Th17 cells, CD8 Treg cells and myeloid-derived suppressor cells (MDSCs) in multiple myeloma.

2. Phenotypic characterizations of regulatory T cells in humans

In mice, CD4 Treg cells can be easily characterized as CD4+FoxP3+ and high expression of CD25 (Sakaguchi et al., 1995). However, identification of human Treg cells is ambiguous because approximately 1-2 % of CD25 expressing T cells are functional Treg cells (Allan et al., 2005; Baecher-Allan et al., 2001). Isolation of CD25hi T cells excludes FoxP3 low and CD25 low/intermediate Treg cells which are found to be naïve Treg cell population (CD45RA+/CD45RO-). Unclear identification of CD25 (intermediate and high) expression on CD4 Treg cells influence the reproducibility of results in various disorders. Several groups suggested that negative expression of CD127 in Treg cells might help in characterization. But it will not ensure the accurate identification of Treg cells because activated CD4 T cells are also CD127- (Liu et al., 2006; Seddiki et al., 2006). Alternatively, CD62L expression could differentiate the recently activated CD4 T cells (CD62L low) and Treg cells (CD25hi+CD62L+CD127low) but CD62L expression is not solely restricted to Treg cells (Hamann et al., 2000). Characterization of Treg cells using the CD127 and CD25 does not exclude the non-regulatory Foxp3 expressing T cells. These cells express CD45RO, lack suppressive ability and secrete pro-inflammatory cytokines IL-2, IFN-γ and IL-17 (Miyara et al., 2009). In conclusion, heterogenic expression of FoxP3 by non-regulatory and Treg cells precludes the inclusion of FoxP3 as a sole marker in humans to characterize the Treg cells.

3. Types and functions of T regulatory cells

The existence of Treg cells was uncovered more than four decades ago in studies showing that neonatally thymectomized mice developed autoimmunity, which could be prevented by reconstitution with CD4 T cells (Nishizuka & Sakakura, 1969; Sakaguchi et al., 1982). Further work characterized these Treg cells as CD4+ T cells expressing high levels of IL-2 receptor α chain (Sakuguchi et al., 1995). Fontenot et al determined that in mice, forkhead transcription factor FoxP3 is a specific marker of Treg cells and a master regulator in development and function of Treg cells (Fontenot et al., 2003). Types and functions of various Treg cells are summarized in Table 1 and Table 2.

Types	Origin	Functions	References
CD4+ natural regulatory T cells	Arise in thymus and disseminate to periphery; constitute about 10%-15% of CD4 cells	In mice, depletion of these cells leads to autoimmunity. In humans, mutation in FoxP3 gene located on X chromosome leads to fatal immune disorder IPEX syndrome (Immune dysregulation, Polyendocrinopathy, Enteropathy, X-linked syndrome)	Gambineri et al., 2003.
CD4+ Tr1 regulatory cells	Periphery	Induced in the periphery from naïve T cells in the presence of IL-10. These cells lack FoxP3 expression but secrete IL-10 and TGF-β.	Groux et al., 1997; Vieira et al., 2004
CD4+ Th3 cells	Periphery	Induced in the periphery from naïve T cells in the presence of TGF-β. Suppression is mediated by TGF-β. Rare Th3 cells express FoxP3 molecule due to induction by TGF-β.	Apostolou & von Boehmer, 2004; Chen et al., 2003.
Double negative Treg cells	Periphery	In mice and humans these cells constitute about 1%-3% and 1%, respectively. Double negative Treg cells inhibit T cell activation and proliferation in an antigen specific manner.	Fischer et al., 2005.
γδ T cells	Infiltrate into tumor site (breast cancer)	Suppress naïve and effector T cell responses and inhibit maturation and function of dendritic cells.	Peng et al., 2007.

Types	Origin	Functions	References
CD8 regulatory T cells	Most of CD8 Treg cells are induced by antigen- specific manner	There are several subsets of CD8 Treg cells: Qa-1 specific CD8 Treg cells suppress autoreactive T cells expressing Qa-1 molecule associated with self peptide. CD8+CD28- Treg cells express FoxP3α molecule and suppress other cells via contact dependent mechanism. CD8+CD25+ Treg cells suppress both naïve CD4 and CD8 T cells by contact dependent or independent (IL-10) mechanisms. CD8+CD25+ Treg cells mostly accumulate in the tumor bed rather than peripheral tissues.	Filaci et al., 2007; Kiniwa et al., 2007; Sarantopoulos et al., 2004; Wang, 2008.

Table 1. Subsets of T regulatory cells

Functions of Treg cells	Mechanism of Suppression	References
Inhibitory cytokines	Mainly cytokines such as IL-10, TGF- β and IL-35 secreted by Treg cells are involved in inhibitory function. Chen et al proved in murine colon carcinoma IL-10 induced suppression of tumor specific CD8 T cell immunity. Peptide inhibitor targeted against the surface TGF-β on Treg cells abrogated their function and enhanced anti-tumor response. In mouse model of inflammatory bowel disease, it was shown that IL-35 played a role in severity of inflammatory bowel disease. In humans IL-35 is not expressed constitutively by Treg cells.	Bardel et al., 2008; Chen et al., 2005; Collison et al., 2007; Gil-Guerrero et al., 2008; Loser et al., 2007.
Cytotoxicity	Perforin/granzyme pathway is well known to be associated with CD8 T cells and NK cells for destruction of intracellular pathogens and tumor cells. Recent studies have shown Treg cells also use the perforin/granzyme pathway. An *in vitro* study demonstrated Treg cells activated with anti CD3 and anti CD46 antibodies expressed granzyme A and B. In murine Treg cells, it was shown that perforin lacking Treg cells also exhibit suppressive function. Cao et al reported in a tumor inoculation system the adoptively transferred Treg cells induced suppression of tumor immunity (CD8 T cells and NK cells) specifically by granzyme B pathway. Fas ligand utilizing Treg cells presence was reported in head and neck squamous cell carcinoma patients and found to suppress CD8 T cells.	Cao et al., 2007; Gondek et al., 2005; Grossman et al, 2004; Lieberman, 2003; Russell & Ley, 2002; Strauss et al., 2009.

Functions of Treg cells	Mechanism of Suppression	References
Inhibition of antigen presenting cells (APCs)	Expression of CTLA-4 under the control of FoxP3 facilitates Treg cells interaction with CD80 and CD86 on APCs and induces the suppression of T cell activation. CTLA-4 mediated interaction between Treg cells and APCs leads to upregulation of indoleamine 2, 3-dioxygenase (IDO) production by the APCs which leads to degradation of the essential amino acid tryptophan. Recently, it was proposed that IDO mediated depletion of tryptophan inhibited T cell proliferation and response against tumors.	Mellor & Munn, 2004; Munn et al., 1999; Oderup et al., 2006; Read et al., 2000.

Table 2. Functions of T regulatory cells

4. Mechanism of migration and induction of tolerance in the tumor bed by regulatory cells

There are several chemokine receptors and ligands are involved in the migration of Treg cells. Before going into detail, we would like to summarize the migration process of Treg cells from thymus to secondary lymphoid organ in normal physiological conditions. Preliminary switch occurs in chemokine receptors CCR8/CCR9 and CXCR4 to CCR7 on thymic precursors of Treg cells. These precursor Treg cells are a homogeneous population and express CD62L, CCR7 and CXCR4^{low} (Lee et al., 2007). After migration from thymus to the periphery, these Treg cells acquire complete expression of CXCR4. Thymic emigrant Treg cells most exclusively migrate to secondary lymphoid organ for antigen contact. After the antigen contact, the second switch occurs in the receptors where they downregulate the CCR7 and CXCR4 expression. Consequently, upregulation of effector/memory chemokine receptors (CCR2, CCR4, CCR6, CCR8, and CCR9) occurs to enhance the heterogenic property of Treg cell population (Lee et al., 2007). It was shown that CCR7 mediated migration of Treg cells into secondary lymphoid organ is an important process for encountering mature dendritic cells and consequent differentiation and proliferation (Schneider et al., 2007). All peripheral blood Treg cells express CCR4 receptor and show chemotactic response to ligands CCL22 and CCL17. In ovarian cancer, Treg cell migration and accumulation at the tumor site is attributed by CCL22 chemokine (Curiel et al., 2004). Secretion of CCL22 by lymphoma cells largely recruits the intratumoral Treg cells that express CCR4 but not CCR8 (Ishida et al., 2006; Yang et al., 2006b). In non-hematological malignancies, it was observed that increased frequency of CCR4 expressing Treg cells associated with CCL22 and CCL17 chemokines. An *in vitro* study in gastric cancer showed that migratory activity of Treg cells was induced by CCL22 and CCL17 chemokines (Mizukami et al., 2008).

Several molecules and receptors contribute the suppressive function of Treg cells in the tumor microenvironment. Suppression mechanism by Treg cells is not solely dependent on cell-cell contact rather it is also supported by soluble IL-10 and TGF-β molecules (Strauss et al., 2007). Treg cells do not depend always on direct inhibition of effector T cells; rather, it impedes function of dendritic cells via IL-10 and TGF-β. This mechanism downregulates NF-kB and subsequently changes downstream molecules (CD80, CD86 and CD40) as well as soluble factors, such as TNF-α, IL-12 and CCL5 (Larmonier et al., 2007). Moreover, Treg cells in tumor bed prevent CD4 T cell mediated generation of CD8 T cell cytotoxic responses (Chaput et al., 2007). Prostaglandin E2 is the effector molecule released by Treg cells; it is also important for activation of Treg cells. This molecule efficiently suppresses the effector T cell responses via COX2 induction. Prostaglandin E2 mediated suppression by Treg cells was observed in colorectal cancer patients (Mahic et al., 2006). Cell-cell contact dependent suppression is partly attributed to CTLA-4 expression by Treg cells (Read et al., 2000). Expression of CTLA-4 also facilitates the TGF-β mediated suppression via intensifying the TGF-β signals at the interaction point of Treg cell and target cell (Oida et al., 2006). Tumor infiltrating Treg cells express ICOS molecule but peripheral Treg cells do not express ICOS. ICOS receptor and its ligand are involved in Treg cell mediated suppression. Treg cells with ICOS low expression did not show strong suppressive function as compared to Treg cells with ICOS high expression (Strauss et al., 2008). Very recently, other novel

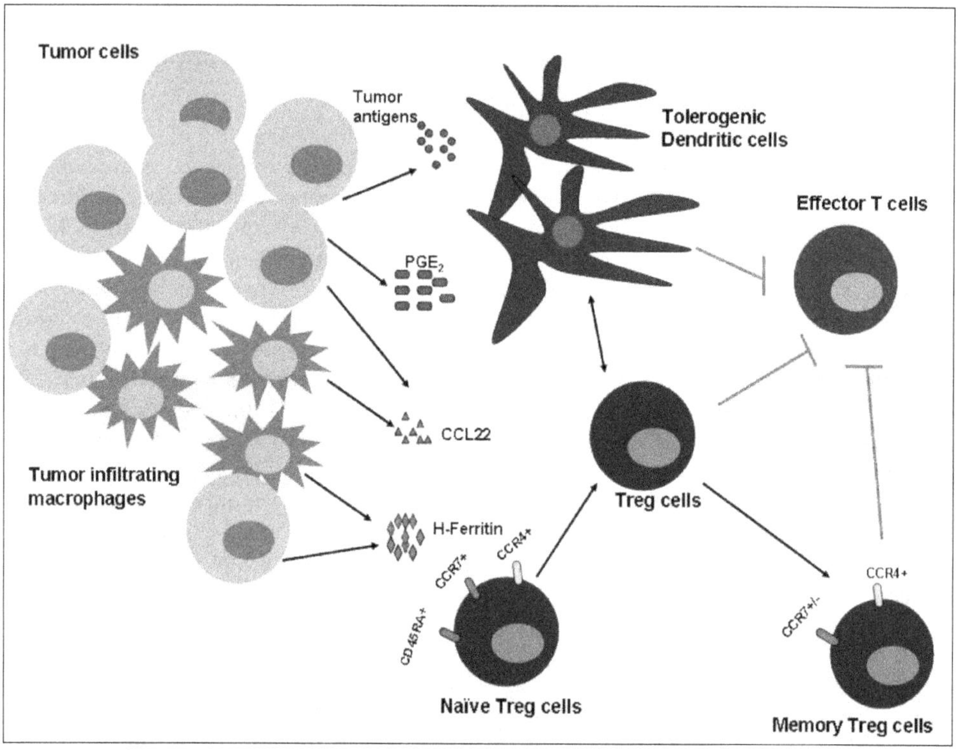

Fig. 1. Mechanism of accumulation and expansion of T regulatory cells in the tumor bed
This schematic diagram represents a mechanism of immune tolerance induced by Treg cells in the tumor microenvironment. CCL22 as well H-ferritin secretion by tumor cells and tumor infiltrating macrophages recruit naïve Treg cells (CCR4+) in the tumor bed. These accumulated naïve Treg cells differentiate and proliferate into memory Treg cells via interaction with prostaglandin E2 (PGE2) induced tolerogenic dendritic cells. These expanded memory Treg cells along with tolerogenic dendritic cells impede the functions of tumor effector T cells.

mechanisms of suppression by Treg cells were revealed. Expression of CD39 in conjunction with CD73 generates the adenosine molecule and its interaction with adenosine A2A receptor on activated T cells creates strong immunosuppressive loops; this suggests one of the important suppressive mechanisms of Treg cells (Deaglio et al., 2007). Transfer of cyclic adenosine monophosphate by Treg cells to effector T cells via cell-cell interaction induces suppression and impedes IL-2 secretion (Bopp et al., 2007). Also, recently it was proven that effector T cells are suppressed via apoptosis induced by deprivation of γ cytokines by Treg cells. Strong association was observed between Treg cell induced apoptosis and increased level of pro-apoptotic proteins Bim and Bad as well as decreased level of pro-survival protein kinase Akt (Pandiyan et al., 2007). Taking all these observations into consideration, the significance of chemokines and their receptors in migration of Treg cells could act as a suitable target for deprivation of Treg cells in the tumor microenvironment; this might also enhance anti-tumor responses. To add more flavors in impeding Treg cell migration, a chimeric monoclonal antibody targeting CCR4 receptor is already under clinical trial. All of the above mentioned mechanisms of suppression collectively work together to induce suppression of immune cells and tolerance in the tumor bed. In some circumstances, these mechanisms might independently act to enforce the suppression of anti-tumor responses.

5. Regulatory T cells and multiple myeloma

Recently, several research groups analyzed Treg cells in multiple myeloma. So far, Treg cells data in multiple myeloma are conflicting. Study from Prabhala et al and Gupta et al reported decreased frequency of peripheral blood Treg cells in multiple myeloma when compared to control group (Gupta et al., 2011; Prabhala et al., 2006). Both studies confirmed that FoxP3 expression was reduced in myeloma patients. In contrast to these studies, Feyler et al and Beyer et al reported increased frequencies of peripheral blood Treg cells in multiple myeloma patients (Feyler et al., 2009; Beyer et al., 2006a). Most of the studies confirmed that peripheral blood and bone marrow Treg cells frequencies were comparable. According to Beyer et al, Treg cells associated markers, such as CTLA-4, GITR, CD62L and OX40 were elevated in myeloma patients compared to healthy subjects (Beyer et al., 2006a). Contrasting to this observation, Prabhala et al showed decreased frequency of CTLA-4 expression on Treg cells of monoclonal gammopathy of undetermined significance and myeloma cohorts than healthy subjects (Prabhala et al., 2006). These opposing results may be due to Treg cells identification strategy. For instance, Prabhala et al identified Treg cells as CD4+FoxP3+, Gupta et al characterized Treg cells with the inclusion of CD127 in their gating, Feyler et al identified Treg cells as CD4+CD25hi+FoxP3+ and Beyer et al identified Treg cells using only CD4 and CD25 markers (Beyer et al., 2006a; Feyler et al., 2009; Gupta et al., 2011; Prabhala et al., 2006). Most of the studies in other cancers including hematological and non-hematological malignancies showed elevated level of Treg cells and these cells are associated with worse prognosis. To support the concept of tumor based expansion of Treg cells, studies clearly showed that established Treg cell clones recognized tumor antigen in MHC class II restricted manner (Wang et al., 2004). In multiple myeloma, no strong conclusions could be made due to the existence of equal number of conflicting results with regard to Treg cells frequency.

5.1 Immunosuppressive function of T regulatory cells in multiple myeloma

Most studies in myeloma agree that Treg cells efficiently suppress both autologous and allogeneic responder cells (CD4+CD25-) similarly to healthy subjects (Beyer et al., 2006a; Brimnes et al., 2010; Feyler et al., 2009; Gupta et al., 2011). Exclusively, Prabhala et al showed that multiple myeloma patients Treg cells lack suppressive function (Prabhala et al., 2006). This contrasting result by Prabhala et al might be due to the use of whole peripheral blood mononuclear cells depleted with CD25+ cells as responder cells (Prabhala et al., 2006). The suppressive nature of Treg cells could be well appreciated by the presence of intracellular cytokines TGF-β and IL-10. Beyer et al confirmed that myeloma patients Treg cells express increased level of TGF-β and IL-10 when compared to healthy subjects (Beyer et al., 2006a). *In vitro* matured dendritic cells using inflammatory cytokines generate functionally active FoxP3+ Treg cells from CD25- T cells. Treg cells derived from dendritic cells are functionally similar in between healthy subjects and myeloma patients. Also, an *in vivo* study showed administration of cytokine matured dendritic cells in myeloma subjects enhanced increase of Treg cell numbers (Banerjee et al., 2006). This study also proposed that use of human dendritic cell vaccination may affect the balance of effector T cells generation because of Treg cell enhancement (Banerjee et al., 2006). In allogeneic stem cell transplanted multiple myeloma patients, donor derived Treg cells reconstituted largely in the bone marrow compartment and prevented graft versus host disease (Atanackovic et al., 2008). This data suggest that *in vivo* inhibitory function of Treg cells and also *in vitro* assay showed reconstituted Treg cells possess complete inhibitory function. Moreover, Atanackovic et al proved that reconstitution of Treg cells in bone marrow positively correlates with time passed since transplantation. Donor derived Treg cells reconstituted in the bone marrow were found to be memory Treg cells, which indicates that Treg cells indeed expanded outside the thymus (Atanackovic et al., 2008). Most of the studies strongly suggest that myeloma patients Treg cells are functional in suppressing the conventional T cell proliferation, and this suppressive function encourages the immune impairments and dysfunctions. However, Treg cells suppressive function could be appreciated in the case of graft versus host disease where donor cells require engraftment to ensure the anti-tumor effects.

5.2 Association of international staging system and myeloma survival status with T regulatory cells

Based on the international staging system (ISS), Treg cells were increased in newly diagnosed multiple myeloma patients. This observation was noticed only in ISS 1 and ISS 2 (Feyler et al., 2009). On the other hand, Gupta et al found a trend of decrease in Treg cells in stages ISS 2 and ISS 3 (Gupta et al., 2011). Apart from ISS, paraprotein level of myeloma patients was positively correlated with frequencies of Treg cells (Feyler et al., 2009).

Giannopoulos et al demonstrated patients with higher level of Treg cells have significantly reduced survival time compared to patients with lower level of Treg cells (21 months vs. median not reached) (Giannopoulos et al., 2010). Our observation also showed that patients with increased peripheral blood Treg cells (≥ 5%) have shorter progression free survival compared to patients with reduced Treg cells (< 5%) cohort (13 months vs. median not reached) (Muthu Raja et al., 2011). These data showing that elevated level of Treg cells correlated unfavorably with progression free survival and overall survival of myeloma patients, so Treg cells could be targeted along with the tumor cells in multiple myeloma.

6. Influence of immunomodulatory drugs on T regulatory cells of multiple myeloma patients

Immunomodulatory drugs are orally bioavailable agents, derived from thalidomide (first generation immunomodulatory drug). The second generation immunomodulatory drugs are lenalidomide and pomalidomide which share similar chemical structure with thalidomide (Galustian et al., 2004). Quach et al recently reviewed the functions of immunomodulatory drugs (Quach et al., 2010). The functions are:

6.1 Immune modulation

Co-stimulation of CD4 and CD8 T cells, activation of NK and NKT cells, production of Th1 cytokines, enhancement of antibody dependent cellular cytotoxicity and Treg cell suppression.

6.2 Hampering tumor microenvironment interactions

Anti-angiogenesis, inhibition of inflammatory effects, anti-osteoclastogenesis and downregulation of adhesion molecules on plasma cells.

6.3 Direct anti-tumor effects

Induction of cyclin dependent kinase inhibitors, such as p15, p21 and p27 which results in cell cycle arrest (G0/G1 phase), increases expression of early growth genes (1, 2), downregulation of NF-kB with subsequent reduction in anti-apoptotic proteins FLIP and cIAP2.

Minnema et al showed that in relapsed myeloma patients (after allogeneic stem cell transplantation), lenalidomide increased frequencies of Treg cells during treatment (Minnema et al., 2009). In contrast, CD4 and CD8 T cells were decreased. This study also showed that ratio of FoxP3+ T cells to IFN-γ secreting T cells was significantly increased during treatment (Minnema et al., 2009). Increased Treg cells always favour allogeneic stem cell transplanted patients because these cells inhibit graft versus host disease (Rezvani et al., 2006). However, Minnema et al study did not show the advantage of increased Treg cells with relevance to graft versus host disease, probably due to small patient numbers (Minnema et al., 2009). Contrasting to this study, an *in vitro* observation demonstrated that lenalidomide and pomalidomide are able to inhibit the proliferation of Treg cells at very low concentrations (10 μM and 1 μM) but thalidomide failed to inhibit the proliferation even at maximum concentration of 200 μM. This study reveals lenalidomide and pomalidomide inhibited the Treg cells mediated suppression of CD4+CD25- cells and also proposes that FoxP3 molecule was targeted efficiently by lenalidomide and pomalidomide but no alterations to GITR were observed (Galustian et al., 2009). Lenalidomide and pomalidomide also inhibit the function of Treg cells by hindering the expression of OX-40 (CD134) molecule (Galustian et al., 2009; Valzasina et al., 2005). Carcinoma animal model study showed Treg cells were depleted after cyclophosphamide treatment; tumor growth was also repressed due to depletion of Treg cells, and tumor clones were cleared followed by immunotherapy. Without administration of cyclophosphamide, no tumor regression or clearance was noticed in the tumor bearing animal (Ghiringhelli et al., 2004). Apart from sensitivity of Treg cells to imunomodulatory drugs and cyclophosphamide, a recent study showed that naturally occurring Treg cells were resistant to pro-apoptotic effect of proteasome inhibitor bortezomib. Long-term culturing of CD4 T cells in the presence of bortezomib promoted the emergence of Treg cells and significantly inhibited proliferation, IFN-γ production and CD40L expression by effector T cells (Blanco et al., 2009). Drug-induced apoptosis resistance by Treg cells is due to the increased expression of BCL-2 and inhibitor of apoptosis protein 1 (IAP1); the expression of IAP1 is in response to TNF induced apoptosis. These BCL-2 and IAP1 protein expression was significantly elevated in Treg cells of B cell leukemic patients than healthy volunteers (Jak et al., 2009). Gupta et al confirmed that multiple myeloma patients treated with immunomodulatory drug combination showed increased Treg cells in relation to irrespective of the response achieved (Gupta et al., 2011). They also showed patients with stable and progressive disease had decreased Treg cells. Taking all these observations into consideration, no strong conclusion can be forwarded because of contrasting results between *in vitro* and *in vivo* studies. However, *in vitro* studies showed promising effects of immunomodulatory drugs on Treg cells when compared to proteasome inhibitor but immunomodulatory drugs effects might be diluted by inclusion of corticosteroid during treatment.

7. Th17 cells in multiple myeloma

Th17 cells are one of the subsets of CD4 T cells. These cells are differentiated in the presence of IL-6, IL-1β, IL-21 and IL-23 with or without TGF-β. Th17 cells secrete IL-17, IL-21, IL-22 and IL-26 cytokines. These cytokines are involved in anti-fungal and anti-parasite responses and participate in inflammatory and autoimmune reactions (Acosta-Rodriguez et al., 2007; Aujla et al., 2008; Bettelli et al., 2006; Ivanov et al., 2006; Veldhoen et al., 2008; Wilson et al., 2007; Zheng et al., 2008). Both Treg cells and Th17 cells originate from naïve CD4 T cells. For Treg cell differentiation, TGF-β is required whereas for Th17 cell differentiation, IL-6 and TGF-β are required (the role of TGF-β in human is unclear) (Bettelli et al., 2006; Veldhoen et al., 2006). Xu et al observed that mature Treg cells can be converted into Th17 cells in the presence of IL-6 (Xu et al., 2007). IL-6 and IL-21 might be involved in transition of Th17/Treg cells to Th17 cells. Some reports show switching of Th17 cells to Th1 cells, but reverse switching is not possible (Annunziato & Romagnani, 2009; Bending et al., 2009; Lee et al., 2009; Shi et al., 2008). Upregulated T-bet expression in Th17 cells resulted in a switch to Th1 cells in the presence of IL-12 or/and IL-23 (Annunziato et al., 2007; Lee et al., 2009).

Recently, a study reported increased Th17 cells and IL-17 in freshly isolated mononuclear cells and sera of myeloma patients compared to healthy subjects. In vitro polarization of CD4 T cells to Th17 cells showed increased Th17 cells in multiple myeloma patients than healthy subjects (Prabhala et al., 2010). Moreover, this study showed expression of IL-17 receptor on myeloma cells which promotes the growth of myeloma cells. IL-21 is a pro-inflammatory cytokine associated with Th17 cells, which is also capable of inducing STAT-3 mediated myeloma growth-promoting effects in synergism with insulin like growth factor-1 (Brenne et al., 2002). Most of the myeloma patients present with bone lytic disorder. In cell culture experiments, Dhodapkar et al showed dendritic cells were efficient inducers of Th17 cells, especially mature dendritic cells. Dendritic cells induced Th17 cells were multifunctional and secreted IL-17 and IFN-γ (Dhodapkar et al., 2008). In myeloma, tumor cells are infiltrated by dendritic cells; Dhodapkar et al demonstrated that Th17 cells were enriched in the tumor microenvironment (Dhodapkar et al., 2008). These IL-17 producing cells were found to enhance the activation of osteoclasts (Noonan et al., 2010). This study also reported significant association between extent of bone lytic lesions and IL-17 cytokine producing Th17 cells (Noonan et al., 2010). These findings suggest that Th17 cells enhance myeloma cell growth and development of bone lytic lesions.

8. CD8 T regulatory cells in multiple myeloma

T cells play an important role in immunosurveillance against cancers. Eventually, these T cells may become CD4/CD8 regulatory T cells due to stimulation by and interaction with tumor cells. Thus, these generated regulatory cells promote the growth of tumor rather than inhibition of tumor (Wang, 2008). Mechanisms of suppression and expansion are well documented for CD4 Treg cells but recent research has been directed to screen the presence of CD8 Treg cells in various tumors and inflammatory conditions.

8.1 Subtypes of CD8 T regulatory cells

8.1.1 Qa-1 restricted CD8 Treg cells

These CD8 Treg cells downregulate autoimmune T cell responses. They are Qa-1 (MHC class 1b molecule) restricted and specifically target self-reactive activated T cells which express Qa-1 molecules associated with self peptide (Jiang & Chess, 2004; Sarantopoulos et al., 2004).

8.1.2 CD8+CD28- Treg cells

These cells are induced by MHC class I peptide antigens. CD8+CD28- Treg cells were found to express FoxP3 α molecule and mediate suppression by cell-cell contact mechanism. CD8+CD28- Treg cells also indirectly target CD4 T cells to become tolerogenic via dendritic cells and non-professional antigen presenting cells. These cells were identified in tumors as well as in the context of transplantation (Cortesini et al., 2001; Filaci & Suciu-Foca, 2002; Filaci et al., 2007; Suciu-Foca et al., 2005).

8.1.3 CD8+CD25hi+ Treg cells

These cells express CD122, Foxp3 and GITR molecules typically associated with CD4 Treg cells (Cosmi et al., 2003; Kiniwa et al., 2007; Lee et al., 2008). They suppress naive CD4 and CD8 T cells via contact dependent mechanism or soluble IL-10. These Treg cells are different from Qa-1 specific CD8 Treg cells but similar to CD4 Treg cells. CD8+CD25hi+ Treg cells are induced by the tumor environment and require antigen stimulation to suppress naïve T cells (Wang, 2008).

8.2 Role of CD8 T regulatory cells

So far, only a few studies have documented the role of CD8 Treg cells (CD8+CD25hi+FoxP3+) in cancers. In prostate and colorectal cancers, elevated levels of CD8

Treg cells have been reported (Chaput et al., 2009; Kiniwa et al., 2007). Both these studies showed that CD8 Treg cells are capable of suppressing naïve T cell proliferation. Additionally, Chaput et al demonstrated suppression of Th1 cytokine production. CD8 Treg cells from colorectal cancer patients were found to correlate with disease stage and micro-invasive status (Chaput et al., 2009). In multiple myeloma, data on CD8 Treg cells are lacking. Our recent observation showed that CD8 Treg cells were significantly elevated in monoclonal gammopathy of undetermined significance and multiple myeloma when compared to healthy subjects (Muthu Raja et al., 2010). However, functional data of CD8 Treg cells are still lacking.

9. Myeloid-derived suppressor cells (MDSCs) in multiple myeloma

Myeloid-derived suppressor cells (MDSCs) are activated immature myeloid cells that have been prevented from differentiation to mature cells. These cells are expanded in pathological conditions (Gabrilovich & Nagaraj, 2009). MDSCs lack the expression of cell surface markers that are specifically expressed by monocytes, macrophages or dendritic cells and comprise a mixture of myeloid cells that have the morphology of granulocytes or monocytes (Youn et al., 2008). They are potent suppressors of T cells. Human MDSCs can be characterized phenotypically as CD14-CD11b+ or by CD33 expression which is a common marker for myeloid cells. Moreover, MDSCs lack the expression of mature lymphoid and myeloid markers as well HLA-DR (MHC class II). Healthy individuals were found to have approximately 0.5% of immature myeloid cells from total peripheral blood mononuclear cells (Gabrilovich & Nagaraj, 2009). In cancer patients and tumor models, accumulation of MDSCs occurs due to release of soluble factors by tumor cells or cells in tumor environment (Almand et al., 2001, Diaz-Montero et al., 2009).

9.1 Mode of suppression

9.1.1 Arginase and inducible nitric oxide synthase

Arginase and inducible nitric oxide synthase enzymes are released by MDSCs. Arginase depletes the non-essential amino acid L-arginine and leads to inhibition of T cell proliferation (Rodriguez et al., 2002). Inducible nitric oxide synthase mediates nitric oxide production. Nitric oxide suppresses the T cell function via induction of apoptosis, inhibition of MHC II expression and inhibition of STAT-5 and JAK3 function in T cells (Gabrilovich & Nagaraj, 2009).

9.1.2 Reactive oxygen species

This is also an important factor from MDSCs that contributes to suppressive activity. Reactive oxygen species release was noticed in tumor bearing mice and cancer patients. Several tumor derived factors including TGF-β, IL-6, IL-3, IL-10 and granulocyte macrophage colony-stimulating factor induce reactive oxygen species synthesis by MDSCs (Gabrilovich & Nagaraj, 2009).

9.1.3 Peroxynitrite

Peroxynitrite induces MDSCs mediated suppression of T cell function. Accumulation of peroxynitrite is noticed where recruitment of MDSCs occurs at the site of inflammation or immunological reactions. In addition, increased peroxynitrite levels associated with tumor progression in several cancers (Gabrilovich & Nagaraj, 2009). Interaction of peroxynitrite producing MDSCs and T cells leads to nitration of T cell receptors and alters specific peptide binding of T cells. This process leads to T cell unresponsiveness (Nagaraj et al., 2007).

9.1.4 Induction of Treg cells

In vivo studies showed that MDSCs can induce *de novo* generation of Treg cells (Huang et al., 2006; Yang et al., 2006a). Induction of Treg cells by MDSCs requires tumor specific T cells together with IFN-γ and IL-10, but independent of nitric oxide production (Huang et al., 2006). In murine models, MDSCs induce generation of Treg cells by CTLA-4 (ovarian tumor) and arginase 1 (lymphoma) molecules (Serafini et al., 2008; Yang et al., 2006a). However, in contrast, other studies report no association of Treg cell generation with MDSCs (Dugast et al., 2008, Movahedi et al., 2008).

9.2 Role of myeloid-derived suppressor cells

Accumulation of MDSCs in cancer patients is an immune evasion mechanism. MDSCs were found to be elevated in peripheral blood of solid tumors including breast, colon, prostrate, hepatocellular and esophageal carcinomas. It was also shown that increase of MDSCs in solid tumors is stage-dependent. Stage IV solid tumor patients showed increased level of MDSCs which correlated with metastatic tumor burden (Diaz-Montero et al., 2009). Early stage breast cancer patients who received cyclophosphamide plus doxorubicin also had increased level of MDSCs. In multiple myeloma, information about MDSCs is lacking. However, a recent study showed significant increase of MDSCs in multiple myeloma patients (Brimnes et al., 2010). This study identified MDSCs as CD14+HLADR-/low, which is contradictory to other studies. In our study, we identified MDSCs as CD33+CD11b+CD14-HLADR-. Cells with this phenotype were elevated in multiple myeloma patients and also an increasing trend was showed in monoclonal gammopathy of undetermined significance patients compared to healthy subjects (Muthu Raja et al., 2011). Due to limited studies on MDSCs of myeloma patients, no strong conclusion could be forwarded. However, studies have shown increased level of MDSCs. Further studies are required to prove their functional activity.

10. Therapeutic targeting of regulatory and suppressor cells to enhance anti-tumor responses

Treg cells favored as a potential target in various cancers to enhance the anti-tumor responses. Chemotherapy agents such as fludarabine and cyclophosphamide were reported to reduce Treg cell numbers in animal models. Cyclophosphamide plus fludarabine and high dose IL-2 treatment was given to metastatic melanoma patients where transient decrease in Treg cells was observed (Powell et al., 2007). Use of chemotherapeutic agents to target Treg cells is relatively unspecific approach but targeting CD25 was found to be more selective in hitting Treg cells than chemotherapies. Various preclinical trials have shown that depletion of Treg cells via specific monoclonal antibodies targeting CD25 in combination with adoptive T cell transfer, denileukin diftitox (a fusion protein of diphtheria toxin and IL-2) and LMB-2 (a fusion protein of a single-chain Fv fragment of an anti-CD25 antibody and the bacterial pseudomonas exotoxin A or 3) enhanced the anti-tumor immunity (Attia et al., 1997; Knutson et al., 2006; Litzinger et al., 2007; Shimizu et al., 1999). Translation of denileukin diftitox and LMB-2 into clinical studies along with vaccination showed efficient improvement in anti-tumor response plus reduced frequency of Treg cells in various cancers, including metastatic renal cell carcinoma, melanoma and colorectal carcinoma. Targeting CTLA-4 molecule is not a precise approach because both effector T cells and Treg cells express CTLA-4. However, a recent animal model study showed CTLA-4 deficient mice lacked the Treg cell mediated immune suppression (Wing et al., 2008). Disadvantage in blockade or depletion of Treg cells is autoimmune toxicity, which was observed in murine models and cancer patients (Dougan & Dranoff, 2009). Recent understanding of MDSCs in cancers provokes to target these suppressor cells. All-trans retinoic acid (ATRA) administration in animal models and *in vitro* study showed decreased number of MDSCs, activated CD4 and CD8 T cells and delayed tumor progression (Kusmartsev et al., 2008). ATRA administration with granulocyte macrophage colony-stimulating factor helped in differentiation of MDSCs into myeloid dendritic cells in tumor-bearing mice (Gabrilovich et al., 2001). In the clinical study ATRA plus IL-2 combination did not have impact on MDSCs of renal cell carcinoma patients. Chemotherapeutic agents, such as gemicitabine and 5-fluorouracil, were reported to reduce the peripheral blood MDSCs in animal models as well as *in vitro* (Le et al., 2009; Vincent et al., 2010). Cyclophosphamide and doxorubicin have negative impact on MDSCs of breast cancer patients (Diaz-Montero et al., 2009). A recent study proposed combination of cyclophosphamide with IL-2 enhanced the clearance of intra-tumoral Treg cells and MDSCs, and enhanced the generation of myeloid inflammatory cells which lack the suppressive function (Medina-Echeverz et al., 2011). STAT-3 is a key regulatory molecule in MDSCs, and this molecule is constitutively expressed by malignant cells. There are several STAT-3 inhibitory molecules under investigation. Sunitinib is one of the STAT-3 inhibitors which influence the phosphorylation of STAT-3 via tyrosine kinase; additionally, it has anti-angiogenic property. Currently, Sunitinib is under investigation for its efficiency on MDSCs (Ko et al., 2009). These observations are showing the efficiency of various inhibitors and chemotherapy agents to hinder the regulatory and suppressor cells *in vitro* and in pre-clinical trials. Unfortunately, clinical trials did not show flourishing impact in all cancers. This might be due to autoimmune toxicities caused by depletion or targeting of Treg cells. Approach of hitting the Treg cells needs further investigation; it is essential to target specifically the tumor associated Treg cells not the global Treg cells which might cause imbalance in the immune homeostasis.

11. Conclusion

Large evidence is available in hematological malignancies and solid tumors for elevated level of various regulatory and suppressor cells which impede anti-tumor responses. Therefore, targeting the regulatory cells could be a useful strategy to enhance the anti-tumor immunity. Approaches of depletion or inhibition of regulatory cells showed countable benefits in pre-clinical and clinical studies of some cancers including renal cell carcinoma, metastatic melanoma and colorectal carcinoma. Targeting regulatory T cells in a non-specific approach might cause detrimental autoimmune toxicities which is the key issue. Further studies are necessary to identify tumor associated regulatory cells which will enhance the depletion of specific regulatory cells but not the global population of regulatory cells.

Moreover, characterization of regulatory cells in humans is an ambiguous aspect due to lack of precise markers. Studies are needed to disclose specific characterization marker for human Treg cells, so that results do not vary between groups. In multiple myeloma, immunotherapeutic targeting of tumor cells at the pre-clinical and clinical studies showed remarkable immunological as well clinical responses in some cohort of patients. When compared to non-hematological malignancies, there are no clinical trials performed to target regulatory cells in myeloma patients. Investigations are required with the inclusion of pre-clinical and clinical studies in myeloma via combinational approach of targeting tumor cells as well regulatory cells. This approach might overcome tumor induced immunosuppression in myeloma patients.

12. Acknowledgement

We kindly thank Dr. Pavel Chrobak for his merit suggestions in preparing this chapter. We also acknowledge the support provided by the research grants MSM0021622434, LC06027, IGA NS10406, IGA NS10408, and GACR P304/10/1395.

13. References

Acosta-Rodriguez, E.V., Rivino, L., Geginat, J., Jarrossay, D., Gattorno, M., Lanzavecchia, A., Sallusto, F. & Napolitani, G. (2007). Surface phenotype and antigenic specificity of human interleukin 17-producing T helper memory cells. *Nature Immunology*, Vol.8, No.6, (June 2007), pp. 639-646, ISSN 1529-2908

Allan, S.E., Passerini, L., Bacchetta, R., Crellin, N., Dai, M., Orban, P.C., Ziegler, S.F., Roncarolo, M.G. & Levings, M.K. (2005). The role of 2 FOXP3 isoforms in the generation of human CD4+ Tregs. *Journal of Clinical Investigation*, vol.115, No.11, (November 2005), pp. 3276-3284, ISSN 0021-9738

Almand, B., Clark, J.I., Nikitina, E., van Beynen, J., English, N.R., Knight, S.C., Carbone, D.P. & Gabrilovich, D.I. (2001). Increased production of immature myeloid cells in cancer patients: a mechanism of immunosuppression in cancer. *Journal of Immunology*, Vol.166, No.1, (January 2001), pp. 678-689, ISSN 0022-1767

Alvaro, T., Lejeune, M., Salvadó, M.T., Bosch, R., García, J.F., Jaén, J., Banham, A.H., Roncador, G., Montalbán, C. & Piris, M.A. (2005). Outcome in Hodgkin's lymphoma can be predicted from the presence of accompanying cytotoxic and regulatory T cells. *Clinical Cancer Research*, Vol.11, No.4, (February 2005), pp. 1467-1473, ISSN 1078-0432

Annunziato, F., Cosmi, L., Santarlasci, V., Maggi, L., Liotta, F., Mazzinghi, B., Parente, E., Filì, L., Ferri, S., Frosali, F., Giudici, F., Romagnani, P., Parronchi, P., Tonelli, F., Maggi, E. & Romagnani, S. (2007). Phenotypic and functional features of human Th17 cells. *Journal of Experimental Medicine*, Vol.204, No.8, (August 2007), pp. 1849-1861, ISSN 0022-1007

Annunziato, F. & Romagnani, S. (2009). Do studies in humans better depict Th17 cells? *Blood*, Vol.114, No.11, (September 2009), pp. 2213-2219, ISSN 0006-4971

Apostolou, I. & von Boehmer, H. (2004). In vivo instruction of suppressor commitment in naive T cells. *Journal of Experimental Medicine*, Vol.199, No.10, (May 2004), pp. 1401-1408, ISSN 0022-1007

Atanackovic, D., Cao, Y., Luetkens, T., Panse, J., Faltz, C., Arfsten, J., Bartels, K., Wolschke, C., Eiermann, T., Zander, A.R., Fehse, B., Bokemeyer, C. & Kroger, N. (2008). CD4+CD25+FOXP3+ T regulatory cells reconstitute and accumulate in the bone marrow of patients with multiple myeloma following allogeneic stem cell transplantation. *Haematologica*, Vol.93, No.3, (March 2008), pp. 423-430, ISSN 0390-6078

Attia, P., Powell, D.J., Maker, A.V., Kreitman, R.J., Pastan, I. & Rosenberg, S.A. (2006). Selective elimination of human regulatory T lymphocytes in vitro with the recombinant immunotoxin LMB-2. *Journal of Immunotherapy*, Vol.29, No.2, (March 2006), pp. 208-214, ISSN 1524-9557

Aujla, S.J., Chan, Y.R., Zheng, M., Fei, M., Askew, D.J., Pociask, D.A., Reinhart, T.A., McAllister, F., Edeal, J., Gaus, K., Husain, S., Kreindler, J.L., Dubin, P.J., Pilewski, J.M., Myerburg, M.M., Mason, C.A., Iwakura, Y. & Kolls, J.K. (2008). IL-22 mediates mucosal host defense against Gram-negative bacterial pneumonia. *Nature Medicine*, Vol.14, No.3, (March 2008), pp. 275-281, ISSN 1078-8956

Azuma, T., Takahashi, T., Kunisato, A., Kitamura, T. & Hirai, H. (2003). Human CD4+ CD25+ regulatory T cells suppress NKT cell functions. *Cancer Research*, Vol.63, No.15, (August 2003), pp. 4516-4520, ISSN 0008-5472

Baecher-Allan, C., Brown, J.A., Freeman, G.J. & Hafler, D.A. (2001). CD4+CD25high regulatory cells in human peripheral *Blood. Journal of Immunology*, Vol.167, No.3, (August 2001), pp. 1245-1253, ISSN 0022-1767

Banerjee, D.K., Dhodapkar, M.V., Matayeva, E., Steinman, R.M. & Dhodapkar, K.M. (2006). Expansion of FOXP3high regulatory T cells by human dendritic cells (DCs) in vitro and after injection of cytokine-matured DCs in myeloma patients. *Blood*, Vol.108, No.8, (October 2006), pp. 2655-2661, ISSN 0006-4971

Bardel, E., Larousserie, F., Charlot-Rabiega, P., Coulomb-L'Herminé, A. & Devergne, O. (2008). Human CD4+ CD25+ Foxp3+ regulatory T cells do not constitutively express IL-35. *Journal of Immunology*, Vol.181, No.10, (November 2008), pp. 6898-6905, ISSN 1550-6606

Bending, D., De la Peña, H., Veldhoen, M., Phillips, J.M., Uyttenhove, C., Stockinger, B. & Cooke, A. (2009). Highly purified Th17 cells from BDC2.5NOD mice convert into Th1-like cells in NOD/SCID recipient mice. *Journal of Clinical Investigation*, Vol.119, No.3, (March 2009), pp. 565-572, ISSN 0021-9738

Bettelli, E., Carrier, Y., Gao, W., Korn, T., Strom, T.B., Oukka, M., Weiner, H.L. & Kuchroo, V.K. (2006). Reciprocal developmental pathways for the generation of pathogenic effector TH17 and regulatory T cells. *Nature*, Vol.441, No.1090, (May 2006), pp. 235-238, ISSN 0028-0836

Beyer, M., Kochanek, M., Giese, T., Endl, E., Weihrauch, M.R., Knolle, P.A., Classen, S. & Schultze, J.L. (2006a). In vivo peripheral expansion of naive CD4+CD25high FoxP3+ regulatory T cells in patients with multiple myeloma. *Blood*, Vol.107, No.10, (May 2006), pp. 3940-3949, ISSN 0006-4971

Beyer, M. & Schultze, J.L. (2006b). Regulatory T cells in cancer. *Blood*, Vol.108, No.3, (August 2006), pp. 804-811.

Blanco, B., Pérez-Simón, J.A., Sánchez-Abarca, L.I., Caballero-Velazquez, T., Gutierrez-Cossío, S., Hernández-Campo, P., Díez-Campelo, M., Herrero-Sanchez, C., Rodriguez-Serrano, C., Santamaría, C., Sánchez-Guijo, F.M., Del Cañizo, C. & San

Miguel, J.F. (2009). Treatment with bortezomib of human CD4+ T cells preserves natural regulatory T cells and allows the emergence of a distinct suppressor T-cell population. *Haematologica*, Vol.94, No.7, (August 2009), pp. 975-983, ISSN 0390-6078

Bopp, T., Becker, C., Klein, M., Klein-Hessling, S., Palmetshofer, A., Serfling, E., Heib, V., Becker, M., Kubach, J., Schmitt, S., Stoll, S., Schild, H., Staege, M.S., Stassen, M., Jonuleit, H. & Schmitt, E. (2007). Cyclic adenosine monophosphate is a key component of regulatory T cell-mediated suppression. *Journal of Experimental Medicine*, Vol.204, No.6, (June 2007), pp. 1303-1310, ISSN 0022-1007

Brenne, A.T., Ro, T.B., Waage, A., Sundan, A., Borset, M. & Hjorth-Hansen, H. (2002). Interleukin-21 is a growth and survival factor for human myeloma cells. *Blood*, Vol.99, No.10, (May 2002), pp. 3756-3762 ISSN 0006-4971

Brimnes, M.K., Vangsted, A.J., Knudsen, L.M., Gimsing, P., Gang, A.O., Johnsen, H.E. & Svane, I.M. (2010). Increased level of both CD4+FOXP3+ regulatory T cells and CD14+HLA-DR?/low myeloid-derived suppressor cells and decreased level of dendritic cells in patients with multiple myeloma. *Scandinavian Journal of Immunology*, Vol.72, No.6, (December 2010), pp. 540-547, ISSN 0300-9475

Cao, X., Cai, S.F., Fehniger, T.A., Song, J., Collins, L.I., Piwnica-Worms, D.R. & Ley, T.J. (2007). Granzyme B and perforin are important for regulatory T cell-mediated suppression of tumor clearance. *Immunity*, Vol.27, No.4, (October 2007), pp. 635-646, ISSN 1074-7613

Carreras, J., Lopez-Guillermo, A., Fox, B.C., Colomo, L., Martinez, A., Roncador, G., Montserrat, E., Campo, E. & Banham, A.H. (2006). High numbers of tumor-infiltrating FOXP3-positive regulatory T cells are associated with improved overall survival in follicular lymphoma. *Blood*, Vol.108, No.9, (November 2006), pp. 2957-2964, ISSN 0006-4971

Chaput, N., Darrasse-Jèze, G., Bergot, A.S., Cordier, C., Ngo-Abdalla, S., Klatzmann, D. & Azogui, O. (2007). Regulatory T cells prevent CD8 T cell maturation by inhibiting CD4 Th cells at tumor sites. *Journal of Immunology*, Vol.179, No.8, (October 2007), pp. 4969-4978, ISSN 0022-1767

Chaput, N., Louafi, S., Bardier, A., Charlotte, F., Vaillant, J.C., Ménégaux, F., Rosenzwajg, M., Lemoine, F., Klatzmann, D. & Taieb, J. (2009). Identification of CD8+CD25+Foxp3+ suppressive T cells in colorectal cancer tissue. *Gut*, Vol.58, No.4, (April 2009), pp. 520-529, ISSN 0017-5749

Chen, W., Jin, W., Hardegen, N., Lei, K.J., Li, L., Marinos, N., McGrady, G. & Wahl, S.M. (2003). Conversion of peripheral CD4+CD25- naive T cells to CD4+CD25+ regulatory T cells by TGF-beta induction of transcription factor Foxp3. *Journal of Experimental Medicine*, Vol.198, No.12, (December 2003), pp. 1875-1886, ISSN 0022-1007

Chen, M.L., Pittet, M.J., Gorelik, L., Flavell, R.A., Weissleder, R., von Boehmer, H. & Khazaie, K. (2005). Regulatory T cells suppress tumor-specific CD8 T cell cytotoxicity through TGF-beta signals in vivo. *Proceedings of the National Academy of Sciences of the United States of America*, Vol.102, No.2, (January 2005), pp. 419-424, ISSN 0027-8424

Chen, W. (2006). Dendritic cells and (CD4+) CD25+ T regulatory cells: crosstalk between two professionals in immunity versus tolerance. *Frontiers in Bioscience*, Vol.11, pp. 1360-1370, ISSN 1093-4715

Collison, L.W., Workman, C.J., Kuo, T.T., Boyd, K., Wang, Y., Vignali, K.M., Cross, R., Sehy, D., Blumberg, R.S. & Vignali, D.A. (2007). The inhibitory cytokine IL-35 contributes to regulatory T-cell function. *Nature*, Vol.450, No. 7169, (November 2007), pp. 566-569, ISSN 1476-4687

Cortesini, R., LeMaoult, J., Ciubotariu, R. & Cortesini, N.S. (2001). CD8+CD28- T suppressor cells and the induction of antigen-specific, antigen-presenting cell-mediated suppression of Th reactivity. *Immunological Reviews*, Vol.182, (August 2001), pp. 201-206, ISSN 0105-2896

Cosmi, L., Liotta, F., Lazzeri, E., Francalanci, M., Angeli, R., Mazzinghi, B., Santarlasci, V., Manetti, R., Vanini, V., Romagnani, P., Maggi, E., Romagnani, S. & Annunziato, F. (2003). Human CD8+CD25+ thymocytes share phenotypic and functional features with CD4+CD25+ regulatory thymocytes. *Blood*, Vol.102, No. 12, (December 2003), pp. 4107-4114, ISSN 0006-4971

Curiel, T.J., Coukos, G., Zou, L., Alvarez, X., Cheng, P., Mottram, P., Evdemon-Hogan, M., Conejo-Garcia, J.R., Zhang, L., Burow, M., Zhu, Y., Wei, S., Kryczek, I., Daniel, B., Gordon, A., Myers, L., Lackner, A., Disis, M.L., Knutson, K.L., Chen, L. & Zou, W. (2004). Specific recruitment of regulatory T cells in ovarian carcinoma fosters immune privilege and predicts reduced survival. *Nature Medicine*, Vol.10, No.9, (September 2004), pp. 942-949, ISSN 1078-8956

Deaglio, S., Dwyer, K.M., Gao, W., Friedman, D., Usheva, A., Erat, A., Chen, J.F., Enjyoji, K., Linden, J., Oukka, M., Kuchroo, V.K., Strom, T.B. & Robson, S.C. (2007). Adenosine generation catalyzed by CD39 and CD73 expressed on regulatory T cells mediates immune suppression. *Journal of Experimental Medicine*, Vol.204, No. 6, (June 2007), pp. 1257-1265, ISSN 0022-1007

Dhodapkar, K.M., Barbuto, S., Matthews, P., Kukreja, A., Mazumder, A., Vesole, D., Jagannath, S. & Dhodapkar, M.V. (2008). Dendritic cells mediate the induction of polyfunctional human IL17-producing cells (Th17-1 cells) enriched in the bone marrow of patients with myeloma. *Blood*, Vol.112, No.7, (October 2008), pp. 2878-2885, ISSN 0006-4971

Dhodapkar, M.V. (2005). Immune response to premalignancy: insights from patients with monoclonal gammopathy. *Annals of New York Academy of Sciences*, Vol.1062, (December 2005), pp. 22-28, ISSN 0077-8923

Dhodapkar, M.V., Krasovsky, J., Osman, K. & Geller, M.D. (2003). Vigorous premalignancy-specific effector T cell response in the bone marrow of patients with monoclonal gammopathy. *Journal of Experimental Medicine*, Vol.198, No.11, (December 2003), pp. 1753-1757, ISSN 0022-1007

Diaz-Montero, C.M., Salem, M.L., Nishimura, M.I., Garrett-Mayer, E., Cole, D.J. & Montero, A.J. (2009). Increased circulating myeloid-derived suppressor cells correlate with clinical cancer stage, metastatic tumor burden, and doxorubicin-cyclophosphamide chemotherapy. *Cancer Immunology Immunotherapy*, Vol.58, No.1, (January 2009), pp. 49-59, ISSN 0340-7004

Dougan, M. & Dranoff, G. (2009). Immune therapy for cancer. *Annual Review of Immunology*, Vol.27, 83-117.

Dugast, A.S., Haudebourg, T., Coulon, F., Heslan, M., Haspot, F., Poirier, N., Vuillefroy de Silly, R., Usal, C., Smit, H., Martinet, B., Thebault, P., Renaudin, K. & Vanhove, B. (2008). Myeloid-derived suppressor cells accumulate in kidney allograft tolerance and specifically suppress effector T cell expansion. *Journal of Immunology*, Vol.180, No.12, (June 2008), pp. 7898-7906, ISSN 0022-1767

Dunn, G.P., Old, L.J. & Schreiber, R.D. (2004). The immunobiology of cancer immunosurveillance and immunoediting. *Immunity*, Vol.21, No.2, (August 2004), pp. 137-148, ISSN 1074-7613

Feyler, S., von Lilienfeld-Toal, M., Jarmin, S., Marles, L., Rawstron, A., Ashcroft, A.J., Owen, R.G., Selby, P.J. & Cook, G. (2009). CD4(+)CD25(+)FoxP3(+) regulatory T cells are increased whilst CD3(+)CD4(-)CD8(-) alphabetaTCR(+) Double Negative T cells are decreased in the peripheral Blood of patients with multiple myeloma which correlates with disease burden. *British Journal of Haematology*, Vol.144, No.5 (March 2009), pp. 686-695, ISSN 1365-2141

Filaci, G., Fenoglio, D., Fravega, M., Ansaldo, G., Borgonovo, G., Traverso, P., Villaggio, B., Ferrera, A., Kunkl, A., Rizzi, M., Ferrera, F., Balestra, P., Ghio, M., Contini, P., Setti, M., Olive, D., Azzarone, B., Carmignani, G., Ravetti, J.L., Torre, G. & Indiveri, F. (2007). CD8+ CD28- T regulatory lymphocytes inhibiting T cell proliferative and cytotoxic functions infiltrate human cancers. *Journal of Immunology*, Vol.179, No.7, (October 2007), pp. 4323-4334, ISSN 0022-1767

Filaci, G. & Suciu-Foca, N. (2002). CD8+ T suppressor cells are back to the game: are they players in autoimmunity? *Autoimmunity Reviews*, Vol.1, No.5, (October 2002), pp. 279-283, ISSN 1568-9972

Fischer, K., Voelkl, S., Heymann, J., Przybylski, G.K., Mondal, K., Laumer, M., Kunz-Schughart, L., Schmidt, C.A., Andreesen, R. & Mackensen, A. (2005). Isolation and characterization of human antigen-specific TCR alpha beta+ CD4(-)CD8- double-negative regulatory T cells. *Blood*, Vol.105, No.7, (April 2005), pp. 2828-2835, ISSN 0006-4971

Fontenot, J.D., Gavin, M.A. & Rudensky, A.Y. (2003). Foxp3 programs the development and function of CD4+CD25+ regulatory T cells. *Nature Immunology*, Vol.4, No.4, (April 2003), pp. 330-336, ISSN 1529-2908

Gabrilovich, D.I. & Nagaraj, S. (2009). Myeloid-derived suppressor cells as regulators of the immune system. *Nature Reviews Immunology*, Vol. 9, No.3, (March 2009), pp.162-174, ISSN 1474-1741.

Gabrilovich, D.I., Velders, M.P., Sotomayor, E.M. & Kast, W.M. (2001). Mechanism of immune dysfunction in cancer mediated by immature Gr-1+ myeloid cells. *Journal of Immunology*, Vol. 166, No.9, (May 2001), pp. 5398-5406, ISSN 0022-1767.

Galustian, C., Labarthe, M.C., Bartlett, J.B. & Dalgleish, A.G. (2004). Thalidomide-derived immunomodulatory drugs as therapeutic agents. *Expert Opinion on Biological Therapy*, Vol.4, No.12, (December 2004), pp. 1963-1970, ISSN 1744-7682

Galustian, C., Meyer, B., Labarthe, M.C., Dredge, K., Klaschka, D., Henry, J., Todryk, S., Chen, R., Muller, G., Stirling, D., Schafer, P., Bartlett, J.B. & Dalgleish, A.G. (2009). The anti-cancer agents lenalidomide and pomalidomide inhibit the proliferation and function of T regulatory cells. *Cancer Immunology Immunotherapy*, Vol.58, No.7, (July 2009), pp. 1033-1045, ISSN 1432-0851

Gambineri, E., Torgerson, T.R. & Ochs, H.D. (2003). Immune dysregulation, polyendocrinopathy, enteropathy, and X-linked inheritance (IPEX), a syndrome of systemic autoimmunity caused by mutations of FOXP3, a critical regulator of T-cell homeostasis. *Current Opinion in Rheumatology*, Vol.15, No.4, (July 2003), pp. 430-435, ISSN 1040-8711

Ghiringhelli, F., Larmonier, N., Schmitt, E., Parcellier, A., Cathelin, D., Garrido, C., Chauffert, B., Solary, E., Bonnotte, B. & Martin, F. (2004). CD4+CD25+ regulatory T cells suppress tumor immunity but are sensitive to cyclophosphamide which allows immunotherapy of established tumors to be curative. *European Journal of Immunology*, Vol.34, No. 2 (February 2004), pp. 336-344, ISSN 0014-2980

Giannopoulous, K., Kameniska, W. & Dmoszynska, A. (2010). The Frequency of T Regulatory Cells Modulates the Survival of Multiple Myeloma Patients: Detailed Characterization of Immune Status in Multiple Myeloma, *American Society of Haematology Meeting*, ISSN 0006-4971, Florida, USA, December 2010

Gil-Guerrero, L., Dotor, J., Huibregtse, I.L., Casares, N., López-Vázquez, A.B., Rudilla, F., Riezu-Boj, J.I., López-Sagaseta, J., Hermida, J., Van Deventer, S., Bezunartea, J., Llopiz, D., Sarobe, P., Prieto, J., Borrás-Cuesta, F. & Lasarte, J.J. (2008). In vitro and in vivo down-regulation of regulatory T cell activity with a peptide inhibitor of TGF-beta1. *Journal of Immunology*, Vol.181, No.1, (July 2008), pp. 126-135, ISSN 0022-1767

Gondek, D.C., Lu, L.F., Quezada, S.A., Sakaguchi, S. & Noelle, R.J. (2005). Cutting edge: contact-mediated suppression by CD4+CD25+ regulatory cells involves a granzyme B-dependent, perforin-independent mechanism. *Journal of Immunology*, Vol.174, No.4, (February 2005), pp.1783-1786, ISSN 0022-1767

Grossman, W.J., Verbsky, J.W., Barchet, W., Colonna, M., Atkinson, J.P. & Ley, T.J. (2004). Human T regulatory cells can use the perforin pathway to cause autologous target cell death. *Immunity*, Vol.21, No.4, (October 2004), pp. 589-601, ISSN 1074-7613

Groux, H., O'Garra, A., Bigler, M., Rouleau, M., Antonenko, S., de Vries, J.E. & Roncarolo, M.G. (1997). A CD4+ T-cell subset inhibits antigen-specific T-cell responses and prevents colitis. *Nature*, Vol.389, No. 6652, (October 1997), pp.737-742, ISSN 0028-0836

Gupta, R., Ganeshan, P., Hakim, M., Verma, R., Sharma, A. & Kumar, L. (2011). Significantly reduced regulatory T cell population in patients with untreated multiple myeloma. *Leukemia Research*, Vol.35, No.7, (July 2011), pp. 874-878, ISSN 1873-5835

Hamann, A., Klugewitz, K., Austrup, F. & Jablonski-Westrich, D. (2000). Activation induces rapid and profound alterations in the trafficking of T cells. *European Journal of Immunology*, Vol.30, No.11, (November 2000), pp. 3207-3218, ISSN 0014-2980

Huang, B., Pan, P.Y., Li, Q., Sato, A.I., Levy, D.E., Bromberg, J., Divino, C.M. & Chen, S.H. (2006). Gr-1+CD115+ immature myeloid suppressor cells mediate the development of tumor-induced T regulatory cells and T-cell anergy in tumor-bearing host. *Cancer Research*, Vol.66, No.2, (January 2006), pp. 1123-1131, ISSN 0008-5472

Ishida, T., Ishii, T., Inagaki, A., Yano, H., Komatsu, H., Iida, S., Inagaki, H. & Ueda, R. (2006). Specific recruitment of CC chemokine receptor 4-positive regulatory T cells in Hodgkin lymphoma fosters immune privilege. *Cancer Research*, Vol. 66, No.11, (June 2006), pp. 5716-5722, ISSN 0008-5472

Ivanov, I.I., McKenzie, B.S., Zhou, L., Tadokoro, C.E., Lepelley, A., Lafaille, J.J., Cua, D.J. & Littman, D.R. (2006). The orphan nuclear receptor RORgammat directs the differentiation program of proinflammatory IL-17+ T helper cells. Cell, Vol.126, No. 6, (September 2006), pp. 1121-1133, ISSN 0092-8674

Jak, M., Mous, R., Remmerswaal, E.B., Spijker, R., Jaspers, A., Yagüe, A., Eldering, E., Van Lier, R.A. & Van Oers, M.H. (2009). Enhanced formation and survival of CD4+ CD25hi Foxp3+ T-cells in chronic lymphocytic leukemia. *Leukemia Lymphoma*, Vol.50, No.5, (May 2009), pp. 788-801, ISSN 1029-2403

Jiang, H. & Chess, L. (2004). An integrated view of suppressor T cell subsets in immunoregulation. *Journal of Clinical Investigation*, Vol.114, No.9, (November 2004), pp. 1198-1208, ISSN 0021-9738

Kay, N.E., Leong, T.L., Bone, N., Vesole, D.H., Greipp, P.R., Van Ness, B., Oken, M.M.& Kyle, R.A. (2001). *Blood* levels of immune cells predict survival in myeloma patients: results of an Eastern Cooperative Oncology Group phase 3 trial for newly diagnosed multiple myeloma patients. *Blood*, Vol.98, No.1, (July 2001), pp. 23-28, ISSN 0006-4971

Kiniwa, Y., Miyahara, Y., Wang, H.Y., Peng, W., Peng, G., Wheeler, T.M., Thompson, T.C., Old, L.J. & Wang, R.F. (2007). CD8+ Foxp3+ regulatory T cells mediate immunosuppression in prostate cancer. *Clinical Cancer Research*, Vol.13, No.23, (December 2007), pp. 6947-6958, ISSN 1078-0432

Knutson, K.L., Dang, Y., Lu, H., Lukas, J., Almand, B., Gad, E., Azeke, E. & Disis, M.L. (2006). IL-2 immunotoxin therapy modulates tumor-associated regulatory T cells and leads to lasting immune-mediated rejection of breast cancers in neu-transgenic mice. *Journal of Immunology*, Vol.177, No.1, (July 2006), pp. 84-91, ISSN 0022-1767

Ko, J.S., Bukowski, R.M. & Fincke, J.H. (2009). Myeloid-derived suppressor cells: a novel therapeutic target. *Current Oncology Reports*, Vol.11, No.2, (March 2009), pp. 87-93, ISSN 1534-6269

Kusmartsev, S., Su, Z., Heiser, A., Dannull, J., Eruslanov, E., Kübler, H., Yancey, D., Dahm, P. & Vieweg, J. (2008). Reversal of myeloid cell-mediated immunosuppression in patients with metastatic renal cell carcinoma. *Clinical Cancer Research*, Vol.14, No.24, (December 2008), pp. 8270-8278, ISSN 1078-0432

Kyle, R.A. & Rajkumar, S.V. (2008). Multiple myeloma. *Blood*, Vol.111, No.6 (March 2008) pp. 2962-2972, ISSN 0006-4971

Larmonier, N., Marron, M., Zeng, Y., Cantrell, J., Romanoski, A., Sepassi, M., Thompson, S., Chen, X., Andreansky, S. & Katsanis, E. (2007). Tumor-derived CD4(+)CD25(+) regulatory T cell suppression of dendritic cell function involves TGF-beta and IL-10. *Cancer Immunology Immunotherapy*, Vol.56, No.1, (January 2007), pp. 48-59, ISSN 0340-7004

Le, H.K., Graham, L., Cha, E., Morales, J.K., Manjili, M.H. & Bear, H.D. (2009). Gemcitabine directly inhibits myeloid derived suppressor cells in BALB/c mice bearing 4T1 mammary carcinoma and augments expansion of T cells from tumor-bearing mice. *International Immunopharmacology*, Vol.9, No.7-8, (July 2009), pp. 900-909, ISSN 1878-1705

Lee, J.H., Kang, S.G. & Kim, C.H. (2007). FoxP3+ T cells undergo conventional first switch to lymphoid tissue homing receptors in thymus but accelerated second switch to nonlymphoid tissue homing receptors in secondary lymphoid tissues. *Journal of Immunology*, Vol.178, No.1, (January 2007), pp. 301-311, ISSN 0022-1767

Lee, Y.H., Ishida, Y., Rifa'i, M., Shi, Z., Isobe, K. & Suzuki, H. (2008). Essential role of CD8+CD122+ regulatory T cells in the recovery from experimental autoimmune encephalomyelitis. *Journal of Immunology*, Vol.180, No.2, (January 2008), pp. 825-832, ISSN 0022-1767

Lee, Y.K., Turner, H., Maynard, C.L., Oliver, J.R., Chen, D., Elson, C.O. & Weaver, C.T. (2009). Late developmental plasticity in the T helper 17 lineage. *Immunity*, Vol.30, No.1, (January 2009), pp. 92-107, ISSN 1097-4180

Lieberman, J. (2003). The ABCs of granule-mediated cytotoxicity: new weapons in the arsenal. *Nature Review Immunology*, Vol.3, No.5, (May 2003), pp. 361-370, ISSN 1474-1733

Lim, H.W., Hillsamer, P., Banham, A.H. & Kim, C.H. (2005). Cutting edge: direct suppression of B cells by CD4+ CD25+ regulatory T cells. *Journal of Immunology*, Vol. 175, No. 7, (October 2005), pp. 4180-4183, ISSN 0022-1767

Litzinger, M.T., Fernando, R., Curiel, T.J., Grosenbach, D.W., Schlom, J. & Palena, C. (2007). IL-2 immunotoxin denileukin diftitox reduces regulatory T cells and enhances vaccine-mediated T-cell immunity. *Blood*, Vol.110, No.9, (November 2007), pp. 3192-3201, ISSN 0006-4971

Liu, W., Putnam, A.L., Xu-Yu, Z., Szot, G.L., Lee, M.R., Zhu, S., Gottlieb, P.A., Kapranov, P., Gingeras, T.R., Fazekas de St Groth, B., Clayberger, C., Soper, D.M., Ziegler, S.F. & Bluestone, J.A. (2006). CD127 expression inversely correlates with FoxP3 and suppressive function of human CD4+ T reg cells. *Journal of Experimental Medicine*, Vol.203, No.7, (July 2006), pp. 1701-1711, ISSN 0022-1007

Loser, K., Apelt, J., Voskort, M., Mohaupt, M., Balkow, S., Schwarz, T., Grabbe, S. & Beissert, S. (2007). IL-10 controls ultraviolet-induced carcinogenesis in mice. *Journal of Immunology*, Vol.179, No.1, (July 2007), pp. 365-371, ISSN 0022-1767

Mahic, M., Yaqub, S., Johansson, C.C., Taskén, K. & Aandahl, E.M. (2006). FOXP3+CD4+CD25+ adaptive regulatory T cells express cyclooxygenase-2 and suppress effector T cells by a prostaglandin E2-dependent mechanism. *Journal of Immunology*, Vol.177, No.1, (July 2006), pp. 246-254, ISSN 0022-1767

Medina-Echeverz, J., Fioravanti, J., Zabala, M., Ardaiz, N., Prieto, J. & Berraondo, P. (2011). Successful colon cancer eradication after chemoimmunotherapy is associated with profound phenotypic change of intratumoral myeloid cells. *Journal of Immunology*, Vol.186, No.2, (January 2011), pp. 807-815, ISSN 1550-6606

Mellor, A.L. & Munn, D.H. (2004). IDO expression by dendritic cells: tolerance and tryptophan catabolism. *Nature Reviews Immunology*, Vol.4, No.10, (October 2004), pp. 762-774, ISSN 1474-1733

Merlo, A., Casalini, P., Carcangiu, M.L., Malventano, C., Triulzi, T., Mènard, S., Tagliabue, E. & Balsari, A. (2009). FOXP3 expression and overall survival in breast cancer. *Journal of Clinical Oncology*, Vol.27, No.11, (April 2009), pp. 1746-1752, ISSN 1527-7755

Minnema, M.C., van der Veer, M.S., Aarts, T., Emmelot, M., Mutis, T. & Lokhorst, H.M. (2009). Lenalidomide alone or in combination with dexamethasone is highly effective in patients with relapsed multiple myeloma following allogeneic stem cell transplantation and increases the frequency of CD4+Foxp3+ T cells. *Leukemia*, Vol.23, No.3, (March 2009), pp. 605-607, ISSN 1476-5551

Miyara, M., Yoshioka, Y., Kitoh, A., Shima, T., Wing, K., Niwa, A., Parizot, C., Taflin, C., Heike, T., Valeyre, D., Mathian, A., Nakahata, T., Yamaguchi, T., Nomura, T., Ono, M., Amoura, Z., Gorochov, G. & Sakaguchi, S. (2009). Functional delineation and differentiation dynamics of human CD4+ T cells expressing the FoxP3 transcription factor. *Immunity*, Vol.30, No.6, (June 2009), pp. 899-911, ISSN 1097-4180

Mizukami, Y., Kono, K., Kawaguchi, Y., Akaike, H., Kamimura, K., Sugai, H. & Fujii, H. (2008). CCL17 and CCL22 chemokines within tumor microenvironment are related to accumulation of Foxp3+ regulatory T cells in gastric cancer. *International Journal of Cancer*, Vol.122, No.10, (May 2008), pp. 2286-2293, ISSN 1097-0215

Movahedi, K., Guilliams, M., Van den Bossche, J., Van den Bergh, R., Gysemans, C., Beschin, A., De Baetselier, P. & Van Ginderachter, J.A. (2008). Identification of discrete tumor-induced myeloid-derived suppressor cell subpopulations with distinct T cell-suppressive activity. *Blood*, Vol.111, No.8, (April 2008), pp. 4233-4244, ISSN 0006-4971

Munn, D.H., Shafizadeh, E., Attwood, J.T., Bondarev, I., Pashine, A. & Mellor, A.L. (1999). Inhibition of T cell proliferation by macrophage tryptophan catabolism. *Journal of Experimental Medicine*, Vol.189, No.9, (May 1999), pp. 1363-1372, ISSN 0022-1007

Murakami, M., Sakamoto, A., Bender, J., Kappler, J. & Marrack, P. (2002). CD25+CD4+ T cells contribute to the control of memory CD8+ T cells. *Proceedings of the National Academy of Sciences of the United States of America*, Vol.99, No.13, (June 2002), pp. 8832-8837, ISSN 0027-8424

Muthu Raja, K.R., Kovarova, L., Buresova, I., Hajek, R. & Michalek, J. (2010). Flow Cytometric Phenotyping and Analysis of CD8 Regulatory and Suppressor Cells In Multiple Myeloma, *American Society of Hematology Meeting*, ISSN 0006-4971, Florida, USA, December 2010

Muthu Raja, K.R., Stossova, J., Kovarova, L. & Hajek, R. (2011). Myeloid derived suppressor cells are elevated in MGUS and MM patients, *International Myeloma Workshop*, ISSN 0390-6078, Paris, France, May 2011

Muthu Raja, K.R., Kovarova, L., Kaisarova, P., Bartonova, J. & Hajek, R. & Michalek. (2011). Regulatory T Cells Predicts Progression in Previously Untreated Myeloma Patients and Treatment by Cyclophosphamide, Thalidomide plus Dexamethasone Reduces Regulatory T Cells, *American Society of Hematology Meeting*, San Diego, CA, USA, December 2011

Nagai, H., Horikawa, T., Hara, I., Fukunaga, A., Oniki, S., Oka, M., Nishigori, C. & Ichihashi, M. (2004). In vivo elimination of CD25+ regulatory T cells leads to tumor rejection of B16F10 melanoma, when combined with interleukin-12 gene transfer. *Experimental Dermatology*, Vol.13, No.10, (October 2004), pp. 613-620, ISSN 0906-6705

Nagaraj, S., Gupta, K., Pisarev, V., Kinarsky, L., Sherman, S., Kang, L., Herber, D.L., Schneck, J. & Gabrilovich, D.I. (2007). Altered recognition of antigen is a mechanism of CD8+ T cell tolerance in cancer. *Nature Medicine*, Vol.13, No.7, (July, 2007), pp. 828-835, ISSN 1078-8956

Nishizuka, Y. & Sakakura, T. (1969). Thymus and reproduction: sex-linked dysgenesia of the gonad after neonatal thymectomy in mice. *Science*, Vol.166, No.906, (November 1969), pp. 753-755, ISSN 0036-8075

Noonan, K., Marchionni, L., Anderson, J., Pardoll, D., Roodman, G.D. & Borrello, I. (2010). A novel role of IL-17-producing lymphocytes in mediating lytic bone disease in multiple myeloma. *Blood*, Vol.116, No.18, (November 2010), pp. 3554-3563, ISSN 1528-0020

Oderup, C., Cederbom, L., Makowska, A., Cilio, C.M. & Ivars, F. (2006). Cytotoxic T lymphocyte antigen-4-dependent down-modulation of costimulatory molecules on dendritic cells in CD4+ CD25+ regulatory T-cell-mediated suppression. *Immunology*, Vol.118, No.2, (June 2006), 240-249, ISSN 0019-2805

Oida, T., Xu, L., Weiner, H.L., Kitani, A. & Strober, W. (2006). TGF-beta-mediated suppression by CD4+CD25+ T cells is facilitated by CTLA-4 signaling. *Journal of Immunology*, Vol.177, No.4, (August 2006), pp. 2331-2339, ISSN 0022-1767

Pandiyan, P., Zheng, L., Ishihara, S., Reed, J. & Lenardo, M.J. (2007). CD4+CD25+Foxp3+ regulatory T cells induce cytokine deprivation-mediated apoptosis of effector CD4+ T cells. *Nature Immunology*, Vol.8, No.12, (December 2007), pp. 1353-1362, ISSN 1529-2916

Pardoll, D. (2003). Does the immune system see tumors as foreign or self? *Annual Review of Immunology*, Vol.21, pp. 807-839, ISSN 0732-0582

Peng, G., Wang, H.Y., Peng, W., Kiniwa, Y., Seo, K.H. & Wang, R.F. (2007). Tumor-infiltrating gammadelta T cells suppress T and dendritic cell function via mechanisms controlled by a unique toll-like receptor signaling pathway. *Immunity*, Vol.27, No.2, (August 2007), pp. 334-348, ISSN 1074-7613

Powell, D.J., Felipe-Silva, A., Merino, M.J., Ahmadzadeh, M., Allen, T., Levy, C., White, D.E., Mavroukakis, S., Kreitman, R.J., Rosenberg, S.A. & Pastan, I. (2007). Administration of a CD25-directed immunotoxin, LMB-2, to patients with metastatic melanoma induces a selective partial reduction in regulatory T cells in vivo. *Journal of Immunology*, Vol.179, No.7, (October 2007), pp. 4919-4928, ISSN 0022-1767

Prabhala, R.H., Neri, P., Bae, J.E., Tassone, P., Shammas, M.A., Allam, C.K., Daley, J.F., Chauhan, D., Blanchard, E., Thatte, H.S., Anderson, K.C. & Munshi, N.C. (2006). Dysfunctional T regulatory cells in multiple myeloma. *Blood*, Vol.107, No.1, (January 2006), pp. 301-304, ISSN 0006-4971

Prabhala, R.H., Pelluru, D., Fulciniti, M., Prabhala, H.K., Nanjappa, P., Song, W., Pai, C., Amin, S., Tai, Y.T., Richardson, P.G., Ghobrial, I.M., Treon, S.P., Daley, J.F., Anderson, K.C., Kutok, J.L. & Munshi, N.C. (2010). Elevated IL-17 produced by TH17 cells promotes myeloma cell growth and inhibits immune function in multiple myeloma. *Blood*, Vol.115, No. 26, (July 2010), pp. 5385-5392, ISSN 1528-0020

Pratt, G., Goodyear, O. & Moss, P. (2007). Immunodeficiency and immunotherapy in multiple myeloma. *British Journal of Haematology*, Vol.138, No.5, (September 2007), pp. 563-579, ISSN 0007-1048

Quach, H., Ritchie, D., Stewart, A.K., Neeson, P., Harrison, S., Smyth, M.J. & Prince, H.M. (2010). Mechanism of action of immunomodulatory drugs (IMiDS) in multiple myeloma. *Leukemia*, Vol.24, No.1 (January 2010), pp. 22-32, ISSN 1476-5551

Raja, K.R., Kovarova, L. & Hajek, R. (2010). Review of phenotypic markers used in flow cytometric analysis of MGUS and MM, and applicability of flow cytometry in other plasma cell disorders. *British Journal of Haematology*, Vol.149, No.3 (May 2010), pp. 334-351, ISSN 1365-2141

Read, S., Malmström, V. & Powrie, F. (2000). Cytotoxic T lymphocyte-associated antigen 4 plays an essential role in the function of CD25(+)CD4(+) regulatory cells that control intestinal inflammation. *Journal of Experimental Medicine*, Vol.192, No.2, (July 2000), pp. 295-302, ISSN 0022-1007

Rezvani, K., Mielke, S., Ahmadzadeh, M., Kilical, Y., Savani, B.N., Zeilah, J., Keyvanfar, K., Montero, A., Hensel, N., Kurlander, R. & Barrett, A.J. (2006). High donor FOXP3-positive regulatory T-cell (Treg) content is associated with a low risk of GVHD following HLA-matched allogeneic SCT. *Blood*, Vol.108, No.4, (August 2006), pp. 1291-1297, ISSN 0006-4971

Rodriguez, P.C., Zea, A.H., Culotta, K.S., Zabaleta, J., Ochoa, J.B. & Ochoa, A.C. (2002). Regulation of T cell receptor CD3zeta chain expression by L-arginine. *Journal of Biological Chemistry*, Vol.277, No.24, (June 2002), pp. 21123-21129, ISSN 0021-9258

Romagnani, C., Della Chiesa, M., Kohler, S., Moewes, B., Radbruch, A., Moretta, L., Moretta, A. & Thiel, A. (2005). Activation of human NK cells by plasmacytoid dendritic cells and its modulation by CD4+ T helper cells and CD4+ CD25hi T regulatory cells. *European Journal of Immunology*, Vol.35, No.8 (August 2005), pp. 2452-2458, ISSN 0014-2980

Russell, J.H. & Ley, T.J. (2002). Lymphocyte-mediated cytotoxicity. Annual Review of Immunology, Vol. 20, pp. 323-370, ISSN 0732-0582

Sakaguchi, S. (2004). Naturally arising CD4+ regulatory t cells for immunologic self-tolerance and negative control of immune responses. Annual Review of Immunology, Vol.22, pp. 531-562, ISSN 0732-0582

Sakaguchi, S., Sakaguchi, N., Asano, M., Itoh, M. & Toda, M. (1995). Immunologic self-tolerance maintained by activated T cells expressing IL-2 receptor alpha-chains (CD25). Breakdown of a single mechanism of self-tolerance causes various autoimmune diseases. *Journal of Immunology*, Vol.155, No.3, (August 1995), pp. 1151-1164, ISSN 0022-1767

Sakaguchi, S., Takahashi, T. & Nishizuka, Y. (1982). Study on cellular events in post-thymectomy autoimmune oophoritis in mice. II. Requirement of Lyt-1 cells in normal female mice for the prevention of oophoritis. *Journal of Experimental Medicine*, Vol.156, No.6, (December 1982), pp. 1577-1586, ISSN 0022-1007

Sakaguchi, S., Yamaguchi, T., Nomura, T. & Ono, M. (2008). Regulatory T cells and immune tolerance. *Cell*, Vol.133, No.5, (May 2008), pp. 775-787, ISSN 1097-4172

Sarantopoulos, S., Lu, L. & Cantor, H. (2004). Qa-1 restriction of CD8+ suppressor T cells. *Journal of Clinical Investigation*, Vol.114, No.9, (November 2004), pp. 1218-1221, ISSN 0021-9738

Sasada, T., Kimura, M., Yoshida, Y., Kanai, M. & Takabayashi, A. (2003). CD4+CD25+ regulatory T cells in patients with gastrointestinal malignancies: possible involvement of regulatory T cells in disease progression. *Cancer*, Vol.98, No.5, (September 2003), pp. 1089-1099, ISSN 0008-543X

Schneider, M.A., Meingassner, J.G., Lipp, M., Moore, H.D. & Rot, A. (2007). CCR7 is required for the in vivo function of CD4+ CD25+ regulatory T cells. *Journal of Experimental Medicine*, Vol.204, No.4, (April 2007), pp. 735-745, ISSN 0022-1007

Seddiki, N., Santner-Nanan, B., Martinson, J., Zaunders, J., Sasson, S., Landay, A., Solomon, M., Selby, W., Alexander, S.I., Nanan, R., Kelleher, A. & Fazekas de St Groth, B. (2006). Expression of interleukin (IL)-2 and IL-7 receptors discriminates between human regulatory and activated T cells. *Journal of Experimental Medicine*, Vol.203, No.7, (July 2006), pp. 1693-1700, ISSN 0022-1007

Serafini, P., Mgebroff, S., Noonan, K. & Borrello, I. (2008). Myeloid-derived suppressor cells promote cross-tolerance in B-cell lymphoma by expanding regulatory T cells. *Cancer Research*, Vol.68, No.13, (July 2008), pp. 5439-5449, ISSN 1538-7445

Shi, G., Cox, C.A., Vistica, B.P., Tan, C., Wawrousek, E.F. & Gery, I. (2008). Phenotype switching by inflammation-inducing polarized Th17 cells, but not by Th1 cells. *Journal of Immunology*, Vol.181, No.10, (November 2008), pp. 7205-7213, ISSN 0022-1767

Shimizu, J., Yamazaki, S. & Sakaguchi, S. (1999). Induction of tumor immunity by removing CD25+CD4+ T cells: a common basis between tumor immunity and autoimmunity. *Journal of Immunology*, Vol.163, No.10, (November 1999), pp. 5211-5218, ISSN 0022-1767

Smyth, M.J., Crowe, N.Y. & Godfrey, D.I. (2001). NK cells and NKT cells collaborate in host protection from methylcholanthrene-induced fibrosarcoma. *International Immunology*, Vol.13, No.4, (April 2001), pp. 459-463, ISSN 0953-8178

Smyth, M.J., Thia, K.Y., Street, S.E., Cretney, E., Trapani, J.A., Taniguchi, M., Kawano, T., Pelikan, S.B., Crowe, N.Y. & Godfrey, D.I. (2000). Differential tumor surveillance by natural killer (NK) and NKT cells. *Journal of Experimental Medicine*, Vol.191, No.4, (February 2000), pp. 661-668, ISSN 0022-1007

Strauss, L., Bergmann, C., Szczepanski, M., Gooding, W., Johnson, J.T. & Whiteside, T.L. (2007). A unique subset of CD4+CD25highFoxp3+ T cells secreting interleukin-10 and transforming growth factor-beta1 mediates suppression in the tumor microenvironment. *Clinical Cancer Research*, Vol.13, No.15, (August 2007), pp. 4345-4354, ISSN 1078-0432

Strauss, L., Bergmann, C., Szczepanski, M.J., Lang, S., Kirkwood, J.M. & Whiteside, T.L. (2008). Expression of ICOS on human melanoma-infiltrating CD4+CD25highFoxp3+ T regulatory cells: implications and impact on tumor-mediated immune suppression. *Journal of Immunology*, Vol.180, No.5, (March 2008), pp. 2967-2980, ISSN 0022-1767

Strauss, L., Bergmann, C. & Whiteside, T.L. (2009). Human circulating CD4+CD25highFoxp3+ regulatory T cells kill autologous CD8+ but not CD4+ responder cells by Fas-mediated apoptosis. *Journal of Immunology*, Vol. 182, No.3, (February 2009), pp. 1469-1480, ISSN 1550-6606

Suciu-Foca, N., Manavalan, J.S., Scotto, L., Kim-Schulze, S., Galluzzo, S., Naiyer, A.J., Fan, J., Vlad, G. & Cortesini, R. (2005). Molecular characterization of allospecific T suppressor and tolerogenic dendritic cells: review. *International Immunopharmacology*, Vol.5, No.1, (January 2005), pp. 7-11, ISSN 1567-5769

Swann, J.B. & Smyth, M.J. (2007). Immune surveillance of tumors. *Journal of Clinical Investigation*, Vol.117, No.5, (May 2007), pp. 1137-1146, ISSN 0021-9738

Trzonkowski, P., Szmit, E., My?liwska, J., Dobyszuk, A. & My?liwski, A. (2004). CD4+CD25+ T regulatory cells inhibit cytotoxic activity of T CD8+ and NK lymphocytes in the direct cell-to-cell interaction. *Clinical Immunology*, Vol.112, No.3, (September 2004), pp. 258-267, ISSN 1521-6616

Valzasina, B., Guiducci, C., Dislich, H., Killeen, N., Weinberg, A.D. & Colombo, M.P. (2005). Triggering of OX40 (CD134) on CD4(+)CD25+ T cells blocks their inhibitory activity: a novel regulatory role for OX40 and its comparison with GITR. *Blood*, Vol.105, No. 7, (April 2005), pp. 2845-2851, ISSN 0006-4971

Veldhoen, M., Hocking, R.J., Atkins, C.J., Locksley, R.M. & Stockinger, B. (2006). TGFbeta in the context of an inflammatory cytokine milieu supports de novo differentiation of IL-17-producing T cells. *Immunity*, Vol.24, No.2, (February 2006), pp. 179-189, ISSN 1074-7613

Vieira, P.L., Christensen, J.R., Minaee, S., O'Neill, E.J., Barrat, F.J., Boonstra, A., Barthlott, T., Stockinger, B., Wraith, D.C. & O'Garra, A. (2004). IL-10-secreting regulatory T cells do not express Foxp3 but have comparable regulatory function to naturally occurring CD4+CD25+ regulatory T cells. *Journal of Immunology*, Vol.172, No.10, (May 2004), pp. 5986-5993, ISSN 0022-1767

Vincent, J., Mignot, G., Chalmin, F., Ladoire, S., Bruchard, M., Chevriaux, A., Martin, F., Apetoh, L., Rébé, C. & Ghiringhelli, F. (2010). 5-Fluorouracil selectively kills tumor-associated myeloid-derived suppressor cells resulting in enhanced T cell-dependent antitumor immunity. *Cancer Research*, Vol.70, No.8, (April 2010), pp. 3052-3061, ISSN 1538-7445

von Boehmer, H. (2005). Mechanisms of suppression by suppressor T cells. *Nature Immunology*, Vol.6, No.4, (April 2005), pp. 338-344, ISSN 1529-2908

Wang, H.Y., Lee, D.A., Peng, G., Guo, Z., Li, Y., Kiniwa, Y., Shevach, E.M. & Wang, R.F. (2004). Tumor-specific human CD4+ regulatory T cells and their ligands: implications for immunotherapy. *Immunity*, Vol.20, No.1, (January 2004), pp. 107-118, ISSN 1074-7613

Wang, R.F. (2008). CD8+ regulatory T cells, their suppressive mechanisms, and regulation in cancer. *Human Immunology*, Vol.69, No.11, (November 2008), pp. 811-814, ISSN 0198-8859

Wilson, N.J., Boniface, K., Chan, J.R., McKenzie, B.S., Blumenschein, W.M., Mattson, J.D., Basham, B., Smith, K., Chen, T., Morel, F., Lecron, J.C., Kastelein, R.A., Cua, D.J., McClanahan, T.K., Bowman, E.P. & de Waal Malefyt, R. (2007). Development, cytokine profile and function of human interleukin 17-producing helper T cells. *Nature Immunology*, Vol.8, No.9, (September 2007), pp. 950-957, ISSN 1529-2908

Wing, K., Onishi, Y., Prieto-Martin, P., Yamaguchi, T., Miyara, M., Fehervari, Z., Nomura, T. & Sakaguchi, S. (2008). CTLA-4 control over Foxp3+ regulatory T cell function. *Science*, Vol.322, No.5899, (October 2008), pp. 271-275, ISSN 1095-9203

Xu, L., Kitani, A., Fuss, I. & Strober, W. (2007). Cutting edge: regulatory T cells induce CD4+CD25-Foxp3- T cells or are self-induced to become Th17 cells in the absence of exogenous TGF-beta. *Journal of Immunology*, Vol.178, No.11, (June 2007), pp. 6725-6729, ISSN 0022-1767

Yamaguchi, T. & Sakaguchi, S. (2006). Regulatory T cells in immune surveillance and treatment of cancer. *Seminars in Cancer Biology*, Vol.16, No.2, (April 2006), pp. 115-123, ISSN 1044-579X

Yang, R., Cai, Z., Zhang, Y., Yutzy, W.H., Roby, K.F. & Roden, R.B. (2006a). CD80 in immune suppression by mouse ovarian carcinoma-associated Gr-1+CD11b+ myeloid cells. *Cancer Research*, Vol.66, No.13, (July 2006), pp. 6807-6815, ISSN 0008-5472

Yang, Z.Z., Novak, A.J., Stenson, M.J., Witzig, T.E. & Ansell, S.M. (2006b). Intratumoral CD4+CD25+ regulatory T-cell mediated suppression of infiltrating CD4+ T cells in B-cell non-Hodgkin lymphoma. *Blood*, Vol.107, No.9, (May 2006), pp. 3639-3646, ISSN 0006-4971

Youn (2), J.I., Nagaraj, S., Collazo, M. & Gabrilovich, D.I. (2008). Subsets of myeloid-derived suppressor cells in tumor-bearing mice. *Journal of Immunology*, Vol.181, No.8, (October 2008), pp. 5791-5802, ISSN 1550-6606

Zheng, S.G., Wang, J. & Horwitz, D.A. (2008). Cutting edge: Foxp3+CD4+CD25+ regulatory T cells induced by IL-2 and TGF-beta are resistant to Th17 conversion by IL-6. *Journal of Immunology*, Vol.180, No.11, (June 2008), pp. 7112-7116, ISSN 0022-1767

3

Effects of Recombinant Human Tumor Necrosis Factor-α and Its Combination with Native Human Leukocyte Interferon-α on P3-X63-Ag8.653 Mouse Myeloma Cell Growth

Andrej Plesničar[1], Gaj Vidmar[2], Borut Štabuc[3] and Blanka Kores Plesničar[4]
[1]*University of Ljubljana, Faculty of Health Sciences, Ljubljana,*
[2]*Institute for Rehabilitation, Ljubljana,*
[3]*University of Ljubljana, Faculty of Medicine, Ljubljana,*
[4]*University of Maribor, Faculty of Medicine, Maribor,*
Slovenia

1. Introduction

Multiple myeloma (MM) is a malignant B-cell disease, characterized by uncontrolled proliferation of differentiated plasma cells in bone marrow (BM), osteolytic bone lesions, monoclonal protein peaks in serum or urine and suppression of normal antibody production. Patients with MM usually present with a number of clinical signs and symptoms, including fatigue, infection, severe bone pain, bone fractures, hypercalcaemia, and renal disease (Bommert et al., 2006; Raman et al., 2007; Redzepovic et al., 2008). Despite clinical responses produced by conventional chemotherapy, radiotherapy, and an increasing number of new compounds and improvements in supportive therapy, MM remains largely incurable (Katzel et al., 2007; Ozdemir et al., 2004; Redzepovic et al., 2008).

Tumor necrosis factor-α (TNF-α) is a known survival and proliferation factor for myeloma cell lines. It is produced by tumor and stromal cells in BM of patients with MM and induces tumor cell proliferation, migration, survival, drug resistance, and blood vessel proliferation (Harrison et al., 2006; Jourdan et al., 1999). Although TNF-α secreted by MM cells does not induce significant growth and drug resistance in tumor cells, it stimulates interleukin-6 (IL-6) secretion in bone marrow stromal cells more potently than vascular endothelial growth factor (VEGF) or transforming growth factor-β (TGF-β) (Yasui et al., 2005). Out of BM environment, circulating TNF-α levels are increased in MM patients with manifest bone disease, whose osteoblasts constitutively overexpress receptors for TNF-related apoptosis-inducing ligand, intercellular adhesion molecule-1 (ICAM-1), and monocyte chemotactic protein-1 (MCP-1) (Silvestris et al., 2004).

In our previous study, treatment with native human leukocyte interferon-α (nhIFN-α), recombinant human interferon-α2a (rhIFN-α2a) and recombinant human interferon-α2b (rhIFN-α2b) in doses of 500 IU/ml, 1000/ml and 2000 IU/ml resulted in differential effects on P3-X63-Ag8.653 mouse myeloma cells. A statistically significant dose-dependent decrease in cell viability was observed in P3-X63-Ag8.653 mouse myeloma cells treated with nhIFN-α in comparison with matched negative controls. Conversely, a statistically significant increase in cell viability was observed in P3-X63-Ag8.653 mouse myeloma cells treated with rhIFN-α2a and rhIFN-α2b. This increase in cell viability occurred only in relation to their matched negative controls and was not dose-dependent (Plesničar et al., 2009). The differences in effects on P3-X63-Ag8.653 mouse myeloma cell viability between nhIFN-α and recombinant interferons probably occurred because nhIFN-α is composed of many subtypes of nhIFN-α and also contains trace amounts of IFN-γ, TNF-α, TNF-β, interleukin (IL)-1α, IL-1β, IL-2, IL-6, granulocyte-macrophage colony-stimulating factor and platelet-derived growth factor. Therefore, the decrease of cell viability in nhIFN-α treated P3-X63-Ag8.653 mouse myeloma cell cultures may have occurred in consequence of a synergistic effect of the various cytokines in nhIFN-α preparation. The quantities and the synergistic effect of the cytokines in nhIFN-α preparation are very small at lower concentrations and probably become active only at higher concentrations, thus accounting for the dose-dependent effects observed on cell growth (Plesničar et al., 2009; Šantak et al., 2007, Zidovec & Mažuran, 1999). In contrast to nhIFN-α, rhIFN-α2a and rhIFN-α2b are each preparations of only one subtype of IFN-α. The increase in cell viability in P3-X63-Ag8.653 mouse myeloma cell culture groups treated with rhIFN-α2a and rhIFN-α2b in our study was in accordance with a number of reports suggesting that IFN-α could induce uncontrolled cell proliferation in some patients with MM (Plesničar et al., 2009; Puthier et al., 2001; Sawamura et al., 1992). Interferon-α has been recognized as a survival factor in MM in some studies, the data supporting this claim are based on the results of studies using recombinant interferons-α (Cheriyath et al., 2007; Ferlin-Bezombes et al., 1998; Puthier et al., 2001).

The P3-X63-Ag8.653 mouse myeloma cell line is routinely cultured in several types of growth media. The cells in P3-X63-Ag8.653 mouse myeloma cell line propagate in suspension and do not secrete immunoglobulin. They can be used as fusion partners for producing hybridomas and show lymphocyte-like morphology (Kearney et al., 1979). Human myeloma blood cells were described as carrying surface membrane monoclonal or idiotypic immunoglobulin structures, and were morphologically classified as atypical small to medium-sized lymphocytes, lymphoblasts, lymphoplasmacytoid, plasmacytoid cells or myeloma cells (Mellstedt et al., 1984). With regard to morphology and despite the differences, it may be possible that P3-X63-Ag8.653 mouse myeloma cells, growing in suspension cell cultures, share at least some common properties with circulating clonogenic CD19 positive and CD138 negative cells, described as phenotypically resembling mature B cells (Cremer et al., 2001; Matsui et al., 2004).

The aim of the present study was to compare the effects of different doses of rTNF-α on the *in-vitro* growth of P3-X63-Ag8.653 mouse myeloma cells. Additionally, in one cell culture study group the aim was also to compare the effect of a combination of rTNF-α and nhIFN-α with the effects of corresponding doses of single cytokines on the *in-vitro* growth of P3-X63-Ag8.653 mouse myeloma cells.

2. Materials and methods

2.1 P3-X63-Ag8.653 mouse myeloma cell preparation

The P3-X63-Ag8.653 mouse myeloma cells were retrieved from the frozen storage at -80 °C and cultured in 25 cm^2 cell culture flasks (Cole Parmer, Vernon Hills, IL, USA) in Dulbecco's modified Eagle's medium (Sigma-Aldrich, St. Louis, MO, USA), supplemented with 10% fetal calf serum (FCS) (Sigma-Aldrich, St. Louis, MO, USA) and gentamycin (Krka, tovarna zdravil, d. d., Novo Mesto, Slovenia). The cells were incubated at 37 °C in a humidified atmosphere of 5% CO_2 for 48 hours.

In preparation for this study, P3-X63-Ag8.653 mouse myeloma cell growth curves on logarithmic scale plots were established when the most convenient seeding density to be used was determined. Various time zero values ranged from 5 X 10^3 to 6 X 10^4 cells/ml and S-shaped growth curves were observed after cell concentrations measured in 24 hour intervals over the 96 hours were plotted on Keuffel & Esser 464970 Semi-Logarithmic Grids general purpose drawing paper. Time zero density of 10^4 P3-X63-Ag8.653 mouse myeloma cells/ml was found to be the most appropriate for the study. With the use of Keuffel & Esser 464970 graph paper it was also possible to observe that P3-X63-Ag8.653 mouse myeloma cells started to enter the log phase in approximately 24 hours (one day) and the plateau phase in approximately 72 hours (three days).

2.2 Recombinant human tumor necrosis factor-α, native human interferon-α and cell culture study groups

Actively growing P3-X63.Ag8.653 mouse myeloma cells were seeded into 35 mm Petri dishes (Becton Dickinson, Franklin Lakes, NJ, USA) and incubated in each study group with three different concentrations of rTNF-α (Prospecbio, East Brunswick, NJ, USA). In the first study group the cells were incubated with 2, 10 and 20 IU/ml of rTNF-α, in the second with 30, 40 and 50 IU/ml of rTNF-α, in the third with 100, 200 and 300 IU/ml of rTNF-α, and in the fourth study group with 400, 800 and 1200 IU/ml of rTNF-α. After the experiments with rTNF-α, in one study group the cells were incubated with a combination of 10 IU/ml of rTNF-α and 2000 IU/ML of nhIFN-α (Institute of Immunology Inc., Zagreb, Croatia). The combination was compared to the corresponding doses of single cytokines. Matched negative controls that consisted of P3-X63-Ag8.653 mouse myeloma cells cultured in the absence of cytokines were established for each of the different cytokine study groups. All experiments were replicated five times and 20 Petri dishes were used for each cytokine cell culture study group and their negative controls. Cell viability was assessed by Trypan blue exclusion in 24 hour intervals (days 1-4).

2.3 Statistical analysis

In proliferating cell lines, it is difficult to distinguish between early cell loss and prolonged lag phase in which cells are still adapting to their new environment (Wilson, 1994). The effects of different concentrations of rTNF-α and its combination with nhIFN-α were thus estimated with the use of whole growth curves to reduce the possibility of misinterpretation. Statistical evaluation was performed using SPSS® software package, version 12.0 (SPSS Inc., Chicago, IL, USA) for Windows®. Analysis of variance (ANOVA) was used to assess the differences between and within different treatment groups and their negative control groups. *P*-values of < 0.05 were considered to be statistically significant.

3. Results

Treatment of P3-X63-Ag8.653 mouse myeloma cells with rTNF-α showed a statistically significant reduction in cell viability in comparison with negative control cells. The reduction in cell viability occurred in dose-dependent manner, with higher doses having a greater effect (Table 1, Figures 1-4). Treatment of P3-X63-Ag8.653 mouse myeloma cells with 400, 800 and 1200 IU/ml of rTNF-α showed a complete cessation of cell growth (Table 1), with the cells being unable to enter the log phase of the S-shaped growth curve (Figure 4). Treatment of P3-X63-Ag8.653 mouse myeloma cells with a combination of rTNF-α and nhIFN-α showed a statistically significant reduction in cell viability in comparison with negative control cells and cells treated exclusively with either rTNF-α or nhIFN-α. The addition of a small dose of rTNF-α (10 IU/ml) to the treatment of P3-X63-Ag8.653 mouse myeloma cells with a relatively high dose of nhIFN-α (2000 IU/ml) resulted in a further, although small, reduction in cell viability (Table 1, Figure 5).

Cell study group	**Cytokine type**	**Cytokine concentration (IU/ml)**	**No. of cells (10^4/ml) Mean +/- SE over days 0-4**	**Statistical significance[1]**
rTNF-α (1)		Negative control	20.400 +/- 0.83306	*P* = 0.001
	rTNF-α	2	20.187 +/- 1.65707	
	rTNF-α	10	16.675 +/- 1.99607	
	rTNF-α	20	13.425 +/- 0.54608	
rTNF-α (2)		Negative control	23.3250 +/- 1.96338	*P* = 0.000
	rTNF-α	30	12.8750 +/- 0.55234	
	rTNF-α	40	10.4250 +/- 0.71709	
	rTNF-α	50	9.3750 +/- 0.20444	
rTNF-α (3)		Negative control	22.9000 +/- 0.79096	*P* = 0.000
	rTNF-α	100	8.5125 +/- 0.32918	
	rTNF-α	200	5.9625 +/- 0.34403	
	rTNF-α	300	1.6750 +/- 0.07500	
rTNF-α (4)		Negative control	22.2000 +/- 1.16011	*P* = 0.000
	rTNF-α	400	1.0375 +/- 0.05078	
	rTNF-α	800	0.9250 +/- 0.06673	
	rTNF-α	1200	0.6750 +/- 0.03644	
rTNF-α and **nhIFN-α**		Negative control	25.9625 +/- 0.62581	*P* = 0.000
	rTNF-α	10	19.6375 +/- 1.07591	
	nhIFN-α	2000	5.8000 +/- 0.10346	
	rTNF-α and **nhIFN-α**	10 and 2000	4.8500 +/- 0.35609	

[1]Comparison between active treatment overall and the corresponding negative control in each cell study group.

Table 1. Effect of recombinant human tumor necrosis factor-α (rTNF-α) at different concentrations, native human interferon-α (nhIFN-α) and the combination of rTNF-α and nhIFN-α on *in-vitro* P3-X63-Ag8.653 mouse myeloma cell growth.

As expected, when the cell numbers for each cell study group of P3-X63-Ag8.653 mouse myeloma cells treated with the different concentrations of rTNF-α and with the combination of rTNF-α and nhIFN-α or their negative controls were plotted on a logarithmic scale for the whole 96 hours (four days) period over which cell viability was measured, the growth curves were S-shaped. P3-X63-Ag8.653 mouse myeloma cells started to enter the log phase at approximately 24 hours (one day) and reached the plateau phase at approximately 72 hours (three days) from incubation with the different concentrations of rTNF-α and with the combination of rTNF-α and nhIFN-α. The intermediate portions (log phase) of the S-shaped growth curves, approximately between 24 and 72 hours, were linear. The slopes of the growth curves in the treated cell culture study groups and their negative controls were not identical (Figures 1-5).

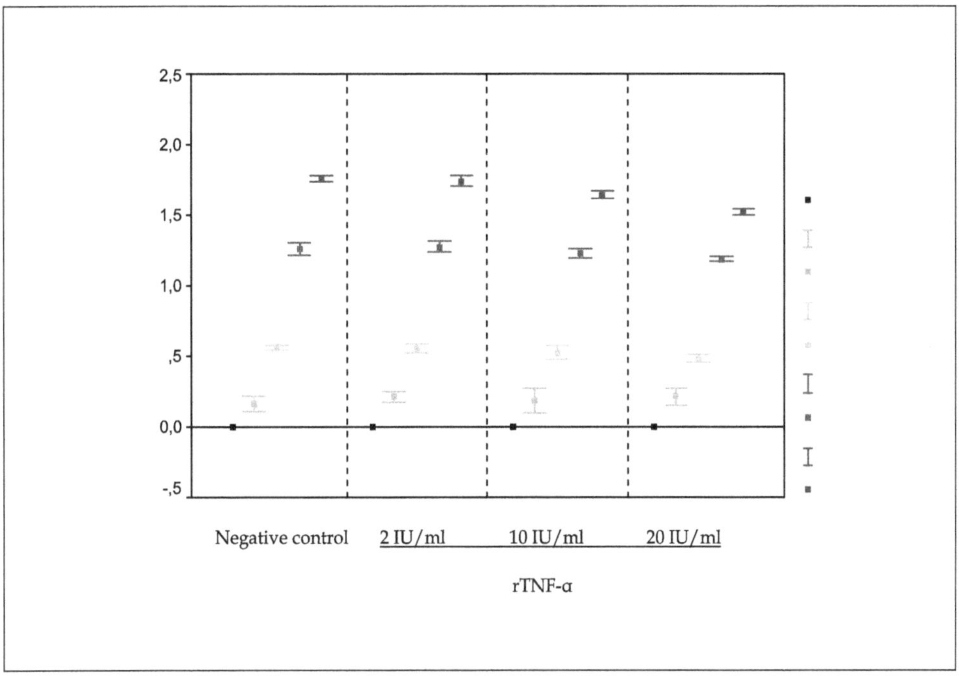

Fig. 1. The effect of 2, 10 and 20 IU/ml of human recombinant TNF-α (rTNF-α) on *in-vitro* P3-X63-Ag8.653 mouse myeloma cell growth plotted on a logarithmic scale (logarithmic number of P3-X63-Ag8.653 cells/ml), showing a dose-dependent reduction in cell viability over four days of treatment. The reduction in cell growth observed with rTNF-α was statistically significant in comparison with negative control ($P = 0.001$). Legend: black, day 0; green, day 1; light blue, day 2; dark blue, day 3; violet, day 4.

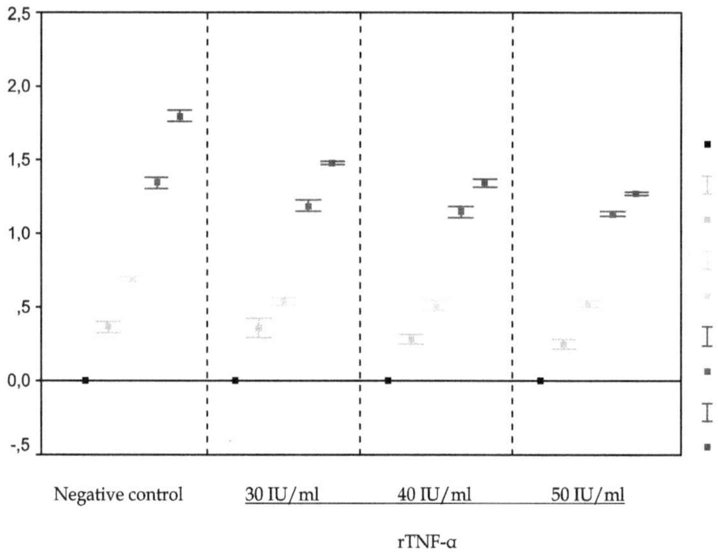

Fig. 2. The effect of 30, 40 and 50 IU/ml of human recombinant tumor necrosis factor-α (rTNF-α) on *in-vitro* P3-X63-Ag8.653 mouse myeloma cell growth plotted on a logarithmic scale (logarithmic number of P3-X63-Ag8.653 cells/ml), showing a dose-dependent reduction in cell viability over four days of treatment. The reduction in cell growth observed with rTNF-α was statistically significant in comparison with negative control ($P = 0.000$). Legend: black, day 0; green, day 1; light blue, day 2; dark blue, day 3; violet, day 4.

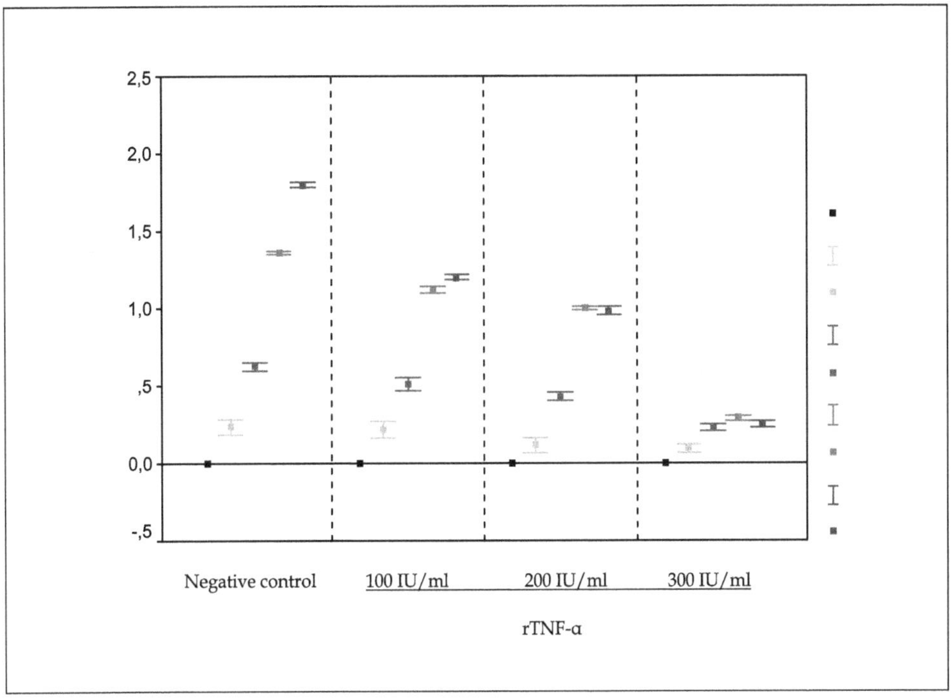

Fig. 3. The effect of 100, 200 and 300 IU/ml of human recombinant TNF-α (rTNF-α) on *in-vitro* P3-X63-Ag8.653 mouse myeloma cell growth plotted on a logarithmic scale (logarithmic number of P3-X63-Ag8.653 cells/ml), showing a dose-dependent reduction in cell viability over four days of treatment. The reduction in cell growth observed with rTNF-α was statistically significant in comparison with negative control *(P* = 0.000). Legend: black, day 0; green, day 1; blue, day 2; light violet, day 3; dark violet, day 4.

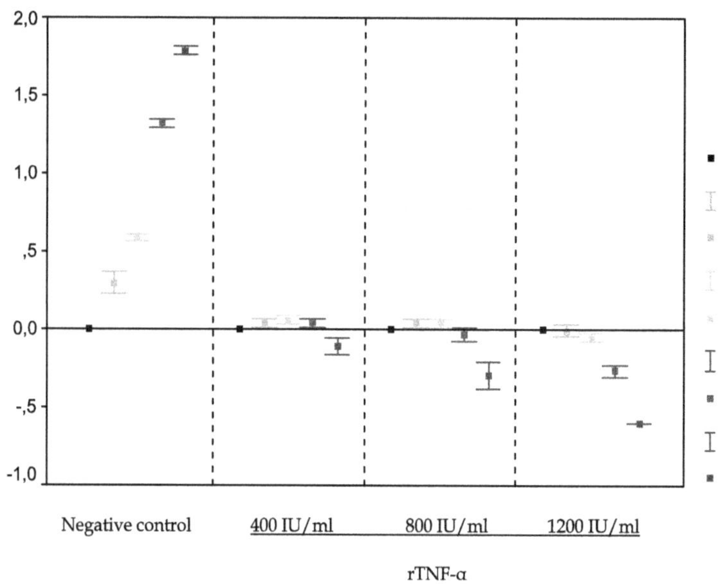

Fig. 4. The effect of 400, 800 and 1200 IU/ml of human recombinant TNF-α (rTNF-α) on *in-vitro* P3-X63-Ag8.653 mouse myeloma cell growth plotted on a logarithmic scale (logarithmic number of P3-X63-Ag8.653 cells/ml), showing a dose-dependent reduction in cell viability over four days of treatment. The reduction in cell growth observed with rTNF-α was statistically significant in comparison with negative control ($P = 0.000$). Legend: black, day 0; green, day 1; light blue, day 2; dark blue, day 3; violet, day 4.

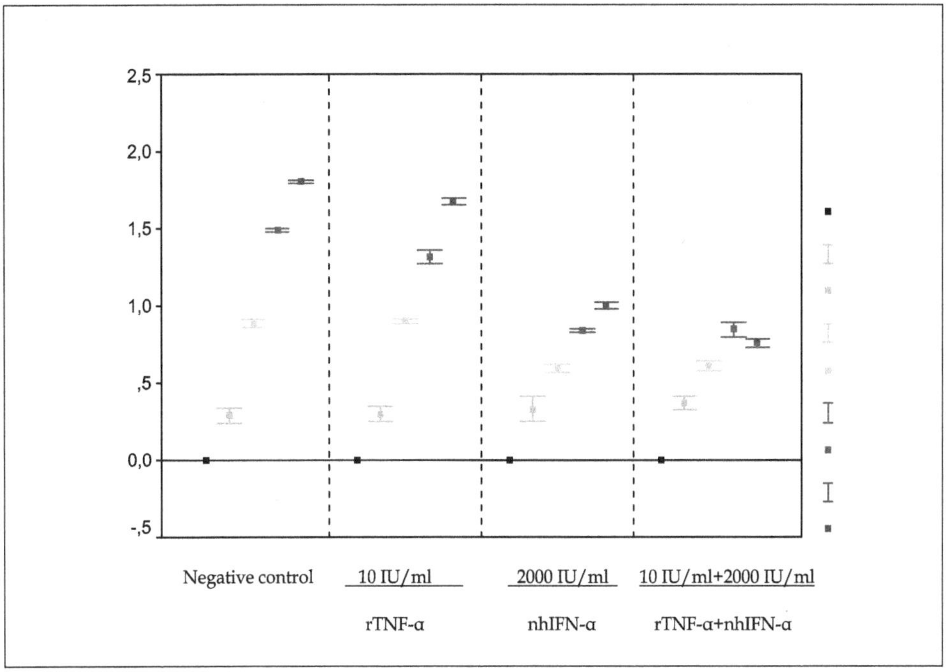

Fig. 5. The effect of 10 IU/ml of human recombinant TNF-α (rTNF-α), 2000 IU/ML of native human leukocyte interferon-α (nhIFN-α), and of a combination of 10 IU/ml of rTNF-α and 2000 IU/ML of nhIFN-α on *in-vitro* P3-X63-Ag8.653 mouse myeloma cell growth plotted on a logarithmic scale (logarithmic number of P3-X63-Ag8.653 cells/ml), showing a reduction in cell viability over four days of treatment. The reduction in cell growth observed after treatment with rTNF-α, nhIFN-α, and with the combination of rTNF-α and nhIFN-α, was statistically significant in comparison with negative control ($P = 0.000$). Legend: black, day 0; green, day 1; light blue, day 2; dark blue, day 3; violet, day 4.

4. Discussion

Treatment with rTNF-α at different doses had a negative effect on *in vitro* P3-X63-Ag8.653 mouse myeloma cell growth. A statistically significant dose-dependent reduction in cell viability was observed in P3-X63-Ag8.653 mouse myeloma cells treated with rTNF-α in comparison with negative controls. Additionally, a slightly enhanced reduction in P3-X63-Ag8.653 mouse myeloma cell viability was observed in cells treated with the combination of rTNF-α and nhIFN-α, in comparison with negative controls and cells treated exclusively with either rTNF-α or nhIFN-α.

The results of this study are surprising, as the treatment of P3-X63-Ag8.653 mouse myeloma with rTNF-α showed statistically significant reduction in cell viability compared with untreated control cells, with higher doses having greater effect. These results are in contradiction with numerous reports describing TNF-α as a survival and proliferation factor in MM (Harrison et al., 2006; Hideshima et al., 2004; Jourdan et al., 1999; Yasui et al., 2006;

Westendorf et al., 1996). However, TNF-α has previously also been described as an apoptotic factor in MM. The TNF-dependent trimerization of TNF receptors may lead to the recruitment of TRADD (TNF-R1 associated death domain protein), FADD (Fas-associated death domain protein) or RIP (receptor interacting protein) adapter proteins, resulting in activation and acceleration of caspase cascade (Baker & Reddy, 1996; Dai et al., 2003; Jourdan et al., 1999). This mechanism may further lead to apoptosis in MM cells (Jourdan et al., 1999).

Treatment of P3-X63-Ag8.653 mouse myeloma cells with the combination of rTNF-α and nHIFN-α resulted in an enhancement of the reduction in cell viability in comparison with negative control cells and cells treated exclusively with either rTNF-α or nhIFN-α. The nHIFN-α used in this study contains traces of a number of other cytokines produced by human peripheral blood leukocytes infected by Sendai virus (Šantak et al., 2007, Zidovec & Mažuran, 1999). The differences between the slopes of the S-shaped growth curves in the rTNF-α treated P3-X63-Ag8.653 mouse myeloma cell cultures and their controls, and equally prominent differences between the slopes of the growth curves of cells treated with the combination of rTNF-α and nHIFN-α and corresponding doses of single cytokines and their controls, may indicate that the active mechanisms associated with rTNF-α and nHIFN-α, and involved in reduction of cell viability, share some similarities and may possibly benefit from the synergy between rTNF-α, various subtypes of IFN-α and the small amounts of a number of other cytokines in the nHIFN-α preparation (Desmyter et al., 1968; Plesničar et al., 2009). In this context, it would be interesting to identify whether TNF-α and IFN-α share any signaling pathways leading to the reduction in MM cell viability and MM cell death.

Contrary to expectations, in this study treatment of P3-X63-Ag8.653 mouse myeloma cells with rTNF-α showed no increase, but a significant dose-dependent reduction in their cell viability. The P3-X63-Ag8.653 mouse myeloma cells propagate in suspension and show lymphocyte-like morphology (Kearney et al., 1979), and with this in mind, these cells may perhaps be useful in assessment of the effects rTNF-α may have on the growth of clonogenic B-cells in blood of patients with MM. Clonogenic B-cells represent the proliferating compartment in MM and possibly also a biologically distinct, drug-resistant MM progenitor population responsible for cell growth in tumor relapse after the treatment (Matsui et al., 2004; Matsui et al., 2008). In comparison to terminally differentiated plasma cells in MM, clonogenic B-cells appear to be relatively resistant to a number of anti-cancer agents, including dexamethasone, bortezomib, lenalidomide, and 4-hydroxycyclophosphamide (Agarwal & Matsui, 2010; Matsui et al., 2008). Possible similarities between P3-X63-Ag8.653 mouse myeloma cells and clonogenic B-cells in patients with MM, and because clonogenic B-cells are insensitive to standard cytotoxic chemotherapy and dexamethasone (Matsui et al., 2008), render the results observed in this study quite intriguing.

It is known that the activity of TNF-α as a survival and proliferation factor for MM is a part of a complex network of interactions between MM plasma cells, stromal cells and other cells in BM (Jourdan et al., 1999; Matsui et al., 2008). In this *in vitro* study, P3-X63-Ag8.653 mouse myeloma cells were grown in suspension culture, probably resembling the circumstances in which clonogenic B-cells in patients with MM grow without influences of BM microenvironment (Matsui et al., 2008). In a number of studies, serum levels of TNF-α were shown to be increased in patients with active MM and manifest bone disease, and to be associated with poor prognosis (Alexandrakis et al., 2004; Fillela et al., 1996; Jourdan et al., 1999). Hypothetically, it may be possible to speculate that the increased serum levels of TNF-α in patients with active MM represent a part of a complex negative control loop mechanism that regulates and negatively affects the quantity of circulating clonogenic B-cells in such patients.

A heterologous system was used to evaluate the effects of rTNF-α and its combination with nHIFN-α on MM cells *in-vitro*. Recombinant human tumor necrosis factor-α and nHIFN-α used in this study were active in P3-X63-Ag8.653 mouse myeloma cells, again confirming the observations that cytokines synthesized in cells of one species may have a considerable effect in cells of another closely related species (Desmyter et al., 1968; Greenberg & Mosny, 1977; Ozdemir et al., 2004). Moreover, MM cells are difficult to grow in vitro (Barker et al., 1993). An important advantage of the P3-X63-Ag8.653 mouse myeloma cell line may also lie in its easy reproducibility, unlimited supply, infinite storability and recoverability, and consequently in important cost savings (Drexler & Matsuo, 2000).

The results of this study point to the importance of the study of differential effects TNF-α may exert on malignant cells in MM during specific phases of their development and differentiation. It is possible that TNF-α may have a role in future carefully planned personalized therapy approaches based on genetic features, age, and other risk factors in patients with MM (Durie, 2008; Ludwig et al., 2008). Such therapy could perhaps include patients' own TNF-α, IFN-α, other substances and their combinations, provided that effective procedures for the establishment and maintenance of *ex vivo* cell cultures of patients' own cytokine-producing cells become available.

5. Conclusion

The results of this study point to the importance of assessing the role of TNF-α in study and therapy of MM. Additional studies with other cytokines and human MM cells are required to obtain further information.

6. References

Agarwal, J.A. & Matsui, W. (2010). Multiple Myeloma: A Paradigm for Translation of the Cancer Stem Cell Hypothesis. *Anti-Cancer Agents in Medicinal Chemistry*, Vol.10, No.2, (February 2010), pp. 116-120, ISSN 1875-5992

Alexandrakis, M.G., Passam, F.J., Ganotakis, E., Dafnis, E., Dambaki, C., Konsolas, J., Kyriakou, D.S. & Stathopoulos, E. (2004). Bone Marrow Microvascular Density and Angiogenic Growth Factors in Multiple Myeloma. *Clinical Chemistry and Laboratory Medicine*, Vol.42, No.10, (October 2004), pp. 1122-1126, ISSN 1434-6621

Baker, S.J. & Reddy, E.P. (1996). Transducers of life and death: TNF Receptor Superfamily and Associated Proteins. *Oncogene*, Vol.12, No.1, (January 1996), pp. 1-9, ISSN 0950-9232

Barker, H.F., Ball, J., Drew, M. & Franklin, I.M. (1993). Multiple Myeloma: The Biology of Malignant Plasma Cells. *Blood Reviews*, Vol.7, No.1 (March 1993), pp.19-23. ISSN 0268-960X

Bommert, K., Bargou, R.C. & Stühmer, T. (2006). Signalling and Survival Pathways in Multiple Myeloma. *European Journal of Cancer*, Vol.42, No.11, (July 2006), pp. 1574-1580, ISSN 0014-2964

Cheriyath, V., Glaser, K.B., Waring, J.F., Baz, R., Hussein, M.A. & Borden, E.C. (2007). G1P3, an IFN-Induced Survival Factor, Antagonizes TRAIL-Induced Apoptosis in Human Myeloma Cells. *Journal of Clinical Investigation*, Vol.117, No.10, (October 2007), pp. 3107-3117, ISSN 0021-9738

Cremer, F.W., Goldschmidt, H. & Moos, M. (2001). Clonotypic B Cells in the Peripheral Blood of Patients with Multiple Myeloma. *Blood*, Vol.97, No.9 (May 2001), pp. 2913-2914, ISSN 1528-0020

Dai, Y., Dent, P. & Grant, S. (2003). Tumor Necrosis Factor-Related Apoptosis-Inducing Ligand (TRAIL) Promotes Mitochondrial dysfunction and Apoptosis Induced by 7-Hydroxystauroporine and Mitogen-Activated Protein Kinase Inhibitors in Human Leukemia Cells That Ectopically Express Bcl-2 and Bcl-xL. *Molecular Pharmacology*, Vol.64, No.6, (December 2003), pp. 1402-1409, ISSN 0026-895X

Desmyter, J., Rawls, W.E. & Melnick, J.L. (1968). A Human Interferon That Crosses the Species Line. *Proceedings of the National Academy of Sciences of the United States of America*, Vol.59, No.1, (January 1968), pp. 69-76, ISSN 0027-8424

Drexler, H.G. & Matsuo, Y. (2000). Malignant Hematopoietic Cell Lines: In Vitro Models for the Study of Multiple Myeloma and Plasma Cell Leukemia. *Leukemia Research*, Vol.24, No.8, (August 2000), pp. 681–703, ISSN 0145-2126

Durie, B.G.M. (2008). Myeloma therapy: 25 Years Forward-Immune Modulation Then and Now. *Journal of Clinical Oncology*, Vol.26, No.29, (October 2008), pp. 4698-4700, ISSN 1527-7755

Ferlin-Bezombes, M., Jourdan, M., Liautard, J., Brochier, B., Rossi, J.F. & Klein, B. (1998). IFN-Alpha is a Survival Factor for Human Myeloma Cells and Reduces Dexamethasone-Induced Apoptosis. *Journal of Immunology*, Vol.161, No.6, (September 1998), pp. 2692-2699, ISSN 0022-1767

Fillela, X., Blade, J., Guillermo, A.L., Molina, R., Rozman, C. & Ballesta, A.M. (1996). Cytokines (IL-6, TNF-alpha, IL-1alpha) and Soluble IL-2 Receptor as Serum Tumor Markers in Multiple Myeloma. *Cancer Detection and Prevention*, Vol.20, No.1, (January 1996), pp. 52-56, ISSN 1525-1500

Greenberg, P.L. & Mosny, S.A. (1977). Cytotoxic Effects of Interferon *In Vitro* on Granulocytic Progenitor Cells. *Cancer Research*, Vol.37, No.6, (June 1977), pp. 1794-1799, ISSN 0008-5472

Harrison, S.J., Cook, G., Nibbs, R.J.B. & Miles Prince, H. (2006). Immunotherapy of Multiple Myeloma: The Start of a Long and Tortuous Journey. *Expert Review of Anticancer Therapy*, Vol.6, No.12, (December 2006), pp. 1769-1785, ISSN 1473-7140

Hideshima, T., Bergsagel P.L., Kuehl W.M. & Anderson, K.C. (2004). Advances in Biology of Multiple Myeloma: Clinical Applications. *Blood*, Vol.104, No.3 (August 2004), pp. 607-618, ISSN 1528-0020

Jourdan, M., Tarte, K., Legouffe, E., Brochier, J., Rossi, J.F. & Klein, B. (1999). Tumor Necrosis Factor is a Survival and Proliferation Factor for Human Myeloma Cells. *European Cytokine Network*, Vol.10, No.1, (March 1999), pp. 65-70, ISSN 1148-5493

Katzel, J.A., Hari, P. & Vesole, D.H. (2007). Multiple Myeloma; Charging Toward Bright Future. *CA Cancer Journal for Clinicians*, Vol.57, No.5, (September/October 2007), pp. 301-318, ISSN 1542-4863

Kearney, J.F., Radbruch A., Liesegang B. & Rajewsky, K. (1979). A New Mouse Myeloma Cell Line That has Lost Immunoglobulin Expression but Permits the Construction of Antibody-Secreting Hybrid Cell Lines. *Journal of Immunology*. Vol.123, No.4, (October 1979), pp. 1548-1550, ISSN 0022-1767

Ludwig, H., Durie, B.G.M., Bolejack, V., Turesson, I., Kyle, R.A., Blade, J., Fonseca, R., Dimopoulos, P., Shimizu, K., San Miguel, J., Westin, J., Harousseau, J.L., Beksac, M., Boccadoro, M., Palumbo, A., Barlogie, B., Shustik, C., Cavo, M., Greipp, P.R., Joshua, D., Attal, M., Sonneveld, P. & Crowley, J. (2008). Myeloma in Patients Younger than Age 50 Years Presents with More Favorable Features and Shows Better Survival: An Analysis of 10,549 Patients from the International Myeloma Working Group. *Blood*, Vol.111, No.8, (April 2008), pp. 4039-4047, ISSN 1528-0020

Matsui, W., Huff, C.A., Wang, Q., Malehorn M.T., Barber, J., Tanhehco, Y., Smith, B.D., Civin, C.I. & Jones, R.J. (2004). Characterization of Clonogenic Multiple Myeloma Cells. *Blood*, Vol.103, No. 6, (March 2004), pp. 2332-2336, ISSN 1528-0020

Matsui, W., Wang, Q., Barber J.P., Brennan, J.P., Brennan, S., Douglas Smith, S., Borrello, I, McNiece, I., Lin, L., Ambinder, R.F., Peacock, C., Watkins, D.N., Huff, C.A. & Jones, R.J. (2008). Clonogenic Multiple Myeloma Progenitors, Stem Cell Properties, and Drug Resistance. *Cancer Research*, Vol.68, No.1, (January 2008), pp. 190-197, ISSN 0008-5472

Mellstedt, H., Holm, G. & Björkholm, M. (1984). Multiple Myeloma, Waldenström's Macroglobulinemia, and Benign Monoclonal Gammopathy; Characteristics of the B Cell Clone, Immunoregulatory Cell Populations and Clinical Implications. *Advances in Cancer Research*, Vol.41, No.00, (Frequency Annual, 1984), pp. 257-289, ISSN 0065-230X

Ozdemir, F., Esen, N., Ovali, E., Tekelioglu, Y., Yilmaz, M., Aydin, F., Kavgaci, H. & Boruban, C. (2004). Effects of Dexamethasone, All-Trans Retinoic Acid, Vitamin D_3 and Interferon-α on FO Myeloma Cells. *Chemotherapy*, Vol.50, No.4 (September 2004), pp. 190-193, ISSN 0009-3157

Plesničar, A., Vidmar, G., Štabuc, B. & Kores Plesničar, B. (2009). Effects of Native Human Leukocyte Interferon-α on P3-X63-Ag8.653 Mouse Myeloma Cell Growth. *The Journal of International Medical Research*, Vol.37, No.5 (September/October 2009), pp. 1570-1576, ISSN 0300-0605

Puthier, D., Thabard, W., Rapp, M., Etrillard, M., Harosseau, J., Bataille, R. & Amiot, M. (2001). Interferon Alpha Extends the Survival of Human Myeloma Cells Through an Upregulation of the Mcl-1 Anti-Apoptotic Molecule. *British Journal of Haematology*, Vol.112, No.2, (February 2001), pp. 358-363, ISSN 1365-2141

Raman, D., Baugher, P.J., Thu, Y.M. & Richmond, A. (2007). Role of Chemokines in Tumor Growth. *Cancer Letters*, Vol.256, No.2, (July 2007), pp. 137-165, ISSN 0304-3835

Redzepovic, J., Weimann, G., Ott, I. & Gust, R. (2008). Current Trends in Multiple Myeloma Management. *The Journal of International Medical Research*, Vol.36, No.3, (May/June 2008), pp. 371-386, ISSN 0300-0605

Sawamura, M., Murayama, K., Ui, G., Matsushima, T., Tamura, J., Murakami, H., Naruse, T. & Tsuchiya, J. (1992). Plasma Cell Leukaemia with Alpha-Interferon Therapy in

Myeloma. *British Journal of Haematology*, Vol.82, No.3, (November 1992), pp. 631, ISSN 1365-2141

Silvestris, F., Cafforio, P., Calvani, N. & Dammaco, M. (2004). Impaired Osteoblastogenesis in Myeloma Bone Disease: Role of Upregulated Apoptosis by Cytokines and Malignant Plasma Cells. *British Journal of Haematology*, Vol.126, No.4, (August 2004), pp. 475-486, ISSN 1365-2141

Šantak, G., Šantak, M. & Forčić, D. (2007). Native Human IFN-α is a More Potent Suppressor of HDF Response to Profibrotic Stimuli Than Recombinant human IFN-α. *Journal of Interferon & Cytokine Research: the Official Journal of the International Society for Interferon and Cytokine Research*, Vol.27, No.6, (June 2007), pp. 481-490, ISSN 1079-9907

Westendorf, J.J., Ahmann G.J., Greipp, J.R., Witzig, T.E., Lust, J.A. & Jelinek, D.F. (1996). Establishment and Characterization of Three Myeloma Cell Lines That Demonstrate Variable Cytokine Responses and Abilities to Produce Autocrine Interleukin-6. *Leukemia*, Vol. 10, No.5, (May 1996), pp. 866-876, ISSN 0887-6924

Wilson, A.P. (1994). Cytotoxicity and Viability Assays. In: *Animal Cell Culture. A Practical Approach, 2nd edn*. Freshney RI Editor, pp. 263-303, Oxford University Press, ISBN 0 19 963212 X (Hbk), Oxford

Yasui, H., Hideshima, T., Richardson P.G. & Anderson, K.C. (2006). Novel Therapeutic Strategies Targeting Growth Factor Signaling Cascades in Multiple Myeloma. *British Journal of Haematology*, Vol.132, No.4, (February 2006), pp. 385-397, ISSN 1365-2141

Zidovec, S. & Mažuran, R. (1999). Sendai Virus Induces Various Cytokines in Human Peripheral Blood Leukocytes: Different Susceptibility of Cytokine Molecules to Low pH. *Cytokine*, Vol.11, No.2, (February 1999), pp. 140–143, ISSN 1043-4666

4

Cellular Immunotherapy Using Dendritic Cells Against Multiple Myeloma

Je-Jung Lee[1,2,3], Youn-Kyung Lee[1,3] and Thanh-Nhan Nguyen-Pham[1,2]

[1]Research Center for Cancer Immunotherapy
[2]Department of Hematology-Oncology,
Chonnam National University Hwasun Hospital, Hwasun, Jeollanamdo,
[3]Vaxcell-Bio Therapeutics, Hwasun, Jeollanamdo,
Republic of Korea

1. Introduction

Multiple myeloma (MM) is a clonal B cell malignant disease that is characterized by the proliferation of plasma cells in the bone marrow (BM) in association with monoclonal protein in the serum and/or urine, immune paresis, skeletal destruction, renal dysfunction, anemia, hypercalcemia and lytic bone diseases (Kyle & Rajkumar, 2004; Sirohi & Powles, 2004). Although the introduction of conventional chemotherapy, high-dose therapy with hematopoietic stem cell transplantation (HSCT), and the development of novel molecular target agents has resulted in a marked improvement in overall survival, the disease still remains incurable (Attal & Harousseau, 2009; Lonial & Cavenagh, 2009). Alternative approaches are clearly needed to prolong the disease-free survival as well as the overall survival of patients with MM. To prolong the survival of patients with MM who are undergoing allogeneic HSCT, donor lymphocyte infusion can be used successfully as a salvage therapy, which is based on the graft-versus myeloma effect in some cases of MM that relapse after allogeneic HSCT (Harrison & Cook, 2005; Perez-Simon et al., 2003). This role of immune effector cells provides the framework for the development of immune-based therapeutic options that use antigen-presenting cells (APCs) with increased potency, such as dendritic cells (DCs), in MM (Harrison & Cook, 2005).

DCs are the most potent APCs for initiating cellular immune responses through the stimulation of naive T cells. Immature DCs are good at antigen uptake and processing, but for a stimulatory T cell response they must mature to become fully activated DCs, which express high levels of cell surface-related major histocompatibility complex (MHC)-antigen and costimulatory molecules. Because of their ability to stimulate T cells, DCs act as a link in antitumor immune responses between innate immunity and adaptive immunity (Banchereau & Steinman, 1998). These DCs play a central role in various immunotherapy protocols by generation of cytotoxic T lymphocytes (CTLs) (Reid, 2001). DC-based vaccines have become the most attractive tool for cancer immunotherapy and have been used in the treatment of more than 20 malignancies, most commonly melanoma, renal cell carcinoma, prostate cancer and colorectal carcinoma (Palucka et al., 2011; Ridgway, 2003). In MM, cellular immunotherapy using DCs is emerging as a useful immunotherapeutic modality to treat MM (Ridgway, 2003). Since tumor antigen-loaded DCs are expected to be able to stimulate tumor-specific CTLs and to overcome T cell tolerance in tumor patients, the development of DC vaccines that can consistently eliminate minimal residual neoplastic disease remains an important goal in the field of tumor immunology (Banchereau & Palucka, 2005).

2. Stream of DC research in MM

MM is believed to induce immunoparesis that interferes with DC function, which diminishes the effective antitumor immune responses in these patients. Usually, *ex vivo* DCs are generated from circulating blood precursors (i.e. monocytes) or bone marrow progenitor cells and are educated with tumor antigens prior to vaccination to patients. *Ex vivo* generated DCs can be loaded with myeloma-associated antigens as vaccines for patients with MM. The use of immature DCs or mature DCs, the way to induce DC maturation, types of tumor antigens, the techniques to load tumor antigens to DCs, routes of administration, dosing schedules are being investigated (Figdor et al., 2004; Nestle et al., 2001).

2.1 Idiotype and idiotype-pulsed DCs in MM

B cell malignancies are distinct from other types of cancer in that a tumor-specific antigen can be defined, namely the variable (V)-regions of the monoclonal immunoglobulin (Ig) that each B cell tumor clone produces. These V-region antigenic determinants are called idiotopes, and the sums of the idiotopes represent the idiotype (Id) of the monoclonal Ig. Id has distinct advantages as a tumor-specific antigen, which can be readily isolated from the plasma of MM patients (Hart & Hill, 1999). The Id protein has been used for immunotherapy both *in vitro* and *in vivo* in MM, and has demonstrated a successful response in follicular lymphoma and a unique expression of Id on the malignant B cell clone (Bergenbrant et al., 1996; Kwak et al., 1995). The first reported in 1971 demonstrated that Id is immunogenic in mice of the same inbred strain in which the myeloma cell originally developed (Sirisinha & Eisen, 1971). In addition, Id vaccination could induce both antibody and Id-specific T cells including $CD4^+$ T cell and $CD8^+$ T cell response by the presentation of Id protein on MHC class I and II of professional APCs. Id-specific $CD4^+$ T cells appeared to be more frequent than $CD8^+$ cells to response against Id protein. Id-specific CTL lines could be generated that killed autologous primary myeloma cells *in vitro*, and killing activity was induced by only MHC class I - restricted (Li et al., 2000), while in the other report both class I - and class II - restriction was observed (Wen et al., 2001). In MM, a number of studies using id vaccination in alone or in combination with cytokines and/or conjugate has been investigated. The Id protein was used as an autologous myeloma protein either alone (Bergenbrant et al., 1996) or combination with cytokine IL-2 with or without granulocyte-macrophage colony-stimulating factor (GM-CSF) (Hansson et al., 2007; Osterborg et al., 1998; Rasmussen et al., 2003) or conjugation with keyhole limpet hemocyanin (KLH) to vaccinate myeloma patients (Coscia et al., 2004; Massaia et al., 1999). In general, Id-specific responses were observed with variable frequency, in which T cell and B cell responses were detected *in vitro* following Id vaccination, but clinical responses were unsatisfactory and the long time response was not observed.

Autologous DCs that were generated from MM patients have been shown to efficiently endocytose different classes of Id protein, and autologous Id-specific CTLs lines containing both $CD4^+$ and $CD8^+$ T cells that were generated by Id-pulsed DCs significantly recognized and killed the autologous primary myeloma cells *in vitro* (Butch et al., 2001; Wen et al., 2001). Until now, the various studies of DC-based Id vaccination in MM have been reported (Bendandi et al., 2006; Lim & Bailey-Wood, 1999; Liso et al., 2000; Reichardt et al., 2003; Rollig et al., 2011; Titzer et al., 2000; Yi et al., 2002, 2010). Although Id-specific CTLs and immune response could be induced in some patients, clinical responses have been observed rarely in few patients after vaccination (Titzer et al., 2000). The Id-pulsed DC in combination with KLH (Liso et al., 2000; Yi et al., 2010), cytokine IL-2 (Yi et al., 2002) were used for vaccination in MM patients to improve the effectiveness of Id-pulsed DC vaccine. However, even both cellular and antibody responses have been observed, the clinical response also was not improvement following vaccinations. The reasons for these results may be attributed mainly to the Id protein as a weak antigen, and the use of immature DCs in some studies (Lim & Bailey-Wood, 1999; Osterborg et al., 1998; Wen et al., 1998).

2.2 Myeloma-associated antigens-based DC immunotherapy

Tumor-associated antigens (TAAs) have been identified in many tumor types including solid tumors and hematological malignancies. The highly specific TAAs such as the antigen that are present in one or only a few individuals and not found in normal cells for a particular tumor, or are only present in a number of related tumors from different patients or overexpress in increasing amounts in malignant cells were the greatest potential for clinically useful assays. Successful immunotherapy requires these sources of TAAs, which provide immune responses against the tumor cells or the cancer tissues that express the TAA on the tumors. A variety of myeloma-associated antigens have been identified in MM patients, which possibility provides an immune response by DC-based vaccine. Many potential TAAs in MM have been investigated including polymorphic epithelial mucin (MUC1), human telomerase reverse transcriptase (hTERT), PRAME, HM1.24, SP17, Wilms' tumor I (WTI), Dickkopf-1 (DKK1), heat shock protein (HSP) gp96 or member of cancer germ-like family (MAGE, GAGE, BAGE, LAGE, NY-ESO-1) (Batchu et al., 2005; Brossart et al., 2001; Hundemer et al., 2006; Lim et al., 2001; Qian et al., 2007; Szmania et al., 2006). T cells from myeloma patients can recognize a variety of TAAs, which suggesting that the T-cell has the capacity to kill myeloma cells selectively if these clonal populations can be activated and expanded effectively by a potent TAA. Among the various TAAs, some have been tested as peptide vaccines and only a few of them has been tested *in vitro* to induce TAA-specific CTLs response via loading the potent TAA to DCs in MM. The first TAAs pulsed with DCs in MM was MUC1, which was expressed on all of MM cell lines and primary myeloma cells and in sera of MM patients. Vaccination with MUC1 antigen has not been studied in MM patients, but MUC1-specific CTLs that were induced *in vitro* using peptide-pulsed DCs or plasma cell RNA-loaded DCs efficiently killed not only target cells pulsed with the antigenic peptide but also MM cells (Brossart et al., 2001; Milazzo et al., 2003). NY-ESO-1 is the most immunogenic of the cancer testis antigens, which are expressed in a variety of tumors, while their presence in normal tissue is limited to the testis and placenta (Szmania et al., 2006). In MM, expression of NY-ESO-1 has been correlated with more advanced disease (van Rhee et al., 2005). Spontaneous humoral and $CD8^+$ T cell-mediated responses to NY-ESO-1 have been identified in patients with advanced disease

(Szmania et al., 2006; van Rhee et al., 2005). Although the clinical trial using NY-ESO-1 with DCs has not been tested, the *in vitro* monocyte-derived DCs transduced with the PTD-NY-ESO-1 protein can induce $CD8^+$ cellular antitumor immunity superior to that achieved with NY-ESO-1 protein alone (Batchu et al., 2005). Sperm protein 17 (Sp17), the other immunogenic TAA, has been used as a tumor antigen to load into DCs. Sp17-specific HLA class I-restricted CTLs were successfully generated by DCs that have been loaded with a recombinant Sp17 protein and the CTLs were able to kill autologous tumor cells that expressed Sp17 (Chiriva-Internati et al., 2002). The over-expression of hTERT on MM compared to normal cells indicated that this telomerase could be used as tumor antigen to induce antitumor immune responses (Vonderheide et al., 1999). hTERT was capable of triggering antitumor CTL responses and kill $hTERT^+$ tumor cells (Vonderheide et al., 1999). Recently, the activated T lymphocytes that were stimulated by DCs loaded with hTERT- and MUC1-derived nonapeptides were successfully able to kill myeloma cell line (Ocadlikova et al., 2010). DKK1, a novel protein that is not expressed in most normal tissues but is expressed in almost myeloma cells, could be a potentially important antigenic target for antimyeloma immunotherapy (Qian et al., 2007). DKK1-specific CTLs that were generated by DCs pulsed with DKK1 peptides were specifically lysed autologous primary myeloma cells and DKK1-positive cell line (Qian et al., 2007). In general, TAAs could be a major interest in immunotherapy in MM. However, problems that should be solved before starting the clinical trials include defining whether a specific TAA is a suitable and safe for immunotherapy of patients with MM. One problem was that TAA susceptible of inducing autoimmunity provided that autoimmunity remains limited to some tissues or is controllable. The other problem was that some members such as Sp17 and MUC1 have been detected in normal tissues; therefore, it remains to be elucidated whether specific CTLs are able to recognize only myeloma cells. Furthermore, although the other TAA such as PRAME and Sp17 could be over-expressed on almost MM cell lines, only a small number of tumor samples from MM patients showed a similar level, limiting its usefulness as an isolated TAA in MM. To overcome the effect of TAAs-based immunotherapy, trials involving more than one TAA need to be designed. Taken together, the data support DC immunotherapy with TAAs as being a promising immunotherapy to support to clinical trials in MM.

2.3 Whole tumor antigen-based DC immunotherapy

An alternative to Id protein- or TAA-based immunotherapy in MM is to use other tumor antigens that derived from whole tumor preparation to improve the efficacy of the DC vaccination in patients with MM. Although a single TAA has the possibility to induce the antitumor immune responses against MM, tumors may escape immune recognition by down-regulating expression of a particular antigen. In contrast, DCs loaded with antigens derived from whole tumor cells can improve the antitumor response and that limits the risk for immunological escape. There have been increasing reports of these alternative approaches, such as DCs pulsed with myeloma lysates (Hayashi et al., 2003; Lee et al., 2007; Wen et al., 2002), DCs pulsed with myeloma apoptotic bodies (Nguyen-Pham et al., 2011; Yang et al., 2010; Yang et al., 2011), DCs transfected with myeloma-derived RNA (Milazzo et al., 2003), DCs pulsed with myeloma-derived HSP gp96 (Qian et al., 2005; Qian et al., 2009), or DC-myeloma cell hybrids (Gong et al., 2002; Hao et al., 2004; Vasir et al., 2005). These techniques have the advantage of allowing the presentation of multiple epitopes to MHC on DCs, therefore can induce polyclonal T cell response from many potentially unknown TAAs and reduce the probability of immune escape by single TAA. The first study reported that bone marrow mononuclear cells from the patients with MM contained more than 90% $CD138^+CD38^+$ myeloma plasma cells and CTLs that were generated by DCs loaded with myeloma cell lysates demonstrated much stronger cytotoxicity against autologous plasma cells than did those by Id protein-pulsed DCs, which suggested the superiority of the myeloma cell itself as a source of a tumor antigen compared with the Id protein (Wen et al., 2002). In other myeloma model, DCs pulsed with purified and optimized myeloma cell lysate were shown to generate CTLs that killed autologous tumor cells but not against mismatch HLA cell lines or K562 cell lines *in vitro* (Lee et al., 2007). The apoptotic bodies derived from either myeloma cell lines or patient's myeloma cells also have been used as tumor antigen to loading with DCs. Interestingly, apoptotic bodies were shown to be more effective than cell lysate at inducing CTLs against autologous myeloma cells (Hayashi et al., 2003). Heat shock proteins (HSPs) are a class of functionally related proteins whose expression is increased when cells are exposed to elevated temperatures or other stress. Tumor-derived HSPs, such as HSP70 and gp96, are immunogenic and potent in stimulating the generation of tumor-specific CTLs. Myeloma-derived gp96 has been obtained and used to pulse DCs to generate the specific CTLs in MM. The specific CTLs was able to lyse myeloma tumor cells but not normal blood cells in a MHC class I-restricted manner and provide a rationale for gp96-based immunotherapy in MM (Qian et al., 2005; Qian et al., 2009). In other way, a promising vaccine strategy in which the autologous DCs were fused with patient-derived tumor cells has been developed. DC fused with tumor can stimulate both helper and cytotoxic T cell responses through the presentation of internalized and newly synthesized antigens (Vasir et al., 2005). In mouse MM models, vaccination with DCs fused with either myeloma cells or tumor cells that were genetically modified to express CD40L resulted in eradication of disease in tumor-bearing animal and protective against subsequent tumor challenge in animals (Gong et al., 2002; Hao et al., 2004). Recently, a phase 1 study in which patients with MM underwent serial vaccination with the DC fused with MM cell fusions in conjunction with GM-CSF (Rosenblatt et al., 2011) resulted in the expansion of circulating $CD4^+$ and $CD8^+$ lymphocytes reactive with autologous myeloma cells in 11 of 15 MM patients and a majority of patients with advanced disease demonstrated disease stabilization. In general, the production of DC vaccine by using whole tumor antigens has become promising in order to induce immunotherapy against MM.

3. Innovative researches in the field of DC vaccination

3.1 Immune disorder in MM

Usually, hematologic malignancies elicit measurable, albeit weak, immunogenic responses that are generally unable to mediate tumor destruction. They are able to escape immune surveillance by down-regulation of immune markers such as costimulatory molecules and MHC class I and II molecules as well as through the production of immunosuppressive cytokines by the tumor cells or by activation of suppressor cells such as regulatory T cells (Treg) and myeloid-derived suppressor cells (MDSCs) (Kim et al., 2007). In particularly, MM induces immune paresis (Quach et al., 2010). Patients with MM have basically dysfunctional DCs that are functionally defective, evidenced by the decreased number of circulating precursors of DCs as well as impaired T cell stimulatory capacity (Brown et al., 2001; Ratta et al., 2002; Tucci et al., 2011). DCs in MM patients are a target of tumor-associated suppressive factors, such as interleukin (IL)-10, transforming growth factor beta (TGF-β), vascular endothelial growth factor (VEGF), and IL-6, resulting in their aberrant functions and impaired development of effector functions in tumor-specific lymphocytes (Brown et al., 2001; Ratta et al., 2002). In addition, the survival and proliferation of tumor cells is partially facilitated by the impaired endogenous immune surveillance against tumor antigens (Zou, 2005). Myeloma cells can produce immunoinhibitory cytokines, such as TGF-β, IL-10, IL-6 and VEGF, which play major roles in the pathogenesis of MM (Brown et al., 2001; Ratta et al., 2002). These tumor-derived factors can also modulate anti-tumor host immune responses, including the abrogation of DC function, by constitutive activation of the signal transducer and activator of transcription 3 (STAT3) (Yu et al., 2007). Impairment in both humoral and cellular immunity in MM is associated with impaired B cell differentiation and antibody responses (Brown et al., 2001), reduced T cell numbers specifically $CD4^+$ T cells and abnormal Th1/Th2 $CD4^+$ T cell ratio (Ogawara et al., 2005), impaired CTL responses (Maecker et al., 2003), and dysfunction of NK cells (Jarahian et al., 2007) and NKT cells (Dhodapkar et al., 2003). In addition, dysregulation of natural $CD4^+CD25^+$T regulatory (Treg) has been reported (Prabhala et al., 2006). Tregs are a group of immuno-suppressive T cells that have been implicated in the suppression of tumor immunity (Curiel, 2007). A higher number of Tregs were reported in myeloma capable of suppressive activity at T cell stimulation (Beyer et al., 2006). Recently, a human study reported that the proportion of $CD4^+FOXP3^+$ Treg cells was increased in MM patients at diagnosis and Treg cells from patients with MM were functionally intact as they were able to inhibit proliferation of both CD4 and CD8 T cells (Brimnes et al., 2010). More recently, the discovery of myeloid-derived suppressor cells (MDSCs) revealed these cells as potent suppressors of tumor immunity and, therefore, a significant impediment to cancer immunotherapy (Ostrand-Rosenberg & Sinha, 2009). MDSCs are a heterogeneous population of cells of myeloid origin, which are present and accumulate in most cancer patients and experimental animals with cancer, and which are considered as a major contributor to the profound immune dysfunction of most patients with sizable tumor burdens (Ostrand-Rosenberg & Sinha, 2009). MDSC levels in cancer patients are driven by tumor burden and by the diversity of factors produced by the tumor and by host cells in the tumor microenvironment (Gabrilovich & Nagaraj, 2009). MDSCs suppress antitumor immunity through a variety of diverse mechanisms (Gabrilovich & Nagaraj, 2009). MDSCs can suppress the activation of T cells, B cells, natural killer (NK) cells and NKT cells. In contrast, MDSCs can enhance the induction of Tregs. Antigen presentation is also limited by the expansion of MDSC at the expense of DCs. Recently, an increase in the proportion of $CD14^+HLA\text{-}DR^{-/low}$ MDSC in patients with MM at diagnosis was described, illustrating that this cell fraction is also distorted in patients with MM (Brimnes et al., 2010). Taken together, the immune paresis in patients with MM suggested that DC-based vaccine therapies in MM need to be boosted with other alternative approaches or potent DCs may be needed to increase the effectiveness of vaccination.

3.2 Key points to improve DC vaccination in MM

For improving clinical outcomes using DC-based immunotherapy, there have been increasing reports of alternative approaches, such as better cytokine combinations to enhance DC function, effective tumor antigens to induce specific CTLs, or modifying signal transcriptions to overcome defective DC function. Our experience in the DC research field has revealed several key points to improve DC vaccination in cancer patients (Fig. 1).

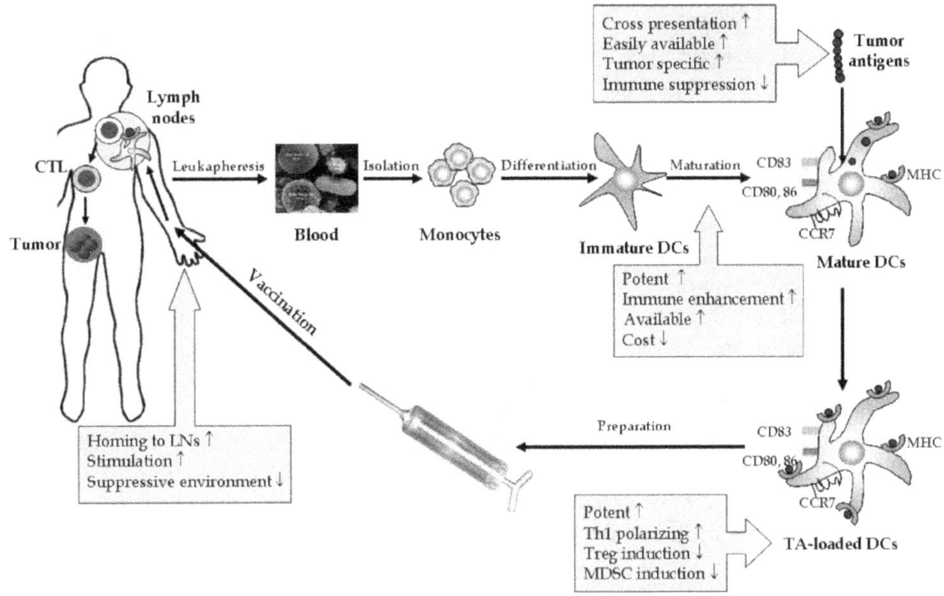

Fig. 1. **Key points to improve DC vaccination in cancer patients.** Abbreviations: CTL, cytotoxic T lymphocyte; DCs, dendritic cells; TA, tumor antigen; LNs, lymph nodes; Treg, regulatory T cell; MDSC, myeloid-derived suppressor cell.

As described above, the results of immunotherapy with Id-pulsed DCs have been unsatisfying. An alternative to Id protein is to use other tumor antigens that improve the efficacy of the DC vaccination in patients with MM. The selected antigen should possess the best characteristics to induce high cross presentation, be tumor specific, be easily available, but be unable to induce immune suppression. Whole tumor antigens is the best tumor antigen, which has been selected by many investigators including myeloma cell lysates (Kortylewski et al., 2005; Lee et al., 2007; Nefedova et al., 2005; Nefedova & Gabrilovich, 2007; Wang et al., 2006; Wang et al., 2006), apoptotic bodies from myeloma cell line (Lee et al., 2007; Nguyen-Pham et al., 2011; Yang et al., 2010), and apoptotic allogeneic myeloma cells from other patients with matched subtype (Yang et al., 2011). In practical terms, there are a number of patients with MM, who have less than 50% of myeloma cells in the bone marrow at the time of diagnosis or during progression of the disease. When mononuclear cells from the bone marrow are used as a source of tumor antigens, there is the potential of contamination with normal cells, especially lymphocytes. Thus, it is necessary to use purified and optimized myeloma cells, if possible, as a source of tumor antigen for the generation of myeloma-specific CTLs stimulated by DCs (Lee et al., 2007). We have shown that the function of the DCs was affected by the concentration of myeloma cell lysates (i.e., higher concentrations of lysates suppress T cell stimulatory capacities more than lower concentration of lysates). Also, the optimization of the lysate concentration did not demonstrate any inferiority in functions, such as T cell stimulatory capacities and cytotoxicities, of the DCs compared with other antigens, such as apoptotic bodies of myeloma cells or formalin-fixed myeloma cells. CTLs that were generated by purified and optimized myeloma cell lysates pulsed with DCs demonstrated much stronger cytotoxicity against autologous plasma cells. These findings indicate that it is important to optimize the concentration of myeloma cell lysates that were loaded onto DCs to potentiate their function.

The use of whole tumor cells, instead of single antigens, may help to enhance antitumor effects but target multiple tumor variants and counteract tumor immune evasion. However, it is impractical to obtain sufficient amounts of purified autologous myeloma cells for tumor antigens in the clinical setting of patients with MM. As an alternative source of tumor-relevant antigens, allogeneic tumor cells or established cancer cell lines have been used to overcome this limitation in various tumors (Koido et al., 2005; Lee et al., 2007; Palucka et al., 2006; Yang et al., 2010). Allogeneic myeloma cell lines used as universal tumor antigens could substitute for an original tumor cell collection and make the culture of tumor cells easier. In clinical practice, allogeneic myeloma cell lines might be an effective source of universal tumor antigen that could be used to load DCs for the generation of myeloma-specific CTLs in MM patients. Tumor antigens that derived from irradiated allogeneic myeloma cell line when loaded with DCs could generate myeloma-specific CTLs against autologous myeloma cells in patients with MM (Nguyen-Pham et al., 2011; Yang et al., 2010). These findings suggest that allogeneic myeloma cell lines are potent immunogens capable of inducing functional CTLs against patients' own tumor cells. The success of using an allogeneic myeloma cell line as tumor antigen led to the possibility that allogeneic myeloma cells could be also used as a viable source of tumor antigen in the context of appropriate major MHC alleles to autologous CTLs. We investigated the possibility of DC therapy using autologous DC loaded with apoptotic allogeneic myeloma cells from the matched monoclonal subtype of myeloma patients and showed that the CTL generated by these tumor antigens loaded-DCs could generate myeloma-specific CTLs against autologous myeloma cells in patients with MM (Yang et al., 2011). These findings suggested that the allogeneic matching monoclonal immunoglobulin subtype of myeloma is an effective tumor antigen capable of inducing functional CTLs against patients' own tumor cells.

The suppressive effects of tumor cells during DC generation have been explained previously by the ability of the tumor microenvironment to suppress DC differentiation (Savill et al., 2002; Yu et al., 2007). The suppression is due to the activation of STAT3 and the production of immunosuppressive factors, such as VEGF, IL-10, and IL-6. These factors can influence STAT3 and extracellular signal-regulated kinase (ERK) phosphorylation, resulting in hyperactivation of STAT3 and ERK, which may be responsible for defective DC differentiation (Kitamura et al., 2005; Yu et al., 2007). In addition to generation of potent and specific tumor antigen-loaded DCs for vaccination, alternative methods have attempted to restore defective DC function and to enhance DC function in MM. Enhanced immune-mediated antitumor effects of DCs have been reported following the inhibition of the janus-activated kinase 2 (JAK2)/STAT3 pathway (Nefedova et al., 2005), inhibition of p38 or activation of the MEK/ERK or mitogen-activated protein kinase (MAPK) pathways, and neutralizion of IL-6 (Wang et al., 2006). Recently, we reported that the inhibitory factors and abnormal signaling pathways of DCs during maturation with tumor antigen might be responsible for the defective activity of DCs in MM, and suggested that the way to overcome these abnormalities is by neutralizing the signaling that would lead to a suppressed immune response (Yang et al., 2009). More recently, we are developing of the strategies that recovering dysfunction of DCs caused from loading tumor antigen through the treatment of a combination of the selective JAK/STAT3 signaling pathway inhibitor (JSI-124) and the proteasome inhibitor (Bortezomib) onto myeloma cells (Lee et al., 2011). We reported that pretreatment of myeloma cells with combination of JSI-124 and bortezomib can recover DC dysfunction from loading the dying myeloma cells through the up-regulation of Hsp90 and the down-regulation of STAT3 phosphorylation and inhibitory cytokines production, and these DCs can generate to potent myeloma-specific CTLs.

For effective induction of tumor-specific immune responses in the field of DC vaccination, the DCs should have potency to stimulate T cells, to produce high levels of Th1 polarized cytokines (IL-12p70), to trigger Th1 polarizing capacity, and to migrate through lymphatic vessels to interact with T cells. Therefore, the strategy to generate the fully functional and potential DCs has been developed. The initial success of the therapeutic vaccines involving immature or partially-mature " first-generation" DCs has been reported (Hsu et al., 1996). However, such DCs express suboptimal levels of co-stimulatory molecules, and constitute a weaker immunogen than the subsequently-implemented mature DCs, constituting the "second generation" of clinically-applied DCs (sDCs). sDC vaccines induced by the IL-1β/TNF-α/IL-6/prostaglandin E_2 (PGE_2) cytokine cocktail have been developed (Jonuleit et al., 1997). Such DCs are fully-mature DCs with high expression of co-stimulatory molecules, high expression of CCR7, and high migratory responsiveness to LN-associated chemokines; they have been widely tested in clinical trials. However, to date, the sDC vaccines have limitations that include the mediation of Th2 polarization, promotion of DC secretion of the immunosuppressive cytokine IL-10, inability to induce effectively the Th1-type response (because PGE_2 abolishes the secretion of IL-12p70), and high activity of such DCs in activating Treg cells (Banerjee et al., 2006; Kalinski et al., 1997, 2001; Yamazaki et al., 2006). Several investigators, including our group, have tried to develop the potent DCs for inducing effective tumor-specific immune responses. In an attempt to increase DC potency using cytokine combinations, α-type-1-polarized DCs (αDC1s) that are induced to mature using the αDC1-inducing cytokine cocktail IL-1β, TNF-α, IFN-α, IFN-γ, and polyinosinic:polycytidylic acid [poly(I:C)]) has been developed to generate strong functional CTLs in several diseases, on average 20-fold higher compared to sDCs (Lee et al., 2008; Mailliard et al., 2004). Recently, we successfully generated αDC1s from a patient with MM with high expression of costimulatory molecules, significant production of IL-12p70, and potent generation of myeloma specific CTLs (Yang et al., 2010, 2011). The potential of polarized αDC1s to produce IL-12 has important implications for the use of DCs as cancer vaccines.

The other strategy to induce potent DCs from patients with MM was the use of a "helper" cell to promote type 1 polarization of DCs. DCs and NK cells reciprocally activate each other during the immune response. Recent data from our and other groups demonstrate that such NK-DC interaction promotes the subsequent induction of tumor-specific responses of $CD4^+$ and $CD8^+$ T cells, allowing NK cells to act as "helper" cells in the development of the type 1 DCs in responses against cancer (Mailliard et al., 2003; Nguyen-Pham et al., 2010, 2011). Resting NK cells that are activated in the presence of TLR agonist, IL-2, and IFN-α can induce DCs from patients with MM maturation and enhance IL-12p70 production *in vitro*. These potent DCs can be developed to generate strong functional CTLs against myeloma cells compared to sDCs (Nguyen-Pham et al., 2011).

Therapeutic DC vaccines against cancer not only need to be highly effective in inducing the expansion of tumor-specific T cells, but they also need to avoid interaction and induction of Tregs. Recently, the type 1-polarized DCs were demonstrated to suppress the secretion of CCL22 (Treg and Th2 type attracting chemokines), enhance the secretion of CCL5 and CXCL10 (Th1 and effector T cell-attracting chemokines), and suppress the induction of Tregs compared to sDCs or PGE_2-matured DCs (Muthuswamy et al., 2008). DCs generated *in vitro* for vaccination protocols that can target a local lymph node are highly sought, but difficult to achieve in practice. Type 1-polarized DCs, with higher levels of IL-12p70 and potent CTL generation targeting, are, however, limited by their migratory capacity to primary lymph organs due to the relatively lower expression of CCR7 compared to sDCs. We recently reported on the nature of the enhancement of the migratory phenotype of DCs. The first important mediator in the mobilization of DCs to lymph nodes is CCR7. However, upregulation of CCR7 alone by DCs is insufficient to drive DC migration toward CCL19 and CCL21. Up-regulation of CD38 and down-regulation of CD74 regulate DC migration *in vitro* and *in vivo* (Faure-Andre et al., 2008; Frasca et al., 2006). By regulating CD38, CD74, and CCR7 expression on DCs, type I and II IFNs have synergistic effects in the presence of TLR agonists on the regulation of DC migration and may provide a novel approach to improving vaccination efficacy (Nguyen-Pham et al., 2011).

Finally, to enhance the antitumor effectiveness of DC-based vaccines in preclinical *in vivo* mouse models, we have developed several models of combination therapy of DCs with an immunomodulatory drugs, such as cyclophosphamide or lenalidomide. Cyclophosphamide is frequently used to enhance or augment the antitumor effects in cancer immunotherapy (Ghiringhelli et al., 2004; Mihalyo et al., 2004). The possible effect of cyclophosphamide to enhance the antitumor efficacy of DC vaccine may be due to the increasing proportion of IFN-γ secreting lymphocytes in combination with the suppressing proportion of $CD4^+CD25^+FoxP3^+$ Treg cells in tumor-bearing mice (Liu et al., 2007). The result of a clinical trial using allogeneic DC vaccine combined with low-dose cyclophosphamide has revealed that the combination therapy could induce stronger antitumor response compared with DC vaccine alone (Holtl et al., 2005). Recently, we developed a combination therapy in mouse cancer model which showed that a single administration of low-dose cyclophosphamide before the first DC vaccination augmented the antitumor effects of DC vaccine to eradicate tumor completely and consequently prolonged the survival of vaccinated mice (Pham et al., 2010). We are now developing a clinical trial in MM patients using this combination therapy.

4. DC-based vaccine in published clinical trials

Clinical trials of DC-based vaccine for MM have been restricted until now. The trial protocol and responses are summarized in Table 1. Almost of the clinical trials were related with using Id-pulsed DC alone or in combination with adjuvant such as cytokines or KLH. In the decade after the first DC-based Id vaccination was started at Stanford University, the results of clinical trials were limited. In general, the majority of clinical trials conducted using Id-pulsed DCs showed immune responses. However, the clinical responses were unsatisfactory, mainly due to the poor immunogenicity of the Id protein. More recent results demonstrated improved clinical response by DC-based Id vaccination (Rollig et al., 2010; Yi et al., 2010). Therefore, DC-based Id vaccination is a possible way to induce the specific T cell responses in myeloma patients. Further trials with increasing numbers of patients are needed to increase the rate of responses.

Most recently, a phase I study was undertaken, in which patients with MM were vaccinated with an autologous DC/tumor cell fusion in combination with GM-CSF administration on the day of DC vaccination (Rosenblatt et al., 2011). Vaccine generation was successful in 17 of the 18 patients. The expansion of circulating $CD4^+$ and $CD8^+$ T cells reactive with autologous myeloma cells in 11 of 15 evaluable patients were detected. A majority of patients (11 of 16) with advanced disease demonstrated disease stabilization, with three patients showing ongoing stable disease at 12, 25, and 41 months. Interestingly, antibody response against some TAAs, such as regulators of G-protein signaling 19 (RGS19), HSP90, BRCA1-associated protein (BRAP) was also detected. So, vaccination with DC/MM fusions was feasible and may provide a new source of DC-based vaccines for the development of immunotherapy against MM.

A commercial product is currently being tested in a phase III trial (Mylovenge™, Dendreon Corp, Seattle, WA, USA). Mylovenge (APC8020) is conducted by pulsing autologous DCs with the patient's Id. A recent report of this commercial product showed that the long-term survival of those receiving the vaccine compared to all other patients with MM who underwent autologous HSCT (Lacy et al., 2009). This approach needs further testing in a phase III trial to confirm the clinical response and define the role of this DC vaccine in MM. We are also conducting a phase I/II clinical trial using type 1-polarized DCs loading with tumor antigens derived either from allogeneic myeloma cell line or patient's autologous-/allogeneic- myeloma cells in combination with chemotherapy in patients with MM after autologous HSCT.

5. Future perspectives

Despite their relative limitations, the data from recent clinical studies have suggested that DC-based vaccine may be a potential therapy in inducing the rate of tumor responses and prolonging the survival of patients with MM. In an attempt to increase DC-based potency and improve immune responses following vaccination, further investigations of additional tools to identify the alternative tumor antigens uniquely or specifically expressed on myeloma cells are needed, to recover or restore the dysfunction of DCs in MM patients, to induce T cells with the desirable effector functions rather than regulatory functions, to migrate into lymph nodes to stimulate T cells, and to clarify the ability of tumor specific CTLs to recognize and kill tumor cells. In our expectation, type 1-polarized DCs can be developed to generate strong functional CTLs. The allogeneic myeloma cell lines or allogeneic myeloma cells might be an effective source of universal tumor antigen that could be used to load to the DC1s for the successful generation of myeloma-specific CTLs. Eventually, the combination therapy, in which a DC vaccine is combined with either alternative therapy including chemotherapy, radiation therapy, molecular target therapy or other immunotherapy (adoptive therapy, NK cells therapy) or with adjuvant, will provide vigorous and maintained immune responses with the benefit clinical efficacy.

Author	DC type	TA	Adjuvant	Immune responses	Clinical responses
Liso et al.	imDC	Id	± KLH	4/24 Id-specific	17/26 SD
Lim et al.	imMo-DC	Id	KLH	5/6 Id-specific; 2/6 Id-specific IFN-γ; 3/6 increase in Id-specific CTL frequency	6/6 PD
Reichardt et al.	imDC	Id	none	2/12 Id-specific proliferation; 1/3 Id-specific CTL	2 relapse; 8/10 PD; 2/10 SD
Titzer et al.	CD34-DC	Id	none	4/10 Id-specific T cell proliferation; 1/10 decreased BM plasmacytosis	1/10 SD; 9/10 PD
Cull et al.	imMo-DC	Id	none	2/2 Id-specific T cell proliferation; no Id-specific CTL response	2/2 PD
Yi et al.	mMo-DC	Id	Il-2	2/5 Id-specific T cell proliferation; 5/5 Id-specific B cell proliferation; 4/5 Id-specific IFN-γ	1/3 PR; 3/5 SD; 1/5 PD
Bendandi et al.	mMo-DC	Id	none	4/4 anti-KLH response; 2/4 Th1 cytokines response	1/4 SD; 3/4 PD
Lacy et al.	APC8020 (Mylovenge)	Id	none	None reported	6/26 CR; 2/26 PR; 19/27 SD Overall survival: 5.3 years of follow-up for alive patients
Lacy et al.	CD40 L-DCs	Id	KLH	9/9 Id-specific IFN-γ; 5/9 Id-specific CTL response; 8/9 anti-KLH response	6/9 SD; 3/9 slowly PD 4/6 continue SD after 5 years
Rosenblatt et al.	DC/tumor fusion		GM-CSF	11/15 CD4 and CD8 response with autologous myeloma cells; 5/5 tested anti-MUC1 response	11/16 SD (3/11 > 1 years SD; 8/11 2.5-5 months SD)
Rollig et al.	mMo-DC	Id	KLH	5/9 Id-specific T cell proliferation; 8/9 Id-specific cytokines response;	3/9 M protein decrease; 5/9 M protein stable

Table 1. **Summary of Clinical trials of DC-based vaccine for MM.** Abbreviations: DC, dendritic cell; TA, tumor antigen; imDC, immature DC; Mo-DC, monocyte-derived DC; Id, idiotype; mMo-DC, mature Mo-DC; KLH, keyhole limpet hemocyanin; CTL, cytotoxic T lymphocyte; PD, progressive disease; PR, partial response; SD, stable disease; CR, complete response

6. Acknowledgements

This study was financially supported by grant no. 2011-0005285 from General Researcher Program Type II of the National Research Foundation of Korea; grant no. RTI05-01-01 from the Regional Technology Innovation Program of the Ministry of Commerce, Industry and Energy; grant no. A000200058 from the Regional Industrial Technology Development program of the Ministry of Knowledge and Economy; grant no. 1120390 from the National R&D Program for Cancer Control, Ministry for Health and Welfare; grant no. 2011-0030034 from Leading Foreign Research Institute Recruitment Program through the National Research Foundation of Korea (NRF) funded by the Ministry of Education, Science and Technology (MEST), Republic of Korea.

7. References

Attal M, Harousseau JL. (2009). The role of high-dose therapy with autologous stem cell support in the era of novel agents. *Semin Hematol,* 46(2), 127-132

Banchereau J, Steinman RM. (1998). Dendritic cells and the control of immunity. *Nature,* 392(6673), 245-252

Banchereau J, Palucka AK. (2005). Dendritic cells as therapeutic vaccines against cancer. Nat Rev Immunol, 5(4), 296-306

Banerjee DK, Dhodapkar MV, Matayeva E, et al. (2006). Expansion of FOXP3high regulatory T cells by human dendritic cells (DCs) in vitro and after injection of cytokine-matured DCs in myeloma patients. *Blood,* 108(8), 2655-2661

Batchu RB, Moreno AM, Szmania SM, et al. (2005). Protein transduction of dendritic cells for NY-ESO-1-based immunotherapy of myeloma. *Cancer Res,* 65(21), 10041-10049

Bendandi M, Rodriguez-Calvillo M, Inoges S, et al. (2006). Combined vaccination with idiotype-pulsed allogeneic dendritic cells and soluble protein idiotype for multiple myeloma patients relapsing after reduced-intensity conditioning allogeneic stem cell transplantation. *Leuk Lymphoma,* 47(1), 29-37

Bergenbrant S, Yi Q, Osterborg A, et al. (1996). Modulation of anti-idiotypic immune response by immunization with the autologous M-component protein in multiple myeloma patients. *Br J Haematol,* 92(4), 840-846

Beyer M, Kochanek M, Giese T, et al. (2006). In vivo peripheral expansion of naive CD4+CD25high FoxP3+ regulatory T cells in patients with multiple myeloma. *Blood,* 107(10), 3940-3949

Brimnes MK, Vangsted AJ, Knudsen LM, et al. (2010). Increased level of both CD4+FOXP3+ regulatory T cells and CD14+HLA-DR/low myeloid-derived suppressor cells and decreased level of dendritic cells in patients with multiple myeloma. *Scand J Immunol,* 72(6), 540-547

Brossart P, Schneider A, Dill P, et al. (2001). The epithelial tumor antigen MUC1 is expressed in hematological malignancies and is recognized by MUC1-specific cytotoxic T-lymphocytes. *Cancer Res,* 61(18), 6846-6850

Brown RD, Pope B, Murray A, et al. (2001). Dendritic cells from patients with myeloma are numerically normal but functionally defective as they fail to up-regulate CD80 (B7-1) expression after huCD40LT stimulation because of inhibition by transforming growth factor-beta1 and interleukin-10. *Blood,* 98(10), 2992-2998

Butch AW, Kelly KA, Munshi NC. (2001). Dendritic cells derived from multiple myeloma patients efficiently internalize different classes of myeloma protein. *Exp Hematol,* 29(1), 85-92

Chiriva-Internati M, Wang Z, Salati E, et al. (2002). Sperm protein 17 (Sp17) is a suitable target for immunotherapy of multiple myeloma. *Blood,* 100(3), 961-965

Coscia M, Mariani S, Battaglio S, et al. (2004). Long-term follow-up of idiotype vaccination in human myeloma as a maintenance therapy after high-dose chemotherapy. *Leukemia,* 18(1), 139-145

Curiel TJ. (2007). Tregs and rethinking cancer immunotherapy. *J Clin Invest,* 117(5), 1167-1174

Dhodapkar MV, Geller MD, Chang DH, et al. (2003). A reversible defect in natural killer T cell function characterizes the progression of premalignant to malignant multiple myeloma. *J Exp Med,* 197(12), 1667-1676

Faure-Andre G, Vargas P, Yuseff MI, et al. (2008). Regulation of dendritic cell migration by CD74, the MHC class II-associated invariant chain. *Science,* 322(5908), 1705-1710

Figdor CG, de Vries IJ, Lesterhuis WJ, et al. (2004). Dendritic cell immunotherapy: mapping the way. *Nat Med,* 10(5), 475-480

Frasca L, Fedele G, Deaglio S, et al. (2006). CD38 orchestrates migration, survival, and Th1 immune response of human mature dendritic cells. *Blood,* 107(6), 2392-2399

Gabrilovich DI, Nagaraj S. (2009). Myeloid-derived suppressor cells as regulators of the immune system. *Nat Rev Immunol,* 9(3), 162-174

Ghiringhelli F, Larmonier N, Schmitt E, et al. (2004). CD4+CD25+ regulatory T cells suppress tumor immunity but are sensitive to cyclophosphamide which allows immunotherapy of established tumors to be curative. *Eur J Immunol,* 34(2), 336-344

Gong J, Koido S, Chen D, et al. (2002). Immunization against murine multiple myeloma with fusions of dendritic and plasmacytoma cells is potentiated by interleukin 12. *Blood,* 99(7), 2512-2517

Hansson L, Abdalla AO, Moshfegh A, et al. (2007). Long-term idiotype vaccination combined with interleukin-12 (IL-12), or IL-12 and granulocyte macrophage colony-stimulating factor, in early-stage multiple myeloma patients. *Clin Cancer Res,* 13(5), 1503-1510

Hao S, Bi X, Xu S, et al. (2004). Enhanced antitumor immunity derived from a novel vaccine of fusion hybrid between dendritic and engineered myeloma cells. *Exp Oncol,* 26(4), 300-306

Harrison SJ, Cook G. (2005). Immunotherapy in multiple myeloma--possibility or probability? *Br J Haematol,* 130(3), 344-362

Hart DN, Hill GR. (1999). Dendritic cell immunotherapy for cancer: application to low-grade lymphoma and multiple myeloma. *Immunol Cell Biol,* 77(5), 451-459

Hayashi T, Hideshima T, Akiyama M, et al. (2003). Ex vivo induction of multiple myeloma-specific cytotoxic T lymphocytes. *Blood,* 102(4), 1435-1442

Holtl L, Ramoner R, Zelle-Rieser C, et al. (2005). Allogeneic dendritic cell vaccination against metastatic renal cell carcinoma with or without cyclophosphamide. *Cancer Immunol Immunother,* 54(7), 663-670

Hsu FJ, Benike C, Fagnoni F, et al. (1996). Vaccination of patients with B-cell lymphoma using autologous antigen-pulsed dendritic cells. *Nat Med,* 2(1), 52-58

Hundemer M, Schmidt S, Condomines M, et al. (2006). Identification of a new HLA-A2-restricted T-cell epitope within HM1.24 as immunotherapy target for multiple myeloma. *Exp Hematol,* 34(4), 486-496

Jarahian M, Watzl C, Issa Y, et al. (2007). Blockade of natural killer cell-mediated lysis by NCAM140 expressed on tumor cells. *Int J Cancer,* 120(12), 2625-2634

Jonuleit H, Kuhn U, Muller G, et al. (1997). Pro-inflammatory cytokines and prostaglandins induce maturation of potent immunostimulatory dendritic cells under fetal calf serum-free conditions. *Eur J Immunol,* 27(12), 3135-3142

Kalinski P, Hilkens CM, Snijders A, et al. (1997). IL-12-deficient dendritic cells, generated in the presence of prostaglandin E2, promote type 2 cytokine production in maturing human naive T helper cells. *J Immunol,* 159(1), 28-35

Kalinski P, Vieira PL, Schuitemaker JH, et al. (2001). Prostaglandin E(2) is a selective inducer of interleukin-12 p40 (IL-12p40) production and an inhibitor of bioactive IL-12p70 heterodimer. *Blood,* 97(11), 3466-3469

Kim R, Emi M, Tanabe K. (2007). Cancer immunoediting from immune surveillance to immune escape. *Immunology,* 121(1), 1-14

Kitamura H, Kamon H, Sawa S, et al. (2005). IL-6-STAT3 controls intracellular MHC class II alphabeta dimer level through cathepsin S activity in dendritic cells. *Immunity,* 23(5), 491-502

Koido S, Hara E, Homma S, et al. (2005). Dendritic cells fused with allogeneic colorectal cancer cell line present multiple colorectal cancer-specific antigens and induce antitumor immunity against autologous tumor cells. *Clin Cancer Res,* 11(21), 7891-7900

Kortylewski M, Kujawski M, Wang T, et al. (2005). Inhibiting Stat3 signaling in the hematopoietic system elicits multicomponent antitumor immunity. *Nat Med,* 11(12), 1314-1321

Kwak LW, Taub DD, Duffey PL, et al. (1995). Transfer of myeloma idiotype-specific immunity from an actively immunised marrow donor. *Lancet,* 345(8956), 1016-1020

Kyle RA, Rajkumar SV. (2004). Multiple myeloma. *N Engl J Med,* 351(18), 1860-1873

Lacy MQ, Mandrekar S, Dispenzieri A, et al. (2009). Idiotype-pulsed antigen-presenting cells following autologous transplantation for multiple myeloma may be associated with prolonged survival. *Am J Hematol,* 84(12), 799-802

Lee JJ, Choi BH, Kang HK, et al. (2007). Induction of multiple myeloma-specific cytotoxic T lymphocyte stimulation by dendritic cell pulsing with purified and optimized myeloma cell lysates. *Leuk Lymphoma,* 48(10), 2022-2031

Lee JJ, Foon KA, Mailliard RB, et al. (2008). Type 1-polarized dendritic cells loaded with autologous tumor are a potent immunogen against chronic lymphocytic leukemia. *J Leukoc Biol,* 84(1), 319-325

Lee YK, Kim MH, Hong CI, et al. (2011). Dendritic cells loaded with pretreating myeloma cells with combination of JSI-124 and bortezomib can generate potent myeloma-specific cytotoxic T lymphocytes through recovering dysfunction of dendritic cells in myeloma. *Haematologica,* 96(Suppl 1), S52. *Proceeding of the 13th International Myeloma Workshop*, Paris, France, May 3-6, 2011

Li Y, Bendandi M, Deng Y, et al. (2000). Tumor-specific recognition of human myeloma cells by idiotype-induced CD8(+) T cells. *Blood,* 96(8), 2828-2833

Lim SH, Bailey-Wood R. (1999). Idiotypic protein-pulsed dendritic cell vaccination in multiple myeloma. *Int J Cancer,* 83(2), 215-222

Lim SH, Wang Z, Chiriva-Internati M, et al. (2001). Sperm protein 17 is a novel cancer-testis antigen in multiple myeloma. *Blood,* 97(5), 1508-1510

Liso A, Stockerl-Goldstein KE, Auffermann-Gretzinger S, et al. (2000). Idiotype vaccination using dendritic cells after autologous peripheral blood progenitor cell transplantation for multiple myeloma. *Biol Blood Marrow Transplant,* 6(6), 621-627

Liu JY, Wu Y, Zhang XS, et al. (2007). Single administration of low dose cyclophosphamide augments the antitumor effect of dendritic cell vaccine. *Cancer Immunol Immunother,* 56(10), 1597-1604

Lonial S, Cavenagh J. (2009). Emerging combination treatment strategies containing novel agents in newly diagnosed multiple myeloma. *Br J Haematol,* 145(6), 681-708

Maecker B, Anderson KS, von Bergwelt-Baildon MS, et al. (2003). Viral antigen-specific CD8+ T-cell responses are impaired in multiple myeloma. *Br J Haematol,* 121(6), 842-848

Mailliard RB, Son YI, Redlinger R, et al. (2003). Dendritic cells mediate NK cell help for Th1 and CTL responses: two-signal requirement for the induction of NK cell helper function. *J Immunol,* 171(5), 2366-2373

Mailliard RB, Wankowicz-Kalinska A, Cai Q, et al. (2004). alpha-type-1 polarized dendritic cells: a novel immunization tool with optimized CTL-inducing activity. *Cancer Res,* 64(17), 5934-5937

Massaia M, Borrione P, Battaglio S, et al. (1999). Idiotype vaccination in human myeloma: generation of tumor-specific immune responses after high-dose chemotherapy. *Blood,* 94(2), 673-683

Mihalyo MA, Doody AD, McAleer JP, et al. (2004). In vivo cyclophosphamide and IL-2 treatment impedes self-antigen-induced effector CD4 cell tolerization: implications for adoptive immunotherapy. *J Immunol,* 172(9), 5338-5345

Milazzo C, Reichardt VL, Muller MR, et al. (2003). Induction of myeloma-specific cytotoxic T cells using dendritic cells transfected with tumor-derived RNA. *Blood,* 101(3), 977-982

Muthuswamy R, Urban J, Lee JJ, et al. (2008). Ability of mature dendritic cells to interact with regulatory T cells is imprinted during maturation. *Cancer Res,* 68(14), 5972-5978

Nefedova Y, Nagaraj S, Rosenbauer A, et al. (2005). Regulation of dendritic cell differentiation and antitumor immune response in cancer by pharmacologic-selective inhibition of the janus-activated kinase 2/signal transducers and activators of transcription 3 pathway. *Cancer Res,* 65(20), 9525-9535

Nefedova Y, Gabrilovich DI. (2007). Targeting of Jak/STAT pathway in antigen presenting cells in cancer. *Curr Cancer Drug Targets,* 7(1), 71-77

Nestle FO, Banchereau J, Hart D. (2001). Dendritic cells: On the move from bench to bedside. *Nat Med,* 7(7), 761-765

Nguyen-Pham TN, Im CM, Thi Nguyen TA, et al. (2011). Induction of myeloma-specific cytotoxic T lymphocytes responses by natural killer cells stimulated-dendritic cells in patients with multiple myeloma. *Leuk Res,* 35(9): 1241-1247

Nguyen-Pham TN, Lim MS, Nguyen TA, et al. (2011). Type I and II interferons enhance dendritic cell maturation and migration capacity by regulating CD38 and CD74 that have synergistic effects with TLR agonists. *Cell Mol Immunol,* 8(4), 341-347

Ocadlikova D, Kryukov F, Mollova K, et al. (2010). Generation of myeloma-specific T cells using dendritic cells loaded with MUC1- and hTERT- drived nonapeptides or myeloma cell apoptotic bodies. *Neoplasma,* 57(5), 455-464

Ogawara H, Handa H, Yamazaki T, et al. (2005). High Th1/Th2 ratio in patients with multiple myeloma. *Leuk Res,* 29(2), 135-140

Osterborg A, Yi Q, Henriksson L, et al. (1998). Idiotype immunization combined with granulocyte-macrophage colony-stimulating factor in myeloma patients induced type I, major histocompatibility complex-restricted, CD8- and CD4-specific T-cell responses. *Blood,* 91(7), 2459-2466

Ostrand-Rosenberg S, Sinha P. (2009). Myeloid-derived suppressor cells: linking inflammation and cancer. *J Immunol,* 182(8), 4499-4506

Palucka AK, Ueno H, Connolly J, et al. (2006). Dendritic cells loaded with killed allogeneic melanoma cells can induce objective clinical responses and MART-1 specific CD8+ T-cell immunity. *J Immunother,* 29(5), 545-557

Palucka K, Ueno H, Banchereau J. (2011). Recent developments in cancer vaccines. *J Immunol,* 186(3), 1325-1331

Perez-Simon JA, Martino R, Alegre A, et al. (2003). Chronic but not acute graft-versus-host disease improves outcome in multiple myeloma patients after non-myeloablative allogeneic transplantation. *Br J Haematol,* 121(1), 104-108

Pham TN, Hong CY, Min JJ, et al. (2010). Enhancement of antitumor effect using dendritic cells activated with natural killer cells in the presence of Toll-like receptor agonist. *Exp Mol Med,* 42(6), 407-419

Prabhala RH, Neri P, Bae JE, et al. (2006). Dysfunctional T regulatory cells in multiple myeloma. *Blood,* 107(1), 301-304

Qian J, Wang S, Yang J, et al. (2005). Targeting heat shock proteins for immunotherapy in multiple myeloma: generation of myeloma-specific CTLs using dendritic cells pulsed with tumor-derived gp96. *Clin Cancer Res,* 11(24 Pt 1), 8808-8815

Qian J, Xie J, Hong S, et al. (2007). Dickkopf-1 (DKK1) is a widely expressed and potent tumor-associated antigen in multiple myeloma. *Blood,* 110(5), 1587-1594

Qian J, Hong S, Wang S, et al. (2009). Myeloma cell line-derived, pooled heat shock proteins as a universal vaccine for immunotherapy of multiple myeloma. *Blood,* 114(18), 3880-3889

Quach H, Ritchie D, Stewart AK, et al. (2010). Mechanism of action of immunomodulatory drugs (IMiDS) in multiple myeloma. *Leukemia,* 24(1), 22-32

Rasmussen T, Hansson L, Osterborg A, et al. (2003). Idiotype vaccination in multiple myeloma induced a reduction of circulating clonal tumor B cells. *Blood,* 101(11), 4607-4610

Ratta M, Fagnoni F, Curti A, et al. (2002). Dendritic cells are functionally defective in multiple myeloma: the role of interleukin-6. *Blood,* 100(1), 230-237

Reichardt VL, Milazzo C, Brugger W, et al. (2003). Idiotype vaccination of multiple myeloma patients using monocyte-derived dendritic cells. *Haematologica,* 88(10), 1139-1149

Reid DC. (2001). Dendritic cells and immunotherapy for malignant disease. *Br J Haematol,* 112(4), 874-887

Ridgway D. (2003). The first 1000 dendritic cell vaccinees. *Cancer Invest,* 21(6), 873-886

Rollig C, Schmidt C, Bornhauser M, et al. (2011). Induction of cellular immune responses in patients with stage-I multiple myeloma after vaccination with autologous idiotype-pulsed dendritic cells. *J Immunother,* 34(1), 100-106

Rosenblatt J, Vasir B, Uhl L, et al. (2011). Vaccination with dendritic cell/tumor fusion cells results in cellular and humoral antitumor immune responses in patients with multiple myeloma. *Blood,* 117(2), 393-402

Savill J, Dransfield I, Gregory C, et al. (2002). A blast from the past: clearance of apoptotic cells regulates immune responses. *Nat Rev Immunol,* 2(12), 965-975

Sirisinha S, Eisen HN. (1971). Autoimmune-like antibodies to the ligand-binding sites of myeloma proteins. *Proc Natl Acad Sci U S A,* 68(12), 3130-3135

Sirohi B, Powles R. (2004). Multiple myeloma. *Lancet,* 363(9412), 875-887

Szmania S, Tricot G, van Rhee F. (2006). NY-ESO-1 immunotherapy for multiple myeloma. *Leuk Lymphoma,* 47(10), 2037-2048

Titzer S, Christensen O, Manzke O, et al. (2000). Vaccination of multiple myeloma patients with idiotype-pulsed dendritic cells: immunological and clinical aspects. *Br J Haematol,* 108(4), 805-816

Tucci M, Stucci S, Strippoli S, et al. (2011). Dendritic Cells and Malignant Plasma Cells: An Alliance in Multiple Myeloma Tumor Progression? *Oncologist,* 16(7): 1040-1048

van Rhee F, Szmania SM, Zhan F, et al. (2005). NY-ESO-1 is highly expressed in poor-prognosis multiple myeloma and induces spontaneous humoral and cellular immune responses. *Blood,* 105(10), 3939-3944

Vasir B, Borges V, Wu Z, et al. (2005). Fusion of dendritic cells with multiple myeloma cells results in maturation and enhanced antigen presentation. *Br J Haematol,* 129(5), 687-700

Vonderheide RH, Hahn WC, Schultze JL, et al. (1999). The telomerase catalytic subunit is a widely expressed tumor-associated antigen recognized by cytotoxic T lymphocytes. *Immunity,* 10(6), 673-679

Wang S, Hong S, Yang J, et al. (2006). Optimizing immunotherapy in multiple myeloma: Restoring the function of patients' monocyte-derived dendritic cells by inhibiting p38 or activating MEK/ERK MAPK and neutralizing interleukin-6 in progenitor cells. *Blood,* 108(13), 4071-4077

Wang S, Yang J, Qian J, et al. (2006). Tumor evasion of the immune system: inhibiting p38 MAPK signaling restores the function of dendritic cells in multiple myeloma. *Blood,* 107(6), 2432-2439

Wen YJ, Ling M, Bailey-Wood R, et al. (1998). Idiotypic protein-pulsed adherent peripheral blood mononuclear cell-derived dendritic cells prime immune system in multiple myeloma. *Clin Cancer Res,* 4(4), 957-962

Wen YJ, Barlogie B, Yi Q. (2001). Idiotype-specific cytotoxic T lymphocytes in multiple myeloma: evidence for their capacity to lyse autologous primary tumor cells. *Blood,* 97(6), 1750-1755

Wen YJ, Min R, Tricot G, et al. (2002). Tumor lysate-specific cytotoxic T lymphocytes in multiple myeloma: promising effector cells for immunotherapy. *Blood,* 99(9), 3280-3285

Yamazaki S, Inaba K, Tarbell KV, et al. (2006). Dendritic cells expand antigen-specific Foxp3+ CD25+ CD4+ regulatory T cells including suppressors of alloreactivity. *Immunol Rev,* 212, 314-329

Yang DH, Kim MH, Hong CY, et al. (2010). Alpha-type 1-polarized dendritic cells loaded with apoptotic allogeneic myeloma cell line induce strong CTL responses against autologous myeloma cells. *Ann Hematol,* 89(8):795-801

Yang DH, Kim MH, Lee YK, et al. (2011) Successful cross-presentation of allogeneic myeloma cells by autologous alpha-type 1-polarized dendritic cells as an effective tumor antigen in myeloma patients with matched monoclonal immunoglobulins. *Ann Hematol,* Apr 5. [Epub ahead of print]

Yang DH, Park JS, Jin CJ, et al. (2009). The dysfunction and abnormal signaling pathway of dendritic cells loaded by tumor antigen can be overcome by neutralizing VEGF in multiple myeloma. *Leuk Res,* 33(5), 665-670

Yi Q, Szmania S, Freeman J, et al. (2010). Optimizing dendritic cell-based immunotherapy in multiple myeloma: intranodal injections of idiotype-pulsed CD40 ligand-matured vaccines led to induction of type-1 and cytotoxic T-cell immune responses in patients. *Br J Haematol,* 150(5), 554-564

Yi Q, Desikan R, Barlogie B, et al. (2002). Optimizing dendritic cell-based immunotherapy in multiple myeloma. *Br J Haematol,* 117(2), 297-305

Yu H, Kortylewski M, Pardoll D. (2007). Crosstalk between cancer and immune cells: role of STAT3 in the tumour microenvironment. *Nat Rev Immunol,* 7(1), 41-51

Zou W. (2005). Immunosuppressive networks in the tumour environment and their therapeutic relevance. *Nat Rev Cancer,* 5(4), 263-274

5

Targeted Inhibition of Multiple Proinflammatory Signalling Pathways for the Prevention and Treatment of Multiple Myeloma

Radhamani Kannaiyan[1], Rohit Surana[1,2], Eun Myoung Shin[2], Lalitha Ramachandran[1], Gautam Sethi[1,2,*] and Alan Prem Kumar[1,2,3,*]

[1]*Department of Pharmacology, Yong Loo Lin School of Medicine, National University of Singapore,*
[2]*Cancer Science Institute of Singapore, National University of Singapore,*
[3]*School of Anatomy and Human Biology, The University of Western Australia, Crawley, Perth, Western Australia*
[1,2]*Singapore*
[3]*Australia*

1. Introduction

Multiple myeloma (MM) is a B cell malignancy involving the post germinal centre B cells. The disease is characterized by the presence of blood and urinary monoclonal proteins, osteolytic bone lesions and infiltration of bone marrow with malignant plasma cells of low proliferative index. Multiple myeloma is mainly a disease of elderly males, but, there is evidence to support that there is increasing incidence in younger individuals as well. American blacks are more prone than American whites. MM is the most common non Hodgkin's haematological malignancy, contributing 13% of all malignancies and 1% of all neoplasias. The median survival is 3-4 years, but with autologous stem cell transplantation and high dose chemotherapy, the median survival has increased to 5-7 years [1].

Most, if not all, multiple myeloma evolve from a premalignant condition known as 'Multiple Gammapathy of Undetermined Significance (MGUS)'. It then progresses via a 'smouldering multiple myeloma' stage, to a full blown disease and finally to an 'extramedullary MM' condition, where the malignant cells are no longer dependent on the bone marrow microenvironment for their proliferation. On a cellular scale, the origin of MM is thought to be post germinal centre B cell or memory B cell, indicated by the presence of hypermutated immunoglobulin gene. Evidence also supports the stem cell origin of the disease, as indicated by activated Wnt and Hedgehog signalling in the subset of cells in MM primary samples [2].

Cornelius Celsus, a Roman physician, first described the features of inflammation (inflammation - to set on fire) with the following signs: heat (calor), pain (dolour), redness (rubor) and swelling (tumour). The main purpose of inflammation is to protect the host

* Corresponding Authors

organism from the microbes and other noxious stimuli. However, when the infection cannot be controlled or when there is a constant presence of the damaging stimuli, inflammatory process gets deregulated, resulting in a condition called chronic inflammation, which is destructive to the host organism. Thus inflammation is aptly termed as a 'double edged sword'. The link between inflammation and cancer was first established in 1897, by a German pathologist named Dr. Rudolf Virchow. He found that leukocytes infiltrate tumour tissue and therefore, termed tumours as 'wounds that do not heal'. Since then there has been much evidence to link inflammation and cancer, so as to be able to add inflammation as one of the hallmarks of cancer [3-5].

In the linking of inflammation and cancer, two pathways are said to exist - extrinsic and intrinsic. In the extrinsic pathway, chronic inflammation leads to autoimmune diseases, which eventually culminate in cancer. For example, H.pylori infection in the stomach, Hepatitis B and Hepatitis C infections in the liver, inflammatory bowel diseases and inflammation of the prostate gland (prostatitis); lead to incidences of gastric cancer, hepatocarcinoma, colon cancer and prostate cancer, respectively. In fact, about 20% of all cancers are said to arise in an inflammatory environment. In the intrinsic pathway, activation of oncogenes or inactivation of the tumour suppressor genes, causing both cancer and inflammation, which complement each other [6, 7]. Irrespective of the pathways involved, the perpetrators of the cancer related inflammation are inflammatory cells and inflammatory mediators, such as cytokines, chemokines, growth factors, all of which finally converge on a few transcription factors [8]. Not surprisingly, agents modulating cancer-related inflammation have been tried in cancer therapeutics [9].

MM cells depend largely on a bone marrow microenvironment for their growth and survival, until the last stage of the disease, where they invade other areas to be termed as extramedullary MM. The bone marrow microenvironment can be broadly divided into cellular and non-cellular components. Cellular components include myeloma cells, bone marrow stromal cells or bone marrow fibroblasts, haematopoietic precursor cells, osteoclasts, osteoblasts, endothelial cells and immune cells. Of these, the supportive role of stromal cells in MM has been studied extensively. The interactions between myeloma cells and osteoclasts have also been studied to an extent. The bone marrow stromal cells and osteoclasts provide the myeloma cells with the ability to grow and survive, either by direct adhesion and/or by secreting growth and survival cytokines.

The non-cellular compartment is comprised of the extracellular matrix and the soluble factors. Extracellular matrix consists of various proteins like collagen, fibronectin and laminin. The extracellular matrix not only acts as depots for the growth factors, but also provides the myeloma cells with the ability to resist cell death induced by chemotherapeutic agents. The survival advantage offered by the bone marrow microenvironment to the MM cells is achieved by 1. the soluble growth factors which are secreted by various cellular components, 2. insoluble growth factors that are bound to the extracellular matrix component and 3. adhesion molecules that help MM cells adhere to the extracellular matrix and the cellular compartment. In fact, in a recent study, 22 out of the 51 multiple myeloma growth factor genes that could be interrogated by affymetrix were found to be significantly overexpressed by at least one bone marrow environment population compared to others [10].

The stromal derived factor (SDF/CXCL12), secreted by the bone marrow stromal cells, plays an important role in the homing of MM cells to the bone marrow, which expresses receptor CXCR4. Moreover, adhesion of MM cells to stromal cells or fibronectin, induces chemoresistance in MM cells, mediated by integrins [11]. The adhesion molecules namely, very late antigen (VLA-4), vascular cell adhesion molecule (VCAM-1) and lymphocyte function–associated antigen 1 (LFA-1), intercellular adhesion molecule (ICAM–1), mediate integrin induced chemoresistance [12]. The resistance is mediated partly due to the activation of NF-κB, which upregulates anti-apoptotic gene products. MM samples are found to have various mutations activating both classical and alternative NF-κB. Apart from the mutations, the NF-κB pathway can also be stimulated by B cell growth factors like BAF and APRIL, which are secreted by the bone marrow microenvironment [13].

Adhesion of MM cells to the stromal cells, induces the latter to secrete IL-6. IL-6 is the main growth factor for the MM cells. IL-6 then induces JAK/STAT 3, PI3/AKT and MAPK survival pathways. STAT 3 transcription factor upregulates its targets, namely, cyclin D1 and Mcl-1, which promote cell proliferation and antiapoptosis respectively. In addition to the IL-6 induced activation of STAT 3, DNA methylation is found to silence the negative regulators of STAT 3. On the other hand, IGF secreted by bone marrow stromal cells induces PI3/AKT pathways [14]. AKT promotes cell proliferation by phosphorilating GSK3β, which regulates cyclin D1 proteolysis. Activated MAPK pathway leads to the activation of ERK, promoting MM growth and survival [15]. The following section will elaborate on the very common and important inflammatory player, involved in the progression of MM.

2. Role of proinflammatory cytokines and growth factors

2.1 Interleukin - 6

Interleukin-6, a pleotropic cytokine, is involved in processes such as haematopoiesis, immunity and inflammation. It was discovered as a factor secreted from mitogen stimulated T cells, which helps mature B cells transform into antibody producing plasma cells [16]. Because of its pleotropic nature, various laboratories were working with its different functions, giving it different names: B cell stimulating factor II (BSF II) as it stimulated B cells to turn into plasma cells and secrete antibodies, interferon-ß2 [17] as it was thought to have the properties of interferon but later it was proven that IL-6 does not have properties of interferon, 26 kDa protein - named after its molecular weight, a hybridoma/plasmacytoma growth factor as it induced plasmacytoma in balb/c mice injected with mineral oil [18] and a hepatocyte-stimulating factor as it stimulated hepatocytes to produce acute phase proteins [19].

IL-6 binds to its receptor, which is either membrane bound or in soluble form. It then activates ubiquitously expressed receptor gp130 [20]. Once gp130 gets activated, IL-6 acts by three of the following signalling pathways: JAK-STAT pathway, MAPK-ERK and PI3-AKT pathway. Most of the actions of IL-6 are executed by JAK-STAT pathway [21]. IL-6 is found to be involved in the growth of many solid tumours like prostate cancer and renal cancer. Pathogenesis of Kaposi sarcoma has been proven to be due to the secretion of IL-6 [22-24]. IL-6 is also involved in the growth of many haematological malignancies.

IL-6 is one of the main growth factors in multiple myeloma [25]. In fact, IL-6 knock out mice failed to develop MM [26]. Moreover, the serum level of IL-6 and soluble IL-6 receptor has been proven to be a prognostic marker for tumour load, disease progression and survival [27-31]. Moreover, serum levels of IL-6 in patients with smouldering MM and monoclonal gammapathy of undetermined significance are comparable with healthy individuals, indicating the important role of IL-6 in the disease progression [32].

Initially, it was thought based on the following findings that myeloma cells secrete and respond to IL-6 in an autocrine manner. Firstly, IL-6 induces in vitro growth of freshly isolated MM cells. Secondly, MM cells express the IL-6 receptor (IL-6R). Thirdly, purified MM cells produce IL-6 and lastly, in vitro growth of MM cells is inhibited by anti-IL-6 antibodies [33]. But, again controversies prevailed among the research laboratories on the autocrine secretion of IL-6 by myeloma cells. Because, though all myeloma derived cell lines and patients cells express IL-6 receptor, only subsets of cell lines express IL-6 mRNA [34]. It was also found that bone marrow stromal cells are the main source of IL-6 [35-37]. Interestingly, when myeloma cells were co-cultured with bone marrow stromal cells, they tend to adhere to each other tightly and the IL-6 secretion by these cells reaches the peak. But, when the bone marrow stromal cells were fixed by paraformaldehyde, there was no increase in the level of IL- 6, confirming that the source of IL-6 was bone marrow stromal cells and not myeloma cells. Moreover, it was found that the stromal cells secrete IL-6 when stimulated by the adhesion of myeloma cells to the stromal cells. This is evident from experimental setup where these cells were cultured in transwell chambers without any physical contact with the myeloma cells. As a result, the bone marrow cells failed to secrete IL-6, emphasising the importance of adhesion molecules in the cross talk between the group of cells and pathophysiology of myeloma [38]. The adhesion mediated secretion of IL-6 was found to be NF-κB dependent [39].

In addition to bone marrow stromal cells, adhesion of myeloma cells to the peripheral blood derived osteoclastic cells protected myeloma cells from serum deprivation induced apoptosis and doxorubicin induced apoptosis. Osteoclasts produced osteopontin (OPN) and IL-6, and adhesion of MM cells to osteocleasts increased IL-6 production from osteoclasts. In addition, IL-6 and osteopontin in combination, enhanced MM cell growth and survival. However, the effects of osteoclasts on MM cell growth and survival were only partially suppressed by a simultaneous addition of anti–IL-6 and anti-osteopontin antibodies and were completely abrogated by inhibition of cellular contact between MM cells and osteoclasts. Osteoclasts enhance MM cell growth and survival through a cell-cell contact-mediated mechanism that is partially dependent on IL-6 and osteopontin [40].

The IL-6 induced survival of myeloma cells is mediated by STAT3, which upregulates anti-apoptotic proteins Bcl-XL and Mcl-1 and cell cycle proteins like cyclin D1, c-Myc and Pim. The IL-6 induced proliferation is mediated by MAPK-ERK pathway [41]. A PI3-AKT pathway mediates proliferation and induces survival by phosphorilating Bad and activating cell cycle proteins and NF-κB. Gene expression profiling studies demonstrated that out of 138 genes shown to be regulated by IL-6 in myeloma cells, 54% regulated cell cycle progression. This finding emphasises the role of IL-6 in myeloma cell proliferation [42]. IL-6 was shown to inhibit Fos induced apoptosis [43]. IL-6 can inhibit dexamethasone induced apoptosis of myeloma cells by gp130 induced activation of SHP2, which deactivates related adhesion focal tyrosine kinase (RAFTK) [44, 45] and activates the PI3/AKT pathway [46]. Partial reduction in the levels of IL-6 can sensitise the myeloma cells to chemotherapeutic agents [47, 48].

Various strategies, including IL-6 antagonist, IL-6 receptor inhibitor (CNTO 328), antisense oligonucleotides against IL-6 and IL-6 super antagonist (SANT7), have been tried for MM, but even after effectively blocking IL-6 receptor by the monoclonal antibody, the results were disappointing in clinical trials [49]. Accordingly, in the presence of bone marrow stromal cells, IL-6 receptor inhibition did not induce apoptosis, indicating the significance of the pleotropism offered by other growth and survival factors present in the bone marrow microenvironment [50, 51].

2.2 TNFα

In 1894, William Coley noticed that an injection of bacterial extracts into the tumour, could induce necrosis of tumours [52]. O'Malley et al. demonstrated that serum from mice injected with bacterial endotoxin can induce tumour regression [53]. The factor that can induce anti-cancer activity in vivo and in vitro, present in the sera of mice treated with endotoxin or LPS, was identified as Tumour Necrosis Factor α [54, 55]. The gene expressing human TNFα was cloned in 1984 [56]. Thereafter, the recombinant TNFα was used for experimental and therapeutic purposes. The therapeutic dose of TNFα induced serious hemodynamic instability and septic shock-like symptoms preclinically. TNFα can induce necrosis of the tumour by selective destruction of the blood vessels, only when injected at higher concentrations loco-regionally [57]. Its induction of apoptosis is highly context dependent. Physiologically, TNFα is an important cytokine regulating inflammation, immunity and haematopoiesis. Its deregulation is involved in lots of inflammatory and autoimmune conditions like rheumatoid arthritis and Crohn's disease. Recent research has realised the potent protumerigenic effect of TNFα [58]. TNFα KO and TNFα-R1 KO mice do not develop chemical carcinogen induced skin cancers [59, 60]. TNFα-R1 KO mice do not develop chemical carcinogen induced liver cancer [61]. TNFα antagonists are in various stages of clinical trials for a variety of cancers.

In MM, TNFα is not a strong growth factor, but it is an important factor secreted from myeloma cells to act on BMSCs to stimulate the secretion of IL-6. TNFα induces the expression of adhesion molecules on both myeloma cells and BMSCs. TNFα secreted by myeloma cells acts both directly and by increasing the adhesion between myeloma cells and the bone marrow stromal cells to secrete IL-6 by an NF-κB mediated mechanism in bone marrow stromal cells. TNFα is very potent when compared to other growth factors [62]. TNFα also participates in transendothelial migration of myeloma cells by acting via TNF-R2 and upregulating the secretion of MCP-1 in myeloma cells [63]. Clinically, the agents which are known to inhibit TNFα; namely, thalidomide and its derivates and bortezomib, have significant anti-myeloma activity.

2.3 BAFF and APRIL

BAFF and APRIL also belong to the TNF family of cytokines. They act by binding to receptors TACI (transmembrane activator and calcium modulator, and cyclophilin ligand interactor), BCMA (B-cell maturation antigen) and BAFF-R (BAFF Receptor) which is specific for BAFF. Myeloma cells express these receptors in a heterogeneous manner [64]. In fact, patient groups whose myeloma cells had low expression of TACI receptor were less differentiated and showed attenuated dependence on the bone marrow and portending poor prognosis; whereas patients whose myeloma cells express high levels of TACI receptor showed mature plasma cell signature exhibiting good prognosis [65]. There is evidence for these cytokines being secreted from myeloma cells [64, 66], bone marrow cells [67] and osteoclastic cells [65]. BAFF and APRIL seem to induce myeloma cell growth and inhibit dexamethasone induced apoptosis. BAFF and APRIL activate NF-κB, PI3kinase/AKT, and MAPK pathways in myeloma cells and induce a strong upregulation of the Mcl-1 and Bcl-2 anti-apoptotic proteins [68, 69]. Cell adhesion induced bone marrow cells secrete BAFF, which acts on myeloma cells to regulate their growth and survival [67]. Interestingly, bortezomib has been found to inhibit BAFF and APRIL induce proliferation of myeloma cells [66].

2.4 Insulin-like Growth Factor 1 (IGF-1)

Recent studies have delineated the role of IGF-1 in MM. IGF-1 was shown to be a strong indicator of prognosis in MM patients [70]. In the bone marrow milieu, IGF-1 is mainly produced and secreted from bone marrow stromal cells and mediates cell growth and survival in MM cells both in vitro [71, 72] and in vivo [73-75]. IGF-1 and its receptor were shown to be acting as growth factors [76] and preferentially expressed in MM cells [77] as compared to B-Lymphoblastoid cell lines.

IGF-1 inhibits Dexametasone-induced apoptosis in MM cell lines [78]. IGF-1 augments the proliferative and anti-apoptotic effects of IL-6 [71, 79] . Although IL-6 has mostly been described as a proliferation factor for MM, it has become clear that IGF-1 has an equally important proliferative and anti-apoptotic effect [80-82]. It could be that IGF-1 plays an even more pivotal role in the survival of MM cells, as IL-6 independent lines still respond to IGF-1 [80, 82]. Another group demonstrates that IGF-1 serves as a chemoattractant for MM cells [73]. In vivo induction of the receptor IGF-1R helps murine multiple myeloma cells in their homing and growth in the bone marrow [83].

IGF-1 transduces its signal by receptor phosphorylation of the insulin response substrate 1 and its activation of PI-3K and subsequently Akt kinase (PI-3K pathway). In fact, IGF-I increases adhesion of MM cell lines to fibronectin (FN) in a time and dose-dependent manner, as a consequence of IGF-1R activation and subsequent activation of β1- integrin and PI3-kinase/AKT signalling [84]. Several important biological characteristics have been associated with this segment of the PI-3K pathway [85]. Akt subsequently phosphorylates Bad, a member of the Bcl-2 family, producing an anti-apoptotic effect. The second pathway associated with IGF-I stimulation signals through the Shc, Grb-2, Sos complex, resulting in activation of Ras and subsequently the mitogen-activated protein kinase (MAPK) signalling cascade.

IGF-1 is also shown to mediate the activation of NF-κB [86], induce the phosphorylation of FKHR (forkhead) transcription factor, upregulate a series of intracellular anti-apoptotic proteins (including FLIP, survivin, cIAP-2, A1/Bfl-1 and XIAP) and decrease drug sensitivity of MM cells [75]. Caveolin-1, which is usually absent in blood cells, is expressed in MM cells and plays a crucial role in IGF-1-mediated signalling cascades [87]. Specifically, IGF-1 induces HIF-1α, which triggers VEGF expression [88, 89]; consequently, inhibition of IGFR-1 activity markedly decreases VEGF secretion in MM/BMSC co-cultures [75].

Therapies targeting IGF-1, such as inhibitors of IGF-1 receptor, have already shown preclinical anti-MM activity and will soon undergo clinical evaluation [75]. IGF-1R inhibition with neutralizing antibody, antagonistic peptide, or the selective kinase inhibitor NVP-ADW742 has in vitro activity against MM cell types and in orthotopic xenograft MM model had synergistic anti-tumour activity in combination with conventional chemotherapy. Another study [90] reports that IGF-1R inhibition blunts tumour cell response to other growth factors, overcomes the drug resistance phenotype conferred by the bone microenvironment and abrogates the production of proangiogenic cytokines. These sets of studies provide in vivo proof of the principle for therapeutic use of selective IGF-1R inhibitors in cancer.

2.5 Fibroblast Growth Factor (FGF)

Besides bone marrow microvessel density (MVD), serum levels of FGF, along with VEGF, are predicted to be prognostic markers of MM disease activity [91, 92]. Expression of bFGF correlates with clinical characteristics of MM and its high level also indicates poor prognosis [93]. However, the levels of bFGF may serve as a predictor for good response to the treatment of MM with Thalidomide [94]. Patients responsive to Thalidomide may have significantly higher concentrations of bFGF than non-responsive patients, but this observation is not consistent even between the same authors [95, 96]. Stimulation of BMSCs with FGF-2 induced a time and dose-dependent increase in IL-6 secretion, a well studied cytokine, which was completely abrogated by anti-bFGF antibodies. Conversely, stimulation with IL-6 enhanced bFGF expression and secretion by myeloma cell lines as well as MM patient cells, suggested a paracrine interaction between the myeloma and the stromal cells with respect to the above cytokines [97].

The FGF receptor 3 (FGFR3) is now recognized as a potential oncogene. Ectopic expression of FGFR3 originates from the translocation t(4;14) occurring in 10-25% of MM patients [98, 99]. Gain of function mutations in FGF receptors, especially FGFR3, have been widely implicated and studied in MM pathogenesis [98]. Suppression of FGFR3 using short hairpin RNAs (shRNAs), lead to apoptosis and anti-tumour effects in MM [100, 101].

FGF binding to the FGFR, results in dimerization of the receptor and autophosphorylation of the FGFR dimer at intracellular tyrosine residues. The activated receptor either binds directly to signalling molecules or recruits adapter molecules to link the activated receptor to downstream targets at the cell membrane.

Three FGF signalling downstream pathways have been identified in MM [102]: the Ras mitogen-activated protein kinase (MAPK) pathway, the phosphoinositol pathway and the signal transducer and activator of transcription (STAT) pathway.

2.6 Transforming Growth Factor (TGF-β)

Transforming Growth Factor beta (TGF-β) is a growth factor that controls proliferation, cellular growth and differentiation [103], and embryonic development [104]. During tumourigenesis, the TGF-β signalling pathway becomes mutated and TGF-β no longer controls the cell cycle [105, 106]. The cancer cells along with the surrounding stromal cells (fibroblasts) proliferate unchecked. Both these cells increase their production of TGF-β, which acts on the surrounding stromal cells, immune cells, endothelial and smooth-muscle cells, causing immunosuppression [106, 107] and tumour angiogenesis, and increasing the invasiveness [108, 109] and motility [110] of cancer.

TGF-β also plays a role in the suppression of bone formation in MM bone lesions [111]. Overproduction of TGF-beta 1 in MM patients was reported by Kroning et al. [112]. TGF-β is mainly produced by BMSCs, but is also secreted by malignant plasma cells and can regulate interleukin-6 (IL-6) secretion [113]. According to Cook et al., TGF-β produced by MM cells plays a significant role in suppressing host T cells and immune responses [114, 115]. TGF-β inhibition was able to suppress MM cell growth within the bone marrow while preventing bone destruction in MM-bearing animal models [116].

3. Role of chemokines

In MM, chemokines mainly help homing the myeloma cells to the bone marrow microenvironment. Their role in proliferation and survival of myeloma cells is only moderate. This effect can be either direct or mediated indirectly by inducing the secretion of IL-6, VEGF, or any other growth factor involved in the growth and survival of myeloma cells. The role of chemokines, especially that of MIPs, in osteolytic bone lesions is well established. Homing is defined by transendothelial migration of cells from the blood stream towards the chemokine gradient. This involves adhesion of cells to the endothelial layer, transendothelial migration and eventually residing in the microenvironment. So, it is apparent that bone marrow endothelial cells play an active role in the migration of plasma cells. They do so by secreting various chemokines and expressing adhesion molecules; thereby helping myeloma cells to migrate towards them. Upon adherence, MM cells will extravasate using their MMP arsenal to move through the basal lamina of bone marrow sinusoids. This process is also aided by the chemokine gradient in the bone marrow microenvironment because certain chemokine are said to be present in higher concentrations in the bone marrow microenvironment than in bone marrow endothelial cells which make sure that the cells are confined to the bone marrow microenvironment.

3.1 Macrophage Inflammatory protein: (MIP-1, CCL3)

MIP1 belongs to the CC family of chemokine and mainly acts via CCR1, CCR5 and CCR9 receptors. Myeloma cells have been shown to express both the receptors (CCR1, CCR5) and the chemokine [117, 118]. Controversial findings on the effect of growth and survival of myeloma cells could be due to usage of different experimental models and design [118, 119], but its role in migration and homing of myeloma cells, and in the progression of the myeloma bone disease, are clearly demonstrated. SCID mice injected with stable MIP1 knock-down clones of ARH cell line showed comparably less adhesion to the bone marrow, reduced survival and less bone pathology when compared to wild type ARH cell line injected group [117]. Suzanne Lentzsch et al. showed in vitro evidence that MIP1α can induce myeloma cell migration. Interestingly, they also showed that MIP1α can induce proliferation and survival of myeloma cells by inducing MAPK/ERK pathway, PI3/AKT pathway [118]. There is a study in which the various effects of MIP1α on 5TMM has been dissected. MIP1α induced migration has been attributed to the CCR5 and CCR1 receptor mediated signalling. Both the receptors mediate the MIP1α induced bone marrow angiogenesis and at least CCR1 mediates this effect directly [119].

3.2 MCP1 (or monocyte chemoattractant protein - CCL2)

As mentioned earlier, endothelial cells play an active role in the extravasation of myeloma cells and eventually their homing to the microenvironment. Murine endothelial cells are shown to secrete CCL2 and murine myeloma cells express the cognate receptor CCR2. Myeloma cells migrated towards the endothelial cell conditioned medium and this migration was inhibited by using antibodies against MCP1 [120]. Human bone marrow stromal cells also secrete MCP1, MCP2 and MCP 3, and myeloma cells migrate towards a stromal cell conditioned medium. This effect was inhibited by using antibodies against the MCPs and maximal inhibition was observed when all the three MCPs were blocked together, suggesting the role of various MCPs in myeloma homing [121].

3.3 CXC chemokines and CXCR3 receptor involvement in MM

CXCR3 receptor is expressed by activated T cells. It binds to CXC chemokines namely,: CXCL11 or Interferon-inducible T-cell Alpha Chemoattractant (I-TAC), Mig (Monocyte/macrophage-activating IFNϒ-inducible protein)/CXCL9 and IP10 (IFNϒ - inducible 10 kDa protein)/CXCL10. Myeloma cells derived from patients with myeloma, as well as myeloma derived cell lines, express CXCR3 receptor and they respond to their ligands by inducing tyrosine kinase phosphorylation and secreting MMP2 and MMP9 [122]. Bone marrow endothelial cells also secrete CXC chemokines and certain myeloma cells expressing their cognate receptors migrate in response to these chemokines [123].

3.4 Stromal Derived Factor (SDF-1α/CXCL12)

Stromal derived factor is a member of CXC family of cytokines and its cognate receptor is CXCR4. CXC12/CXCR4 is the most extensively studied chemokine/receptor system with respect to cancer. It has been implicated in progression, migration, invasion and metastasis of various cancers. The role of CXC12/CXCR4 has been well established in the homing of haematopoietic progenitor cells. Bone marrow plasma and bone marrow stromal cells secrete this chemokine, with the myeloma cells from the patient sample and myeloma derived cell lines expressing the cognate receptors. The chemokine mediates the secretion of IL-6 and VEGF, and induces proliferation, migration and inhibits dexamethasone induced cell death [124]. In the 5TMM model, bone marrow stromal cells and endothelial cells secrete SDF-1α and myeloma cells express the receptor. In vitro, SDF-1α induces moderate proliferation of myeloma cells, which was abrogated by blocking antibodies. 5T myeloma cells migrated towards a stromal cells conditioned medium which was partially inhibited by CXCR4 inhibitor. SDF also stimulated myeloma cells to secrete MMP9, demonstrated by zymography. Accordingly, SDF induces invasion and the CXCR4 inhibitor inhibits SDF induced invasion. In vivo, CXCR4 inhibitor inhibited the tumour burden and the immediate homing to about 40% [125].

When the myeloma cells were mobilized, the CXCL12/CXCR4 axis is downregulated. There is a downregulation of very late antigen (VLA4) in the peripheral blood myeloma cells after mobilization. This results in a suppression of the adhesion of myeloma cells to the bone marrow stromal cells, which can be rescued by induction with IL-6 [126]. Moreover, bone marrow endothelial cells are also shown to secrete CXCL12 and induce migration of myeloma cells towards the bone marrow endothelial cells. Thus, angiogenesis induced migration of myeloma cells is also mediated by CXCL12 chemokine [123]. The expression of CXCR4 was higher in bone marrow plasma cells of patients with myeloma than patients with MGUS. Moreover, the bone marrow plasma of myeloma patients has higher SDF-1α levels than that of peripheral blood of myeloma cells and bone marrow plasma of healthy individuals [127]. Consistent with its effect on migration, invasion, homing, proliferation and survival, CXCL12/CXCR4 axis induced MAPK/ERK, AKT, PKC and NF-kB pathways [124, 127].

4. Role of proinflammatory transcription factors

4.1 STAT3

STAT3 is a member of the STAT family of transcription factors. STAT family proteins were first discovered in the context of the specificity of the IFN signalling [128]. STAT3 was first described as a DNA-binding factor, in IL-6 stimulated hepatocytes, capable of selectively interacting with an enhancer element in the promoter region of acute-phase genes [129].

STAT3 is constitutively phosphorylated in v-Src–transformed cells and has been found to be necessary for the v-Src induced carcinogenesis. Expression of a constitutively active version of STAT3 on its own can lead to fibroblast transformation, showing that STAT3 is an oncogene [130]. Consistent with its role in various cancers, STAT3 regulates various genes involved in different aspects of cancer progression. Genes regulated by STAT3 that are involved in proliferation and growth include c-myc, cyclinD3, cyclin A, cdc25a, p21, cyclinD1, Pim-1 and Pim-2. Genes regulated by STAT3 that are involved in survival include proteins belonging to the family of Bcl-2 and IAPs, namely, Bcl-2, Bcl-xL, Mcl-1 and survivin. STAT3 has also been shown to downregulate the Fas cytokine. STAT3 mediated angiogenesis is mediated by VEGF; STAT3 also regulates MMP family members MMP2 and MMP9 [131]. STAT3 is vital for development, seen from STAT3 knock out mice which succumb to embryonic lethality [132]. However, disruption of STAT3 function either by deleting the gene or by introducing the dominant negative form of STAT3, leads to only a few phenotypical changes [133]. These findings are critical for the development of therapeutic strategies with high therapeutic index. In MM, STAT3 plays an important role in survival. It upregulates anti-apoptotic proteins like Bcl2, Bcl-XL and Mcl-1 [134-136]. Constitutive expression of STAT3 confers myeloma cells resistance to apoptosis [137]. Out of all the anti-apoptotic proteins regulated by STAT3, Mcl-1 seems to be more important. While antisense inhibition of Bcl-xL did not inhibit survival, knock down of Mcl-1 was sufficient to inhibit survival in myeloma cells. Overexpression of Mcl-1 was able to promote proliferation of multiple myeloma cells lines, even in the absence of IL-6 [138].

Knock down of Bcl-2 can augment dexamethasone induced apoptosis [139], but again, the importance of STAT3 in regulating the anti-apoptotic proteins and thereby the survival of myeloma cells remains controversial in the light of a lack of correlation between the constitutive expression of STAT3 and the anti-apoptotic proteins [140]. However, it is clear that STAT3 is not the only factor which regulates the survival of myeloma cells because myeloma cells become independent of a IL-6-gp130-STAT3 pathway in the presence of bone marrow stromal cells [51]. Almost 48% of MM patients have constitutively activated STAT3 [140]. There has been no activating mutations of STAT3 detected in MM. But, there has been epigenetic silencing of negative regulators of STAT3, namely, SHP1 and SOCS in MM. 27 of

34 (79.4%) myeloma samples showed SHP1 hypermethylation. At least in U266 MM cells, methylation of SHP1 may be responsible for constitutive STAT3 activation, because treatment with 5-azacytidine, a DNA demethylator, led to a progressive demethylation of SHP1 and a parallel downregulation of phosphorylated STAT3 [15]. SOCS-1 is hypermethylated in 23 out of 35 (62.9%) MM patient samples and consistently expression of this protein is upregulated after treatment with demethylators. So, it can be concluded that suppression of the expression of negative regulators of IL6-JAK-S TAT pathway by epigenetic silencing increases the sensitivity of myeloma cells to IL-6 induced proliferation and survival [141]. Moreover, overexpression of SOCS using adenoviral vector inhibited the IL-6 induced proliferation in IL-6 dependent multiple myeloma cells, hinting at another strategy to inhibit IL-6 induced downstream signal transduction pathways [142].

There are lots of therapeutic strategies that are being developed to target JAK-STAT3 pathway in MM. In fact, the novel agents that are being used nowadays namely, thalidomide and its derivatives and bortezomib, act partially to disrupt the NF-κB induced activation of IL-6 and thereby STAT3 activation. Numerous drugs that inhibit IL-6-JAK-STAT3 pathway at various levels induce apoptosis, both in vitro and in vivo [143-175].

4.2 NF-κB pathway

NF-κB is a Rel family of transcription factors consisting of p50, p52, c-Rel, p65/RelA and RelB subunits [176, 177]. It was discovered by Dr. Baltimore and colleagues in 1986 as a DNA binding protein, recognising specific sequences in the immunoglobulin kappa light chain joining (J) segment gene region in B cells [178].

Various inflammatory stimuli activate the NF-κB pathway. There are two pathways involved in the activation of the NF-κB pathway: the classical pathway and the alternative pathway.

NF-κB is a main transcription factor regulating various genes involved in inflammation. NF-κB has been casually implicated in various types of tumours [179]. Selective deletion of NF-κB in hepatocytes or inhibition of TNF-α production by neighbouring parenchymal cells, induced programmed cell death of transformed hepatocytes and reduced the incidence of liver tumours. Paracrine activation of NF-κB in initiated cells was not important in the early stages of liver tumour development, but it was crucial for malignant conversion [180]. In colitis associated cancer model of mice, selective deletion of IKK-β in inflammatory cells that are surrounding the enterocytes reduced the mRNA of inflammatory cytokine levels and subsequently decreased the tumour formation. However, selective deletion of IKK-β in enterocytes did not reduce inflammatory features, but it induced enhanced cell death in enterocytes leading to a decrease in the incidence of colon cancer [181]. It is quite obvious from these experiments that NF-κB affects both tumour cells and inflammatory stromal cells to induce and promote cancer. NF-κB acts on enteroctyes to inhibit apoptosis and also acts on inflammatory cells to stimulate the secretion of various mediators of inflammation which inturn acts on the enteroctyes to induce cancer. However, in some tissues, NF-κB acts to prevent cancer. For example, inhibition of NF-κB in keratinocytes leads to squamous cell carcinoma of skin [182]. In MM, patient samples show a constitutive activation of NF-κB to a variable degree [183]. How these cells activate NF-κB in a constitutive manner is still under investigation. Soluble cytokines belonging to TNFα super family including TNF-α, BAFF,

APRIL, lymphotoxin b, are known to activate NF-κB and are present in the bone marrow microenvironment. Adhesion of myeloma cells to the bone marrow stromal cells and osteoclasts also activates the NF-κB pathway in both myeloma cells and osteoclasts, and bone marrow stromal cells.

Moreover, around 15-20% of myeloma samples and 40% of the cell lines show activating mutations in the NF-κB pathway [13, 184, 185]. There could be some unidentified genetic mutations or epigenetic modifications that might explain the constitutive activation in the remaining tumours. Gain of function mutations include ones encoding receptors known to activate NF-κB namely, CD40, LTβR, TAC1, NIK (NF-κB-inducing kinase), and direct mutations involving NF-κB1 p50/p105 and NF-κB2 p52/ p100. Loss of function mutations include those that involve negative regulators of NF-κB activation namely, TRAF3, TRAF2, CYLD and cIAP1/cIAP2, inactivation of TRAF3 being the most common. These mutations activate both classical and alternative pathways of NF-κB. CD40, LTβR, TAC1 and receptor overexpression may be sufficient to activate the NF-κB pathway or might enhance the sensitivity of MM cells to factors in the tumour microenvironment. Overexpression of NIK or NF-κB1 p105 directly leads to constitutive activation of NF-κB. Deletion of sequences in the p100 IκB-like domain of NF-KB2 promotes processing of p100 to p52 and activation of the alternative NF-κB pathway [184, 185]. Activating mutations of the NF-κB pathway helps the myeloma cells become independent of the bone marrow, as they overcome the need for external cytokines activating the pathway [13].

Activation of NF-κB in myeloma cells induces proliferation, survival and chemoresistance. When compared to chemosensitive myeloma cell lines, chemoresistant myeloma cells express higher levels of NF-κB, suggesting a link between NF-κB and development of chemoresistance [186, 187]. Moreover, dexamethasone induced apoptosis is associated with a decrease in the NF-κB DNA binding activity. Interestingly, NF-κB can also serve as a prognostic indicator for response to dexamethasone. Only patients who responded to dexamethasone, demonstrated decreased NF-κB DNA binding activity in their samples. Enforced ectopic expression of Bcl-2 in myeloma cells conferred resistance to dexamethasone induced apoptosis, and this was also associated with enhanced NF-κB DNA binding [187]. Inhibition of NF-κB by IKK inhibitor abrogates the protective effect of IL-6 on dexamethesone induced apoptosis. It also potentiated TNFα induced apoptosis in myeloma cells. NF-κB inhibition abrogated the TNFα induced upregulation of ICAM-1, both in myeloma cells and in bone marrow stromal cells. It also inhibited the myeloma cell adhesion induced IL-6 secretion by bone marrow stromal cells and resulting proliferation of myeloma cells. These findings indicate that pro-survival functions of the bone marrow microenvironment are abrogated upon NF-κB inhibition. The novel therapeutic agents namely, bortezomib and thalidomide and its derivatives, act at least partially by inhibiting NF-κB [188].

5. Role of matrix proteinases, angiogneic and adhesion molecules

5.1 Matrix metalloproteinase

Matrix metalloproteinase belong to a family of proteases, capable of degrading all kinds of extracellular matrix proteins. In 1962, Gross et al. discovered MMP, when they found collagenase activity in the tail of a tadpole during metamorphogenesis [189]. These proteins function not only to remodel the extracellular matrix, but also are involved in the cleavage and thereby activation and inactivation of various biologically significant proteins like chemokines and growth factors. In the context of cancer, both the cancer cells and stromal cells secrete MMPs. Their involvement in invasion and metastasis was examined in various clinical models. Recent evidence suggests the role of MMPs in various hallmarks of cancer progression [190]. Culture supernatants of bone marrow derived stromal cells from multiple myeloma patients were found to have higher levels of MMP-1 and MMP-2 than control samples [191]. Moreover, endothelial cells secrete hepatocyte growth factor, which acts on myeloma cells to stimulate the secretion of MMP-9 [192]. 5T MM bone marrow expresses various MMPs, such as MMP2, MMP8, MMP9 and MMP13. Adequate inhibition of these MMPs by a broad spectrum MMP inhibitor SC-964 suppresses angiogenesis, reduces tumour load and osteolytic lesions [193].

5.2 Vascular Endothelial Growth Factor (VEGF)

VEGF is a signal protein that stimulates formation of new blood vessels, through vasculogenesis and angiogenesis. The activity of VEGF is mediated through three receptor tyrosine kinases: VEGFR-1 (Flt-1), VEGFR-2 (KDR/Flk-1) and VEGFR-3 [194]. Dysregulation of VEGF has been shown to be a major contributor to tumour angiogenesis as well, promoting tumour growth, invasion and metastasis [195]. Upon stimulation by VEGF, bovine capillary endothelial cells were shown to proliferate and show signs of capillary-like tube structures [196]. Significantly elevated levels of VEGF are observed in a variety of haematologic malignancies [197-201]. Several studies link VEGF inactivation to anti-tumour effects [202]. Angiogenesis appears to play a role in haematological malignancies [203]. There is growing evidence that increased bone marrow angiogenesis occurs in myeloma [204, 205] and is related to disease activity [206, 207]. Angiogenesis in myeloma also appears to be correlated with the Plasma Cell Labelling Index, PCLI [206]. Micro vessel density (MVD) increases five-to-six fold in magnitude with progression from gammopathy of undetermined significance (MGUS) or non-active MM to the active MM [93, 208]. Moreover, after chemotherapy, MVD decreases significantly in patients in complete or partial remission [209]. MM cells release angiogenic factors, such as FGF and VEGF [93, 210], and are shown to induce angiogenesis in vivo in the Chick Chorioallantoic Membrane assay [93]. They secrete matrix metalloproteinase-2 and -9 (MMP-2 and MMP-9) and urokinase-type plasminogen activator [93] and cytokines recruiting inflammatory cells, such as mast cells, that then induce angiogenesis through secretion of angiogenic factors in their granules [211]. A better understanding of some of the above angiogenic factors would help in developing novel therapeutic targets against MM. A few of the widely prominent angiogenic factors are reviewed in detail in the following section.

A number of studies implicate dysregulation of VEGF in MM pathogenesis and associated clinical features, including lytic lesions of the bone and immune deficiency. VEGF protein was found in malignant cells from 75% of MM patients studied [212]. Increased serum levels of VEGF have been correlated with a poor prognosis in patients with advanced stages of MM [213]. In fact, Iwasaki T et al. report predicting treatment responses and disease progression in myeloma using serum vascular endothelial growth factor [214]. Another patient study claims that the levels of VEGF, along with FGF, parallel disease activity [210]. VEGF may also affect the immune response in MM patients. Sera from MM patients' bone marrow inhibits antigen presentation by dendritic cells (DCs); conversely, anti-VEGF antibodies neutralized this inhibitory effect, confirming that VEGF mediates immunosuppression in MM patients [215]. The cytokine is probably involved in the progression of MM to plasma cell leukaemia (PCL) [216]. Not just the ligand, its receptor VEGFR-1 is also widely expressed on both MM cell lines and patient MM cells, confirmed both by reverse-transcriptase polymerase chain reaction (RT-PCR) analyses and immunoprecipitation [217-219]. VEGF is generally present in the bone marrow (BM) microenvironment of patients with MM and associated with neovascularization at sites of MM cell infiltration [220]. The induction of VEGF enhances the microvascular density of bone marrow and accounts for the abnormal structure of myeloma tumour vessels [221]http://www.nejm.org.libproxy1.nus.edu.sg/doi/full/10.1056/NEJMra1011442 - ref12. VEGF increases both osteoclastic bone-resorbing activity [222] and osteoclast chemotaxis [223], and inhibits maturation of dendritic cells [224]. As marrow neovascularization parallels disease activity in MM, it is reasonable to postulate that the vascular growth factor is acting in an autocrine fashion. However, MM cells express VEGF receptors only weakly, if at all. Therefore, the mechanism may be paracrine and result from a VEGF-induced time and dose-dependent increase in stromal cell secretion of interleukin-6 (IL-6), a known MM growth factor [225]. Another cytokine, TNFα, has been reported to be involved in the control of VEGF production by myeloma cells [226]. Moreover, VEGF directly, or indirectly through its stimulatory activity on TNF-α and IL-β1, stimulates the activation of osteoclasts and thus contributes to the lytic lesions in MM [222].

Other factors modulating VEGF secretion include Interleukins: IL-1β [227], IL-10 and IL-13 [228]; secretion of IL-6 [218, 225, 229] or VEGF by both BMSCs and tumour cells (paracrine/autocrine loop); hypoxia and the presence of mutant oncogenes (i.e., mutant Ras [mutRas] or Bcr-Abl, which up-regulate VEGF expression via HIF-1α protein); secretion of growth factors, such as insulin-like growth factor-1 (IGF-1) [88, 230], fibroblast growth factor- 4 (FGF-4) [231], platelet-derived growth factor (PDGF) [232], TGF-β [233], TNF-α [234] and gonadotropins [235]; c-maf–driven expression of tumour integrin β7 [236]; tumour cell expression of ICAM1 and LFA1 modulating adhesion to ECM and BMSCs, thereby increasing VEGF production and secretion; and CD40 activation, which induces p53-dependent VEGF secretion. Binding of VEGF to MM cells triggers VEGFR tyrosine phosphorylation, activating several downstream signalling pathways, particularly involving phosphatidyl-inositol-3 kinase [237, 238]. PI3-kinase- dependent cascade mediates MM cell migration on fibronectin, evidenced by using the PI3-kinase inhibitor bis-indolylmaleimide I and LY294002 [237]. This signal transduction pathway is mediated by focal adhesion proteins [239], such as FAK, paxillin and cortactin, which are responsible for the stabilization of focal adhesion plaques and the reorganization of actin fibres [240]. VEGF also regulates MM cell survival by modulating the expression of Mcl-1 and survivin [241].

MAP kinases (MAPK) are the final effectors of the signal to the nucleus, thereby activating genes for proliferation, migration and survival [242]. This increased migration and cell proliferation is because of the activation of VEGFR-2, since it is totally inhibited by a VEGFR-2 blocking antibody [243]. In fact, MEK-extracellular signal-regulated protein kinase (ERK) pathway is shown to mediate MM cell proliferation, evidenced by use of anti-VEGF antibody and PD098059 [217]. Approaches to disrupt the VEGF/VEGF receptor signalling pathways range from small molecule VEGF/VEGFR inhibitors, anti-VEGF and anti-VEGF receptor antibodies, such as bevacizumab [244, 245], and VEGF transcription inhibitors. Of interest are various kinase inhibitors that block the signal transduction mediated by VEGF. The VEGF receptor tyrosine kinase inhibitor PTK787 is active preclinically and undergoing clinical protocol testing in MM [246, 247]. It acts directly on MM cells to inhibit VEGF-induced MM cell growth and migration, and inhibits paracrine IL-6–mediated MM cell growth in the BM milieu. Pazopanib [248], another VEGF receptor tyrosine kinase inhibitor, has been studied for cancer therapy.

5.3 Adhesion molecules

Cell adhesion is a key physiological event involved in morphogenesis and histogenesis. Adhesion molecules mediate cell-cell and cell-ECM interactions [249], and are also involved in intracellular signalling after engagement with their receptors. Broadly, there are five groups of adhesion molecules. They are 1) the integrins-mediating cell-ECM and cell-cell adhesion 2) the cadherin family-mediating homotypic cell-cell adhesion 3) the selectin family-mediating heterotypic cell-cell adhesion 4) the immunoglobulin superfamily-mediating cell-cell adhesion and 5) other transmembrane proteoglycans, such as CD44 adhesion molecules and syndecan that mediate cell-extracellular matrix adhesion [12]. Dysregulated expression or function of adhesion molecules are involved in various steps of cancer progression.

In MM, there is evidence that adhesion molecules mediate homing of MM cells to the bone marrow, secretion of cytokines and growth factors, and development of chemoresistance. Out of all the adhesion molecules, VLA-4 and VLA-5 expressed by the myeloma cells play a crucial role in the myeloma pathogenesis [250]. VCAM-1 and fibronectin are the receptors for VLA. VLA adheres to the bone marrow stromal cells by binding to VCAM, CS-1 fragment and H1 region of fibronectin [251]. Inhibition of VLA using blocking antibodies inhibit the adhesion of myeloma cells to the bone marrow stromal cells and fibronectin [252]. VLA dependent adhesion to the bone marrow is regulated by the CXCL12/CXCR4 axis [253]. This is further supported by the finding that disruption of CXCL12/CXCR4 axis results in downregulation of VLA-4 and decreased adhesive capacity in the mobilised myeloma cells when compared to premobilisation bone marrow myeloma cells [126].

VLA dependent adhesion of MM cells to the bone marrow stromal cells induces secretion of IL-6 by an NF-κB mediated mechanism [38, 39]. Drug-sensitive 8226 human myeloma cells, expressing both VLA-4 and VLA-5 receptors, are relatively resistant to the apoptotic effects of doxorubicin and melphalan, when pre-adhered to FN and compared with cells grown in suspension. Upon exposure to chemotherapeutic agents, myeloma cells expressing high levels of VLA-4 have survival advantage over those that express them at low levels. When the cells were removed from a chronic drug exposure, the VLA-4 expression decreased. However, there was no upregulation of common mediators of drug resistance like anti-apoptotic proteins and drug exporting glycoproteins in the cells. It was concluded that though the survival advantage offered by VLA-4 induced adhesion to fibronectin is less, it is significant in helping them survive the acute drug exposure and gives them adequate time to employ the classic mechanisms of drug resistance [254]. How adhesion of cells to fibronecin is rendering the cells resistance to chemotherapy, is still not completely understood. It was shown that adhesion of myeloma cells to fibronectin activates NF-κB and its regulated gene products, leading to drug resistance [255]. Moreover, it seems that IL-6 and fibronectin collaborate to stimulate STAT3 and fibronectin augments IL-6 induced STAT3 activation [256].

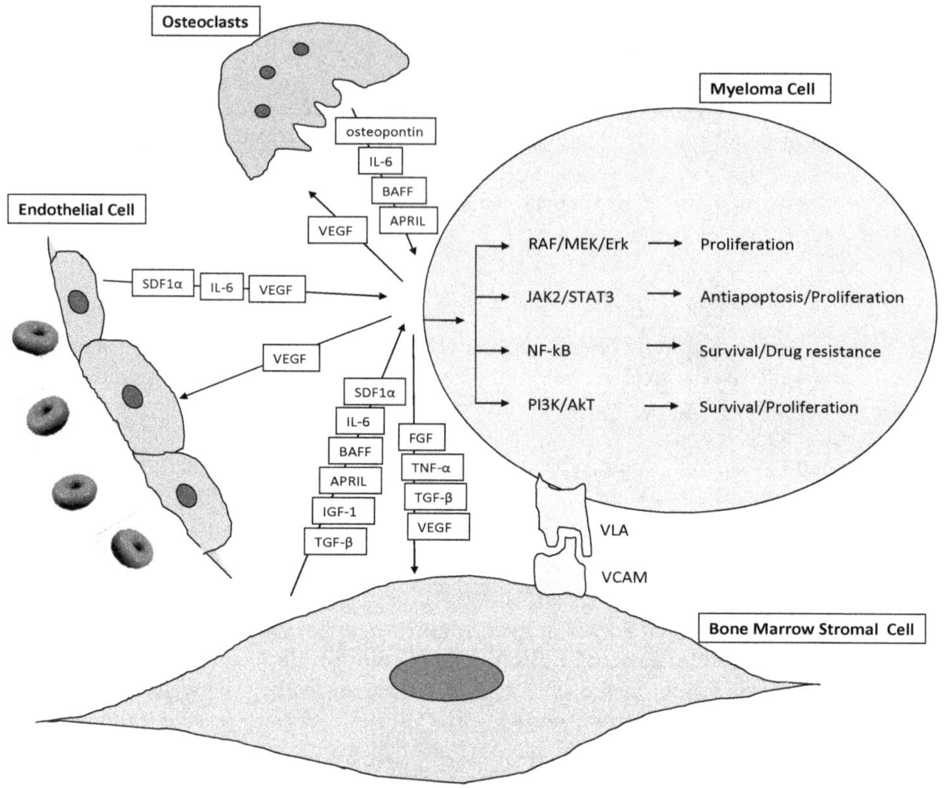

Fig. 1. Comprehensive representation of the role(s) of various inflammatory mediators in MM

	Pharmacological/ Biological Blockers	*Mechanism(s) of Action*	**References**
IL-6	1339	high-affinity fully humanized anti-IL-6 mAb	[257]
	6-amino-4-quinazoline	inhibits IL-6 signalling	[166]
	Bortezomib		
	CHIR-12.12 (Human anti-CD40 antagonist antibody)	downregulates gp130 inhibits CD-40 enhanced IL-6 secretion	[258] [259]
	CNTO 328 (siltuximab)	IL-6 neutralizing monoclonal antibody	[260-262]
	ITF2357 histone deacetylase inhibitor	down-modulates the interleukin-6 receptor α (CD126)	[263]
	Novel indolinone BIBF 1000	abrogates stroma-derived IL-6 secretion	[264]
	Sant7	IL-6 receptor superantagonist	[265]

	Pharmacological/ Biological Blockers	*Mechanism(s) of Action*	References
TNFα	Rituximab	monoclonal antibody	[266]
	Thalidomide and its analogues	suppresses the expression of TNFα	[267]
BAFF & APRIL	Atacicept	blocks the binding of BAFF and APRIL	[268]
VEGF	CHIR-12.12 (Human anti-CD40 antagonist antibody)	inhibits CD-40 enhanced VEGF secretion	[259]
	Bevacizumab	humanized murine anti--VEGF monoclonal antibody	[269]
	PTK787/ZK222584, SU6668, SU5416	VEGF receptor tyrosine kinase inhibitors	[203, 270-272] [273]
	Sorafenib	dual Raf kinase/VEGF-R inhibitor	
IGF	α-IR3	neutralizing monoclonal antibody to IGF-1R	[274]
	JB-1	IGF-1 like competitive peptide antagonist	[275, 276]
	NVP-ADW742	IGF-1R tyrosine kinase inhibitor	[277]
TGF-β	SD-208	TGF-β receptor I kinase inhibitor	[278]
CXCL12	4F-benzoyl-TN14003 AMD3100	CXCR4 antoganist	[279]
	Thalidomide	CXCR4 inhibitor	[267, 280]
		immnunomodulator- downregulates CXCL12 and CXCR4	[281]
STAT3	AR-42	downregulates gp130	[175]
	Atiprimod	inhibits STAT3 activation	[143]
	Auranofin	inhibits activation of JAK2	[162]
	Avicin D	activates protein phosphatase-1	[282]
	Azaspirane	inhibits STAT3	[283]
	AZD1480	JAK-2 inhibitor	[174]
	Baicalein	Inhibits IL-6-mediated phosphorylation of signalling proteins	[157]
	Betulinic acid	inhibits the activation of Src kinase, JAK1 and JAK2	[165]
	Butein	inhibits the activation of Src kinase, JAK1 and JAK2; and upregulates SHP-1	[164]
	Cantharidin	inhibits phosphorylation of STAT3	[172]
	Capsaicin	inhibits the activation of Src kinase, JAK1	[146]
	Celastrol	inhibits JAK2 and Src kinase phosphorylation upregulates SHP-1	[284]

	Pharmacological/ Biological Blockers	*Mechanism(s) of Action*	**References**
	Compound K	inhibits constitutive and IL-6-inducible	[167]
	Curcumin	STAT3 phosphorylation	[145]
		inhibits activation of JAK2	
	Decursin	upregulates PTEN	[150]
	Embelin	inhibitor of JAK-2	[149]
	Emodin	inhibits the activation of c-src	[161]
	Genipin	induces protein tyrosine phosphatase	[152]
	Guggulsterone	SHP-1	[172]
		inhibits the activation of c-src and	
	Icariside II	JAK-2 and upregulates the expression of SHP-1 and PTEN	[151]
		JAK1/2 selective inhibitor	
	INCB16562	Janus kinase inhibitor	[155]
	INCB20	forced overexpression of SOCS	[285]
	Infectivity-enhanced adenoviral vector of SOCS		[142]
		inhibits Aurora kinase A, Aurora	
	Multitargeted kinase inhibitor, AT9283	kinase B, and Janus kinase 2/3	[173]
		reduces Jak kinase auto-	
	Nifuroxazide	phosphorylation	[163]
		induces the expression of the protein	
	Plumbagin	tyrosine phosphatase, SHP-1	[286]
		pan-Janus-activated kinase inhibitor	
	Pyridone 6	inhibits both constitutive and IL-6	[169]
	Resveratrol	induced activation of STAT3	[287]
		inhibits activation JAK2	
	TG101209	inhibits of c-Src and JAK2 activation	[171]
	Thymoquinone	JAK2 tyrosine kinase inhibitor	[154]
	Tyrphostin AG490	inhibits the activation of Src kinase,	[148]
	Ursolic acid	JAK1 and JAK2, and upregulates SHP-1	[168]
NF-κB	Azacitidine	inhibits both NF-κB nuclear translocation and DNA binding	[288]
	Azaspirane	inhibits IκBα NFκB- p65 phosphorylation TNF-α	[283]
	Bay 11-7082	pharmacological NF-κB inhibitors	[289]
	Celastrol	inhibits JAK2 and Src kinase phosphorylation	[284]
	Curcumin	suppresses NF-κB activation	[183]
	Genistein	suppresses constitutively active NF-κB	[290]
		IκB kinase β inhibitor	
	MLN120B	suppresses NF-κB activation	[291]
	Parthenolide	suppresses constitutively active NF-κB	[292]
	Resveratrol	through inhibition of IκBα kinase and	[287]

	Pharmacological/ Biological Blockers	*Mechanism(s) of Action*	**References**
		the phosphorylation of IκBα and of p65	
MMPs	Chitosan	a marine phospholipid that inhibits the activity of MMP-2 and MMP-9	[293]
	SST0001	a chemically modified heparin with antiheparanase activity	[294]
Integrins	Anti-alpha4 Ab	monoclonal antibody to alpha4 integrin	[295, 296]
	QLT0267	integrin-linked kinase inhibitor	[297297]

Table 1. List of various pharmacological/biological agents modulating inflammatory mediators in MM

6. Conclusions

Understanding the various growth and survival pathways activated in both myeloma cells and various components of the bone marrow microenvironment is of paramount importance, not only to the basic understanding of the biology of MM, but also to effectively produce efficacious and safer anti-myeloma agents. In essence, myeloma is initiated by the primary genetic abnormalities and supported by the bone marrow microenvironment induced growth and survival. The secondary genetic mutations and epigenetic abnormalities emancipate myeloma cells of their dependence on the bone marrow microenvironment, which is when they progress to extramedullary MM. There are multiple signalling pathways activated, which serve overlapping functions. Combined inhibition of multiple signalling pathways offers better effects.

7. Acknowledgements

This work was supported by grants from the National Medical Research Council of Singapore [Grant R-713-000-124-213] and Cancer Science Institute of Singapore, Experimental Therapeutics I Program [Grant R-713-001-011-271] to APK; NUS Academic Research Fund [Grants R-184-000-170-112 and R-184-000-177-112], National kidney Foundation [Grant R-184-000-196-592] and National Medical Research Council of Singapore [Grant R-184-000-201-275] to GS.

8. References

[1] Raab, M.S., et al., *Multiple myeloma.* The Lancet, 2009. 374(9686): p. 324-339.

[2] Agarwal, J.R. and W. Matsui, *Multiple myeloma: A paradigm for translation of the cancer stem cell hypothesis.* Anti-Cancer Agents in Medicinal Chemistry, 2010. 10(2): p. 116-120.

[3] Colotta, F., et al., *Cancer-related inflammation, the seventh hallmark of cancer: Links to genetic instability.* Carcinogenesis, 2009. 30(7): p. 1073-1081.

[4] Hanahan, D. and R.A. Weinberg, *Hallmarks of cancer: The next generation.* Cell, 2011. 144(5): p. 646-674.

[5] Balkwill, F. and A. Mantovani, *Inflammation and cancer: Back to Virchow?* Lancet, 2001. 357(9255): p. 539-545.

[6] Mantovani, A., *Molecular pathways linking inflammation and cancer.* Current Molecular Medicine, 2010. 10(4): p. 369-373.

[7] Porta, C., et al., *Cellular and molecular pathways linking inflammation and cancer.* Immunobiology, 2009. 214(9-10): p. 761-777.

[8] Mantovani, A., et al., *Cancer-related inflammation.* Nature, 2008. 454(7203): p. 436-444.

[9] Balkwill, F. and A. Mantovani, *Cancer and inflammation: Implications for pharmacology and therapeutics.* Clinical Pharmacology and Therapeutics, 2010. 87(4): p. 401-406.

[10] Mahtouk, K., et al., *Growth factors in multiple myeloma: A comprehensive analysis of their expression in tumor cells and bone marrow environment using Affymetrix microarrays.* BMC Cancer, 2010. 10.

[11] Katz, B.Z., *Adhesion molecules-The lifelines of multiple myeloma cells.* Seminars in Cancer Biology, 2010. 20(3): p. 186-195.

[12] Bewick, M.A. and R.M. Lafrenie, *Adhesion dependent signalling in the tumour microenvironment: The future of drug targeting.* Current Pharmaceutical Design, 2006. 12(22): p. 2833-2848.

[13] Demchenko, Y.N., et al., *Classical and/or alternative NF-κB pathway activation in multiple myeloma.* Blood, 2010. 115(17): p. 3541-3552.

[14] Kawauchi, K., et al., *The PI3K/Akt pathway as a target in the treatment of hematologic malignancies.* Anti-Cancer Agents in Medicinal Chemistry, 2009. 9(5): p. 550-559.

[15] Chim, C.S., et al., *SOCS1 and SHP1 hypermethylation in multiple myeloma: Implications for epigenetic activation of the Jak/STAT pathway.* Blood, 2004. 103(12): p. 4630-4635.

[16] Hirano, T., T. Taga, and N. Nakano, *Purification to homogeneity and characterization of human B-cell differentiation factor (BCDF or BSFp-2).* Proceedings of the National Academy of Sciences of the United States of America, 1985. 82(16): p. 5490-5494.

[17] Van Damme, J., G. Opdenakker, and R.J. Simpson, *Identification of the human 26-kD protein, interferon β2 (IFN-β2), as a B cell hybridoma/plasmacytoma growth factor induced by interleukin 1 and tumor necrosis factor.* Journal of Experimental Medicine, 1987. 165(3): p. 914-919.

[18] Aarden, L.A., *Hybridoma growth factor.* Annals of the New York Academy of Sciences, 1989. 557: p. 192-199.

[19] Van Damme, J. and J. Van Snick, *Induction of hybridoma growth factor (HGF) identical to IL-6, in human fibroblasts by IL-1: Use of HGF activity in specific and sensitive biological assays for IL-1 and IL-6.* Developments in Biological Standardization, 1988. 69: p. 31-38.

[20] Nishimoto, N., et al., *Oncostatin M, leukemia inhibitory factor, and interleukin 6 induce the proliferation of human plasmacytoma cells via the common signal transducer, GP130.* Journal of Experimental Medicine, 1994. 179(4): p. 1343-1347.

[21] Hirano, T., K. Ishihara, and M. Hibi, *Roles of STAT3 in mediating the cell growth, differentiation and survival signals relayed through the IL-6 family of cytokine receptors.* Oncogene, 2000. 19(21): p. 2548-2556.

[22] Nishimoto, N. and T. Kishimoto, *Interleukin 6: From bench to bedside.* Nature Clinical Practice Rheumatology, 2006. 2(11): p. 619-626.

[23] Barton, B.E., *Interleukin-6 and new strategies for the treatment of cancer, hyperproliferative diseases and paraneoplastic syndromes.* Expert Opinion on Therapeutic Targets, 2005. 9(4): p. 737-752.

[24] Adachi, Y., N. Yoshio-Hoshino, and N. Nishimoto, *The blockade of IL-6 signaling in rational drug design.* Current Pharmaceutical Design, 2008. 14(12): p. 1217-1224.

[25] Barut, B.A., et al., *Role of interleukin 6 in the growth of myeloma-derived cell lines.* Leukemia Research, 1992. 16(10): p. 951-959.

[26] Hilbert, D.M., et al., *Interleukin 6 is essential for in vivo development of B lineage neoplasms.* Journal of Experimental Medicine, 1995. 182(1): p. 243-248.

[27] Pulkki, K., et al., *Soluble interleukin-6 receptor as a prognostic factor in multiple myeloma.* British Journal of Haematology, 1996. 92(2): p. 370-374.

[28] Kyrtsonis, M.C., et al., *Soluble interleukin-6 receptor (sIL-6R), a new prognostic factor in multiple myeloma.* British Journal of Haematology, 1996. 93(2): p. 398-400.

[29] Stasi, R., et al., *The prognostic value of soluble interleukin-6 receptor in patients with multiple myeloma.* Cancer, 1998. 82(10): p. 1860-1866.

[30] Pelliniemi, T.T., et al., *Immunoreactive interleukin-6 and acute phase proteins as prognostic factors in multiple myeloma.* Blood, 1995. 85(3): p. 765-771.

[31] Bataille, R., et al., *Serum levels of interleukin 6, a potent myeloma cell growth factor, as a reflection of disease severity in plasma cell dyscrasias.* Journal of Clinical Investigation, 1989. 84(6): p. 2008-2011.

[32] Bataille, R., et al., *Serum levels of interleukin 6, a potent myeloma cell growth factor, as a reflection of disease severity in plasma cell dyscrasias.* The Journal of Clinical Investigation, 1989. 84(6): p. 2008-2011.

[33] Kawano, M., et al., *Autocrine generation and requirement of BSF-2/IL-6 for human multiple myelomas.* Nature, 1988. 332(6159): p. 83-84.

[34] Anderson, K.C., et al., *Response patterns of purified myeloma cells to hematopoietic growth factors.* Blood, 1989. 73(7): p. 1915-1924.

[35] Caligaris-Cappio, F., et al., *'Role of bone marrow stromal cells in the growth of human multiple myeloma.* Blood, 1991. 77(12): p. 2688-2693.

[36] Klein, B., et al., *Paracrine rather than autocrine regulation of myeloma-cell growth and differentiation by interleukin-6.* Blood, 1989. 73(2): p. 517-526.

[37] Lichtenstein, A., et al., *Production of cytokines by bone marrow cells obtained from patients with multiple myeloma.* Blood, 1989. 74(4): p. 1266-1273.

[38] Uchiyama, H., et al., *Adhesion of human myeloma-derived cell lines to bone marrow stromal cells stimulates interleukin-6 secretion.* Blood, 1993. 82(12): p. 3712-3720.

[39] Chauhan, D., et al., *Multiple myeloma cell adhesion-induced interleukin-6 expression in bone marrow stromal cells involves activation of NF-κB.* Blood, 1996. 87(3): p. 1104-1112.

[40] Abe, M., et al., *Osteoclasts enhance myeloma cell growth and survival via cell-cell contact: A vicious cycle between bone destruction and myeloma expansion.* Blood, 2004. 104(8): p. 2484-2491.

[41] Ogata, A., et al., *IL-6 triggers cell growth via the ras-dependent mitogen-activated protein kinase cascade.* Journal of Immunology, 1997. 159(5): p. 2212-2221.

[42] Croonquist, P.A., et al., *Gene profiling of a myeloma cell line reveals similarities and unique signatures among IL-6 response, N-ras-activating mutations, and coculture with bone marrow stromal cells.* Blood, 2003. 102(7): p. 2581-2592.

[43] Chauhan, D., et al., *Interleukin-6 inhibits Fas-induced apoptosis and stress-activated protein kinase activation in multiple myeloma cells.* Blood, 1997. 89(1): p. 227-234.

[44] Chauhan, D., et al., *RAFTK/PYK2-dependent and -independent apoptosis in multiple myeloma cells.* Oncogene, 1999. 18(48): p. 6733-6740.

[45] Chauhan, D., et al., *SHP2 mediates the protective effect of interleukin-6 against dexamethasone-induced apoptosis in multiple myeloma cells.* Journal of Biological Chemistry, 2000. 275(36): p. 27845-27850.

[46] Hideshima, T., et al., *Biologic sequelae of interleukin-6 induced PI3-K/Akt signaling in multiple myeloma.* Oncogene, 2001. 20(42): p. 5991-6000.

[47] Salem, M., et al., *Identification of predictors of disease status and progression in patients with myeloma (MM).* Hematology, 2000. 5(1): p. 41-45.

[48] Thavasu, P.W., et al., *Multiple myeloma: An immunoclinical study of disease and response to treatment.* Hematological Oncology, 1995. 13(2): p. 69-82.

[49] Trikha, M., et al., *Targeted Anti-Interleukin-6 Monoclonal Antibody Therapy for Cancer: A Review of the Rationale and Clinical Evidence.* Clinical Cancer Research, 2003. 9(13): p. 4653-4665.

[50] Chatterjee, M., et al., *Combined disruption of both the MEK/ERK and the IL-6R/STAT3 pathways is required to induce apoptosis of multiple myeloma cells in the presence of bone marrow stromal cells.* Blood, 2004. 104(12): p. 3712-3721.

[51] Chatterjee, M., et al., *In the presence of bone marrow stromal cells human multiple myeloma cells become independent of the IL-6/gp130/STAT3 pathway.* Blood, 2002. 100(9): p. 3311-3318.

[52] Wiemann, B. and C.O. Starnes, *Coley's toxins, tumor necrosis factor and cancer research: A historical perspective.* Pharmacology and Therapeutics, 1994. 64(3): p. 529-564.

[53] O'Malley, W.E., B. Achinstein, and M.J. Shear, *ACTION OF BACTERIAL POLYSACCHARIDE ON TUMORS. III. REPEATED RESPONSE OF.* Cancer research, 1963. 23: p. 890-895.

[54] Carswell, E.A., L.J. Old, and R.L. Kassel, *An endotoxin induced serum factor that causes necrosis of tumors.* Proceedings of the National Academy of Sciences of the United States of America, 1975. 72(9): p. 3666-3670.

[55] Oettgen, H.F., et al., *Endotoxin-induced tumor necrosis factor.* Recent results in cancer research. Fortschritte der Krebsforschung. Progres dans les recherches sur le cancer, 1980. 75: p. 207-212.

[56] Pennica, D., G.E. Nedwin, and J.S. Hayflick, *Human tumour necrosis factor: Precursor structure, expression and homology to lymphotoxin.* Nature, 1984. 312(5996): p. 724-729.

[57] Lejeune, F.J., *Clinical use of TNF revisited: Improving penetration of anti-cancer agents by increasing vascular permeability.* Journal of Clinical Investigation, 2002. 110(4): p. 433-435.

[58] Balkwill, F., *TNF-a in promotion and progression of cancer.* Cancer and Metastasis Reviews, 2006. 25(3): p. 409-416.

[59] Moore, R.J., et al., *Mice deficient in tumor necrosis factor-a are resistant to skin carcinogenesis.* Nature Medicine, 1999. 5(7): p. 828-831.

[60] Arnott, C.H., et al., *Expression of both TNF-a receptor subtypes is essential for optimal skin tumour development.* Oncogene, 2004. 23(10): p. 1902-1910.

[61] Knight, B., et al., *Impaired preneoplastic changes and liver tumor formation in tumor necrosis factor receptor type 1 knockout mice.* Journal of Experimental Medicine, 2000. 192(12): p. 1809-1818.

[62] Hideshima, T., et al., *The role of tumor necrosis factors in the pathophysiology of human multiple myeloma: Therapeutic applications.* Oncogene, 2001. 20(33): p. 4519-4527.

[63] Johrer, K., et al., *Transendothelial Migration of Myeloma Cells Is Increased by Tumor Necrosis Factor (TNF)-a via TNF Receptor 2 and Autocrine Up-Regulation of MCP-1.* Clinical Cancer Research, 2004. 10(6): p. 1901-1910.

[64] Novak, A.J., et al., *Expression of BCMA, TACI, and BAFF-R in multiple myeloma: A mechanism for growth and survival.* Blood, 2004. 103(2): p. 689-694.

[65] Moreaux, J., et al., *The level of TACI gene expression in myeloma cells is associated with a signature of microenvironment dependence versus a plasmablastic signature.* Blood, 2005. 106(3): p. 1021-1030.

[66] Li, W., et al., *New targets of PS-341: BAFF and APRIL.* Medical Oncology, 2010. 27(2): p. 439-445.

[67] Tai, Y.T., et al., *Role of B-cell-activating factor in adhesion and growth of human multiple myeloma cells in the bone marrow microenvironment.* Cancer research, 2006. 66(13): p. 6675-6682.

[68] Moreaux, J., et al., *BAFF and APRIL protect myeloma cells from apoptosis induced by interleukin 6 deprivation and dexamethasone.* Blood, 2004. 103(8): p. 3148-3157.

[69] Quinn, J., et al., *APRIL promotes cell-cycle progression in primary multiple myeloma cells: Influence of D-type cyclin group and translocation status.* Blood, 2011. 117(3): p. 890-901.

[70] Standal, T., et al., *Serum insulin-like growth factor is not elevated in patients with multiple myeloma but is still a prognostic factor.* Blood, 2002. 100(12): p. 3925-3929.

[71] Jelinek, D.F., T.E. Witzig, and B.K. Arendt, *A Role for Insulin-Like Growth Factor in the Regulation of IL-6-Responsive Human Myeloma Cell Line Growth.* Journal of Immunology, 1997. 159(1): p. 487-496.

[72] Ogawa, M., et al., *Cytokines prevent dexamethasone-induced apoptosis via the activation of mitogen-activated protein kinase and phosphatidylinositol 3-kinase pathways in a new multiple myeloma cell line1.* Cancer Research, 2000. 60(15): p. 4262-4269.

[73] Vanderkerken, K., et al., *Insulin-Like Growth Factor-1 Acts as a Chemoattractant Factor for 5T2 Multiple Myeloma Cells.* Blood, 1999. 93(1): p. 235-241.

[74] Ge, N.-L. and S. Rudikoff, *Insulin-like growth factor I is a dual effector of multiple myeloma cell growth.* Blood, 2000. 96(8): p. 2856-2861.

[75] Mitsiades, C.S., et al., *Inhibition of the insulin-like growth factor receptor-1 tyrosine kinase activity as a therapeutic strategy for multiple myeloma, other hematologic malignancies, and solid tumors.* Cancer cell, 2004. 5(3): p. 221-230.

[76] Georgii-Hemming, P., et al., *Insulin-like growth factor I is a growth and survival factor in human multiple myeloma cell lines.* Blood, 1996. 88(6): p. 2250-2258.

[77] Freund, G.G., et al., *Functional Insulin and Insulin-like Growth Factor-1 Receptors Are Preferentially Expressed in Multiple Myeloma Cell Lines as Compared to B-Lymphoblastoid Cell Lines.* Cancer Research, 1994. 54(12): p. 3179-3185.

[78] Xu, F., et al., *Multiple myeloma cells are protected against dexamethasone-induced apoptosis by insulin-like growth factors.* British Journal of Haematology, 1997. 97(2): p. 429-440.

[79] Abroun, S., et al., *Receptor synergy of interleukin-6 (IL-6) and insulin-like growth factor-I that highly express IL-6 receptor a myeloma cells.* Blood, 2004. 103(6): p. 2291-2298.

[80] Ferlin, M., et al., *Insulin-like growth factor induces the survival and proliferation of myeloma cells through an interleukin-6-independent transduction pathway.* British Journal of Haematology, 2000. 111(2): p. 626-634.

[81] Tu, Y., A. Gardner, and A. Lichtenstein, *The Phosphatidylinositol 3-Kinase/AKT Kinase Pathway in Multiple Myeloma Plasma Cells: Roles in Cytokine-dependent Survival and Proliferative Responses.* Cancer Research, 2000. 60(23): p. 6763-6770.

[82] Qiang, Y.-W., E. Kopantzev, and S. Rudikoff, *Insulin-like growth factor-I signaling in multiple myeloma: downstream elements, functional correlates, and pathway cross-talk.* Blood, 2002. 99(11): p. 4138-4146.

[83] Asosingh, K., et al., *In Vivo Induction of Insulin-like Growth Factor-I Receptor and CD44v6 Confers Homing and Adhesion to Murine Multiple Myeloma Cells.* Cancer Research, 2000. 60(11): p. 3096-3104.

[84] Tai, Y.T., et al., *Insulin-like growth factor-1 induces adhesion and migration in human multiple myeloma cells via activation of β1-integrin and phosphatidylinositol 3'-kinase/AKT signaling.* Cancer Research, 2003. 63(18): p. 5850-5858.

[85] Ge, N.L. and S. Rudikoff, *Insulin-like growth factor I is a dual effector of multiple myeloma cell growth.* Blood, 2000. 96(8): p. 2856-2861.

[86] Akiyama, M., et al., *Cytokines modulate telomerase activity in a human multiple myeloma cell line.* Cancer Research, 2002. 62(13): p. 3876-3882.

[87] Podar, K., et al., *Essential role of caveolae in interleukin-6- and insulin-like growth factor I-triggered Akt-1-mediated survival of multiple myeloma cells.* Journal of Biological Chemistry, 2003. 278(8): p. 5794-5801.

[88] Fukuda, R., et al., *Insulin-like Growth Factor 1 Induces Hypoxia-inducible Factor 1-mediated Vascular Endothelial Growth Factor Expression, Which is Dependent on MAP Kinase and Phosphatidylinositol 3-Kinase Signaling in Colon Cancer Cells.* Journal of Biological Chemistry, 2002. 277(41): p. 38205-38211.

[89] Miele, C., et al., *Insulin and Insulin-like Growth Factor-I Induce Vascular Endothelial Growth Factor mRNA Expression via Different Signaling Pathways.* Journal of Biological Chemistry, 2000. 275(28): p. 21695-21702.

[90] Mitsiades, C.S., et al., *Inhibition of the insulin-like growth factor receptor-1 tyrosine kinase activity as a therapeutic strategy for multiple myeloma, other hematologic malignancies, and solid tumors.* Cancer cell, 2004. 5(3): p. 221-230.

[91] Sucak, G.T., et al., *Prognostic value of bone marrow microvessel density and angiogenic cytokines in patients with multiple myeloma undergoing autologous stem cell transplant.* Leukemia & Lymphoma, 2011. 52(7): p. 1281-1289.

[92] Sezer, O., et al., *Serum levels of the angiogenic cytokines basic fibroblast growth factor (bFGF), vascular endothelial growth factor (VEGF) and hepatocyte growth factor (HGF) in multiple myeloma.* European Journal of Haematology, 2001. 66(2): p. 83-88.

[93] Vacca, A., et al., *Bone Marrow Neovascularization, Plasma Cell Angiogenic Potential, and Matrix Metalloproteinase-2 Secretion Parallel Progression of Human Multiple Myeloma.* Blood, 1999. 93(9): p. 3064-3073.

[94] Bertolini, F., et al., *Thalidomide in multiple myeloma, myelodysplastic syndromes and histiocytosis. Analysis of clinical results and of surrogate angiogenesis markers.* Annals of Oncology, 2001. 12(7): p. 987-990.

[95] Neben, K., et al., *High Plasma Basic Fibroblast Growth Factor Concentration Is Associated with Response to Thalidomide in Progressive Multiple Myeloma.* Clinical Cancer Research, 2001. 7(9): p. 2675-2681.

[96] Neben, K., et al., *Response to thalidomide in progressive multiple myeloma is not mediated by inhibition of angiogenic cytokine secretion.* British Journal of Haematology, 2001. 115(3): p. 605-608.

[97] Bisping, G., et al., *Paracrine interactions of basic fibroblast growth factor and interleukin-6 in multiple myeloma.* Blood, 2003. 101(7): p. 2775-2783.

[98] Chesi, M., et al., *Frequent translocation t(4;14)(p16.3;q32.3) in multiple myeloma is associated with increased expression and activating mutations of fibroblast growth factor receptor 3.* Nat Genet, 1997. 16(3): p. 260-264.

[99] Richelda, R., et al., *A Novel Chromosomal Translocation t(4; 14)(p16.3; q32) in Multiple Myeloma Involves the Fibroblast Growth-Factor Receptor 3 Gene.* Blood, 1997. 90(10): p. 4062-4070.

[100] Zhu, L., et al., *Fibroblast growth factor receptor 3 inhibition by short hairpin RNAs leads to apoptosis in multiple myeloma.* Molecular Cancer Therapeutics, 2005. 4(5): p. 787-798.

[101] Hadari, Y. and J. Schlessinger, *FGFR3-targeted mAb therapy for bladder cancer and multiple myeloma.* The Journal of Clinical Investigation, 2009. 119(5): p. 1077-1079.

[102] Eswarakumar, V.P., I. Lax, and J. Schlessinger, *Cellular signaling by fibroblast growth factor receptors.* Cytokine & Growth Factor Reviews, 2005. 16(2): p. 139-149.

[103] Alexandrow, M.G. and H.L. Moses, *Transforming Growth Factor β and Cell Cycle Regulation.* Cancer Research, 1995. 55(7): p. 1452-1457.

[104] Pepper, M.S., *Transforming growth factor-beta: Vasculogenesis, angiogenesis, and vessel wall integrity.* Cytokine & Growth Factor Reviews, 1997. 8(1): p. 21-43.

[105] Taipale, J., J. Saharinen, and J. Keski-Oja, *Extracellular Matrix-Associated Transforming Growth Factor-[beta]: Role in Cancer Cell Growth and Invasion*, in *Advances in Cancer Research*, F.V.W. George and K. George, Editors. 1998, Academic Press. p. 87-134.

[106] Norgaard, P., et al., *Transforming growth factor β and cancer.* Cancer treatment reviews, 1995. 21(4): p. 367-403.

[107] Letterio, J.J. and A.B. Roberts, *Regulation of immune responses by TGF-beta.* Annual Review of Immunology, 1998. 16: p. 137-161.

[108] Maehara, Y., et al., *Role of Transforming Growth Factor-β1 in Invasion and Metastasis in Gastric Carcinoma.* Journal of Clinical Oncology, 1999. 17(2): p. 607.

[109] Picon, A., et al., *A subset of metastatic human colon cancers expresses elevated levels of transforming growth factor beta1.* Cancer Epidemiology Biomarkers & Prevention, 1998. 7(6): p. 497-504.

[110] Hojo, M., et al., *Cyclosporine induces cancer progression by a cell-autonomous mechanism.* Nature, 1999. 397(6719): p. 530-534.

[111] Matsumoto, T. and M. Abe, *TGF-β-related mechanisms of bone destruction in multiple myeloma.* Bone, 2011. 48(1): p. 129-134.

[112] Kroning, H., et al., *Overproduction of IL-7, IL-10 and TGF-beta 1 in multiple myeloma.* Acta Haematologica, 1997. 98(2): p. 116-118.

[113] Urashima, M., et al., *Transforming growth factor-beta1: differential effects on multiple myeloma versus normal B cells.* Blood, 1996. 87(5): p. 1928-1938.

[114] Cook, G., et al., *Transforming growth factor beta from multiple myeloma cells inhibits proliferation and IL-2 responsiveness in T lymphocytes.* Journal of Leukocyte Biology, 1999. 66(6): p. 981-988.

[115] Cook, G. and J.D.M. Campbell, *Immune regulation in multiple myeloma: the host-tumour conflict.* Blood reviews, 1999. 13(3): p. 151-162.

[116] Takeuchi, K., et al., *TGF-β Inhibition Restores Terminal Osteoblast Differentiation to Suppress Myeloma Growth.* PLoS ONE, 2010. 5(3): p. e9870.

[117] Choi, S.J., et al., *Antisense inhibition of macrophage inflammatory protein 1-a blocks bone destruction in a model of myeloma bone disease.* Journal of Clinical Investigation, 2001. 108(12): p. 1833-1841.

[118] Lentzsch, S., et al., *Macrophage inflammatory protein 1-alpha (MIP-1a) triggers migration and signaling cascades mediating survival and proliferation in multiple myeloma (MM) cells.* Blood, 2003. 101(9): p. 3568-3573.

[119] Menu, E., et al., *Role of CCR1 and CCR5 in homing and growth of multiple myeloma and in the development of osteolytic lesions: A study in the 5TMM model.* Clinical and Experimental Metastasis, 2006. 23(5-6): p. 291-300.

[120] Vanderkerken, K., et al., *Monocyte chemoattractant protein-1 (MCP-1), secreted by bone marrow endothelial cells, induces chemoattraction of 5T multiple myeloma cells.* Clinical and Experimental Metastasis, 2002. 19(1): p. 87-90.

[121] Vande Broek, I., et al., *Chemokine receptor CCR2 is expressed by human multiple myeloma cells and mediates migration to bone marrow stromal cell-produced monocyte chemotactic proteins MCP-1, -2 and -3.* British Journal of Cancer, 2003. 88(6): p. 855-862.

[122] Pellegrino, A., et al., *CXCR3-binding chemokines in multiple myeloma.* Cancer Letters, 2004. 207(2): p. 221-227.

[123] Pellegrino, A., et al., *Bone marrow endothelial cells in multiple myeloma secrete CXC-chemokines that mediate interactions with plasma cells.* British Journal of Haematology, 2005. 129(2): p. 248-256.

[124] Hideshima, T., et al., *The biological sequelae of stromal cell-derived factor-1alpha in multiple myeloma.* Molecular cancer therapeutics, 2002. 1(7): p. 539-544.

[125] Menu, E., et al., *The involvement of stromal derived factor 1a in homing and progression of multiple myeloma in the 5TMM model.* Haematologica, 2006. 91(5): p. 605-612.

[126] Gazitt, Y. and C. Akay, *Mobilization of Myeloma Cells Involves SDF-1/CXCR4 Signaling and Downregulation of VLA-4.* Stem Cells, 2004. 22(1): p. 65-73.

[127] Alsayed, Y., et al., *Mechanisms of regulation of CXCR4/SDF-1 (CXCL12)-dependent migration and homing in multiple myeloma.* Blood, 2007. 109(7): p. 2708-2717.

[128] Darnell Jr, J.E., I.M. Kerr, and G.R. Stark, *Jak-STAT pathways and transcriptional activation in response to IFNs and other extracellular signaling proteins.* Science, 1994. 264(5164): p. 1415-1421.

[129] Akira, S., et al., *Molecular cloning of APRF, a novel IFN-stimulated gene factor 3 p91-related transcription factor involved in the gp130-mediated signaling pathway.* Cell, 1994. 77(1): p. 63-71.

[130] Bromberg, J., *Stat proteins and oncogenesis.* Journal of Clinical Investigation, 2002. 109(9): p. 1139-1142.

[131] Alvarez, J.V. and D.A. Frank, *Genome-wide analysis of STAT target genes: Elucidating the mechanism of STAT-mediated oncogenesis.* Cancer Biology and Therapy, 2004. 3(11): p. 1045-1050.

[132] Takeda, K., et al., *Targeted disruption of the mouse Stat3 gene leads to early embryonic lethality.* Proceedings of the National Academy of Sciences of the United States of America, 1997. 94(8): p. 3801-3804.

[133] Akira, S., *Roles of STAT3 defined by tissue-specific gene targeting.* Oncogene, 2000. 19(21): p. 2607-2611.

[134] Puthier, D., R. Bataille, and M. Amiot, *IL-6 up-regulates Mcl-1 in human myeloma cells through JAK/STAT rather than Ras/MAP kinase pathway.* European Journal of Immunology, 1999. 29(12): p. 3945-3950.

[135] Puthier, D., et al., *Mcl-1 and Bcl-X(L) are co-regulated by IL-6 in human myeloma cells.* British Journal of Haematology, 1999. 107(2): p. 392-395.

[136] Spets, H., et al., *Expression of the bcl-2 family of pro- and anti-apoptotic genes in multiple myeloma and normal plasma cells: Regulation during interleukin-6 (IL-6)-induced growth and survival.* European Journal of Haematology, 2002. 69(2): p. 76-89.

[137] Catlett-Falcone, R., et al., *Constitutive activation of Stat3 signaling confers resistance to apoptosis in human U266 myeloma cells.* Immunity, 1999. 10(1): p. 105-115.

[138] Song, L., et al., *Mcl-1 mediates cytokine deprivation induced apoptosis of human myeloma cell line XG-7.* Chinese Medical Journal, 2002. 115(8): p. 1241-1243.

[139] Chanan-Khan, A.A., *Bcl-2 antisense therapy in multiple myeloma.* Oncology (Williston Park, N.Y.), 2004. 18(13 Suppl 10): p. 21-24.

[140] Quintanilla-Martinez, L., et al., *Analysis of signal transducer and activator of transcription 3 (Stat 3) pathway in multiple myeloma: Stat 3 activation and cyclin D1 dysregulation are mutually exclusive events.* American Journal of Pathology, 2003. 162(5): p. 1449-1461.

[141] Galm, O., et al., *SOCS-1, a negative regulator of cytokine signaling, is frequently silenced by methylation in multiple myeloma.* Blood, 2003. 101(7): p. 2784-2788.

[142] Yamamoto, M., et al., *Suppressor of cytokine signaling-1 expression by infectivity-enhanced adenoviral vector inhibits IL-6-dependent proliferation of multiple myeloma cells.* Cancer Gene Therapy, 2006. 13(2): p. 194-202.

[143] Amit-Vazina, M., et al., *Atiprimod blocks STAT3 phosphorylation and induces apoptosis in multiple myeloma cells.* British Journal of Cancer, 2005. 93(1): p. 70-80.

[144] Bai, L.Y., et al., *OSU-03012 sensitizes TIB-196 myeloma cells to imatinib mesylate via AMP-activated protein kinase and STAT3 pathways.* Leukemia Research, 2010. 34(6): p. 816-820.

[145] Bharti, A.C., N. Donato, and B.B. Aggarwal, *Curcumin (diferuloylmethane) inhibits constitutive and IL-6-inducible STAT3 phosphorylation in human multiple myeloma cells.* Journal of Immunology, 2003. 171(7): p. 3863-3871.

[146] Bhutani, M., et al., *Capsaicin is a novel blocker of constitutive and interleukin-6 - Inducible STAT3 activation.* Clinical Cancer Research, 2007. 13(10): p. 3024-3032.

[147] Che, Y., et al., *Serenoa repens induces growth arrest and apoptosis of human multiple myeloma cells via inactivation of STAT 3 signaling.* Oncology Reports, 2009. 22(2): p. 377-383.

[148] De Vos, J., et al., *JAK2 tyrosine kinase inhibitor tyrphostin AG490 downregulates the mitogen-activated protein kinase (MAPK) and signal transducer and activator of transcription (STAT) pathways and induces apoptosis in myeloma cells.* British Journal of Haematology, 2000. 109(4): p. 823-828.

[149] Heo, J.Y., et al., *Embelin suppresses STAT3 signaling, proliferation, and survival of multiple myeloma via the protein tyrosine phosphatase PTEN.* Cancer Letters, 2011. 308(1): p. 71-80.

[150] Kim, H.J., et al., *Decursin chemosensitizes human multiple myeloma cells through inhibition of STAT3 signaling pathway.* Cancer Letters, 2011. 301(1): p. 29-37.

[151] Kim, S.H., et al., *Janus activated kinase 2/signal transducer and activator of transcription 3 pathway mediates icariside II-induced apoptosis in U266 multiple myeloma cells.* European Journal of Pharmacology, 2011. 654(1): p. 10-16.

[152] Kim, S.H., et al., *Signal transducer and activator of transcription 3 pathway mediates genipin-induced apoptosis in U266 multiple myeloma cells.* Journal of Cellular Biochemistry, 2011. 112(6): p. 1552-1562.

[153] Kunnumakkara, A.B., et al., *Boswellic acid blocks signal transducers and activators of transcription 3 signaling, proliferation, and survival of multiple myeloma via the protein tyrosine phosphatase SHP-1.* Molecular Cancer Research, 2009. 7(1): p. 118-128.

[154] Li, F., P. Rajendran, and G. Sethi, *Thymoquinone inhibits proliferation, induces apoptosis and chemosensitizes human multiple myeloma cells through suppression of signal transducer and activator of transcription 3 activation pathway.* British Journal of Pharmacology, 2010. 161(3): p. 541-554.

[155] Li, J., et al., *INCB16562, a JAK1/2 selective inhibitor, is efficacious against multiple myeloma cells and reverses the protective effects of cytokine and stromal cell support.* Neoplasia, 2010. 12(1): p. 28-38.

[156] Lin, L., et al., *A novel small molecule inhibits STAT3 phosphorylation and DNA binding activity and exhibits potent growth suppressive activity in human cancer cells.* Molecular Cancer, 2010. 9.

[157] Liu, S., et al., *Inhibitory effect of baicalein on IL-6-mediated signaling cascades in human myeloma cells.* European Journal of Haematology, 2010. 84(2): p. 137-144.

[158] Ma, J., et al., *Therapeutic potential of cladribine in combination with STAT3 inhibitor against multiple myeloma.* BMC Cancer, 2011: p. 255.

[159] Ma, J., et al., *Mechanism of MS-275 blocking STAT3 and NF-κB signaling, inducing apoptosis in U266 cells.* Chinese Journal of Cancer Prevention and Treatment, 2009. 16(16): p. 1234-1237.

[160] Malara, N., et al., *Simultaneous inhibition of the constitutively activated nuclear factor κB and of the Interleukin-6 pathways is necessary and sufficient to completely overcome apoptosis resistance of human U266 myeloma cells.* Cell Cycle, 2008. 7(20): p. 3235-3245.

[161] Muto, A., et al., *Emodin has a cytotoxic activity against human multiple myeloma as a Janus-activated kinase 2 inhibitor.* Molecular cancer therapeutics, 2007. 6(3): p. 987-994.

[162] Nakaya, A., et al., *The gold compound auranofin induces apoptosis of human multiple myeloma cells through both down-regulation of STAT3 and inhibition of NF-κB activity.* Leukemia Research, 2011. 35(2): p. 243-249.

[163] Nelson, E.A., et al., *Nifuroxazide inhibits survival of multiple myeloma cells by directly inhibiting STAT3.* Blood, 2008. 112(13): p. 5095-5102.

[164] Pandey, M.K., et al., *Butein suppresses constitutive and inducible signal transducer and activator of transcription (stat) 3 activation and stat3-regulated gene products through the induction of a protein tyrosine phosphatase SHP-1.* Molecular Pharmacology, 2009. 75(3): p. 525-533.

[165] Pandey, M.K., B. Sung, and B.B. Aggarwal, *Betulinic acid suppresses STAT3 activation pathway through induction of protein tyrosine phosphatase SHP-1 in human multiple myeloma cells.* International Journal of Cancer, 2010. 127(2): p. 282-292.

[166] Park, J., et al., *Blockage of interleukin-6 signaling with 6-amino-4-quinazoline synergistically induces the inhibitory effect of bortezomib in human U266 cells.* Anti-Cancer Drugs, 2008. 19(8): p. 777-782.

[167] Park, S., et al., *Inhibition of JAK1/STAT3 signaling mediates compound K-induced apoptosis in human multiple myeloma U266 cells.* Food and Chemical Toxicology, 2011. 49(6): p. 1367-1372.

[168] Pathak, A.K., et al., *Ursolic acid inhibits STAT3 activation pathway leading to suppression of proliferation and chemosensitization of human multiple myeloma cells.* Molecular Cancer Research, 2007. 5(9): p. 943-955.

[169] Pedranzini, L., et al., *Pyridone 6, a Pan-Janus-activated kinase inhibitor, induces growth inhibition of multiple myeloma cells.* Cancer research, 2006. 66(19): p. 9714-9721.

[170] Peng, J., et al., *Patrinia scabiosaefolia extract suppresses proliferation and promotes apoptosis by inhibiting the STAT3 pathway in human multiple myeloma cells.* Molecular Medicine Reports, 2011. 4(2): p. 313-318.

[171] Ramakrishnan, V., et al., *TG101209, a novel JAK2 inhibitor, has significant in vitro activity in multiple myeloma and displays preferential cytotoxicity for CD45+ myeloma cells.* American Journal of Hematology, 2010. 85(9): p. 675-686.

[172] Sagawa, M., et al., *Cantharidin induces apoptosis of human multiple myeloma cells via inhibition of the JAK/STAT pathway.* Cancer Science, 2008. 99(9): p. 1820-1826.

[173] Santo, L., et al., *Antimyeloma activity of a multitargeted kinase inhibitor, AT9283, via potent Aurora kinase and STAT3 inhibition either alone or in combination with lenalidomide.* Clinical Cancer Research, 2011. 17(10): p. 3259-3271.

[174] Scuto, A., et al., *The novel JAK inhibitor AZD1480 blocks STAT3 and FGFR3 signaling, resulting in suppression of human myeloma cell growth and survival.* Leukemia, 2011. 25(3): p. 538-550.

[175] Zhang, S., et al., *The novel histone deacetylase inhibitor, AR-42, inhibits gp130/Stat3 pathway and induces apoptosis and cell cycle arrest in multiple myeloma cells.* International Journal of Cancer, 2011. 129(1): p. 204-213.

[176] Sethi, G., B. Sung, and B.B. Aggarwal, *Nuclear factor-κB activation: From bench to bedside.* Experimental Biology and Medicine, 2008. 233(1): p. 21-31.

[177] Sethi, G. and V. Tergaonkar, *Potential pharmacological control of the NF-κB pathway.* Trends in Pharmacological Sciences, 2009. 30(6): p. 313-321.

[178] Weaver, D. and D. Baltimore, *B lymphocyte-specific protein binding near an immunoglobulin κ-chain gene J segment (DNA binding protein/B cell-specific protein/DNA rearranggement).* Proceedings of the National Academy of Sciences of the United States of America, 1987. 84(6): p. 1516-1520.

[179] Aggarwal, B.B., *Nuclear factor-κB: The enemy within.* Cancer Cell, 2004. 6(3): p. 203-208.

[180] Pikarsky, E., et al., *NF-κB functions as a tumour promoter in inflammation-associated cancer.* Nature, 2004. 431(7007): p. 461-466.

[181] Greten, F.R., et al., *IKKβ links inflammation and tumorigenesis in a mouse model of colitis-associated cancer.* Cell, 2004. 118(3): p. 285-296.

[182] Seitz, C.S., et al., *Alterations in NF-κB function in transgenic epithelial tissue demonstrate a growth inhibitory role for NF-κB.* Proceedings of the National Academy of Sciences of the United States of America, 1998. 95(5): p. 2307-2312.

[183] Bharti, A.C., et al., *Nuclear factor-κB and STAT3 are constitutively active in CD138 + cells derived from multiple myeloma patients, and suppression of these transcription factors leads to apoptosis.* Blood, 2004. 103(8): p. 3175-3184.

[184] Keats, J.J., et al., *Promiscuous Mutations Activate the Noncanonical NF-κB Pathway in Multiple Myeloma.* Cancer Cell, 2007. 12(2): p. 131-144.

[185] Annunziata, C.M., et al., *Frequent Engagement of the Classical and Alternative NF-κB Pathways by Diverse Genetic Abnormalities in Multiple Myeloma.* Cancer Cell, 2007. 12(2): p. 115-130.

[186] Berenson, J.R., H.M. Ma, and R. Vescio, *The role of nuclear factor-κB in the biology and treatment of multiple myeloma.* Seminars in Oncology, 2001. 28(6): p. 626-633.

[187] Feinman, R., et al., *Role of NF-κB in the rescue of multiple myeloma cells from glucocorticoid-induced apoptosis by bcl-2.* Blood, 1999. 93(9): p. 3044-3052.

[188] Hideshima, T., et al., *NF-κB as a therapeutic target in multiple myeloma.* Journal of Biological Chemistry, 2002. 277(19): p. 16639-16647.

[189] Brinckerhoff, C.E. and L.M. Matrisian, *Matrix metalloproteinases: A tail of a frog that became a prince.* Nature Reviews Molecular Cell Biology, 2002. 3(3): p. 207-214.

[190] Egeblad, M. and Z. Werb, *New functions for the matrix metalloproteinases in cancer progression.* Nature Reviews Cancer, 2002. 2(3): p. 161-174.

[191] Zdzisińska, B., et al., *Matrix metalloproteinase and cytokine production by bone marrow adherent cells from multiple myeloma patients.* Archivum Immunologiae et Therapiae Experimentalis, 2006. 54(4): p. 289-296.

[192] Vande Broek, I., et al., *Bone marrow endothelial cells increase the invasiveness of human multiple myeloma cells through upregulation of MMP-9: Evidence for a role of hepatocyte growth factor.* Leukemia, 2004. 18(5): p. 976-982.

[193] Van Valckenborgh, E., et al., *Multifunctional role of matrix metalloproteinases in multiple myeloma: A study in the 5T2MM mouse model.* American Journal of Pathology, 2004. 165(3): p. 869-878.

[194] Klagsbrun, M. and P. A. D'Amore, *Vascular endothelial growth factor and its receptors.* Cytokine & Growth Factor Reviews, 1996. 7(3): p. 259-270.

[195] Dvorak, H.F., *Vascular Permeability Factor/Vascular Endothelial Growth Factor: A Critical Cytokine in Tumor Angiogenesis and a Potential Target for Diagnosis and Therapy.* Journal of Clinical Oncology, 2002. 20(21): p. 4368-4380.

[196] Asahara, T., et al., *Synergistic Effect of Vascular Endothelial Growth Factor and Basic Fibroblast Growth Factor on Angiogenesis In Vivo.* Circulation, 1995. 92(9): p. 365-371.

[197] Aguayo, A., et al., *Angiogenesis in acute and chronic leukemias and myelodysplastic syndromes.* Blood, 2000. 96(6): p. 2240-2245.

[198] Salven, P., et al., *Simultaneous elevation in the serum concentrations of the angiogenic growth factors VEGF and bFGF is an independent predictor of poor prognosis in non-Hodgkin lymphoma: a single-institution study of 200 patients.* Blood, 2000. 96(12): p. 3712-3718.

[199] Molica, S., et al., *Increased serum levels of vascular endothelial growth factor predict risk of progression in early B-cell chronic lymphocytic leukaemia.* British Journal of Haematology, 1999. 107(3): p. 605-610.

[200] Aguayo, A., et al., *Clinical relevance of intracellular vascular endothelial growth factor levels in B-cell chronic lymphocytic leukemia.* Blood, 2000. 96(2): p. 768-770.

[201] *A Predictive Model for Aggressive Non-Hodgkin's Lymphoma.* New England Journal of Medicine, 1993. 329(14): p. 987-994.

[202] Inoue, M., et al., *VEGF-A has a critical, nonredundant role in angiogenic switching and pancreatic ² cell carcinogenesis.* Cancer cell, 2002. 1(2): p. 193-202.

[203] Moehler, T.M., et al., *Angiogenesis in hematologic malignancies.* Critical reviews in oncology/hematology, 2003. 45(3): p. 227-244.

[204] Rajkumar, S.V. and R.A. Kyle, *Angiogenesis in multiple myeloma.* Seminars in oncology, 2001. 28(6): p. 560-564.

[205] Jakob, C., et al., *Angiogenesis in multiple myeloma.* European journal of cancer (Oxford, England : 1990), 2006. 42(11): p. 1581-1590.

[206] Vacca, A., et al., *Bone marrow angiogenesis and progression in multiple myeloma.* British Journal of Haematology, 1994. 87(3): p. 503-508.

[207] Vacca, A., et al., *Angiogenesis in B Cell Lymphoproliferative Diseases. Biological and Clinical Studies.* Leukemia & Lymphoma, 1995. 20(1-2): p. 27-38.

[208] Rajkumar, S.V., et al., *Prognostic Value of Bone Marrow Angiogenesis in Multiple Myeloma.* Clinical Cancer Research, 2000. 6(8): p. 3111-3116.

[209] Sezer, et al., *Relationship between bone marrow angiogenesis and plasma cell infiltration and serum ß2-microglobulin levels in patients with multiple myeloma.* Annals of Hematology, 2001. 80(10): p. 598-601.

[210] Di Raimondo, F., et al., *Angiogenic factors in multiple myeloma: higher levels in bone marrow than in peripheral blood.* Haematologica, 2000. 85(8): p. 800-805.

[211] Ribatti, D., et al., *Bone marrow angiogenesis and mast cell density increase simultaneously with progression of human multiple myeloma.* Br J Cancer, 1999. 79(3-4): p. 451-455.

[212] Bellamy, W.T., *Expression of vascular endothelial growth factor and its receptors in multiple myeloma and other hematopoietic malignancies.* Seminars in oncology, 2001. 28(6): p. 551-559.

[213] Ugurel, S., et al., *Increased Serum Concentration of Angiogenic Factors in Malignant Melanoma Patients Correlates With Tumor Progression and Survival.* Journal of Clinical Oncology, 2001. 19(2): p. 577-583.

[214] Iwasaki, T. and H. Sano, *Predicting Treatment Responses and Disease Progression in Myeloma using Serum Vascular Endothelial Growth Factor and Hepatocyte Growth Factor Levels.* Leukemia & Lymphoma, 2003. 44(8): p. 1347-1351.

[215] Hayashi, T., et al., *Ex vivo induction of multiple myeloma-specific cytotoxic T lymphocytes.* Blood, 2003. 102(4): p. 1435-1442.

[216] Hideshima, T., et al., *Novel therapies targeting the myeloma cell and its bone marrow microenvironment.* Seminars in oncology, 2001. 28(6): p. 607-612.

[217] Podar, K., et al., *Vascular endothelial growth factor triggers signaling cascades mediating multiple myeloma cell growth and migration.* Blood, 2001. 98(2): p. 428-435.

[218] Bellamy, W.T., et al., *Expression of Vascular Endothelial Growth Factor and Its Receptors in Hematopoietic Malignancies.* Cancer Research, 1999. 59(3): p. 728-733.

[219] Kumar, S., et al., *Expression of VEGF and its receptors by myeloma cells.* Leukemia, 0000. 17(10): p. 2025-2031.

[220] Yaccoby, S., B. Barlogie, and J. Epstein, *Primary Myeloma Cells Growing in SCID-hu Mice: A Model for Studying the Biology and Treatment of Myeloma and Its Manifestations.* Blood, 1998. 92(8): p. 2908-2913.

[221] Hideshima, T., et al., *Understanding multiple myeloma pathogenesis in the bone marrow to identify new therapeutic targets.* Nature Reviews Cancer, 2007. 7(8): p. 585-598.

[222] Nakagawa, M., et al., *Vascular endothelial growth factor (VEGF) directly enhances osteoclastic bone resorption and survival of mature osteoclasts.* Febs Letters, 2000. 473(2): p. 161-164.

[223] Henriksen, K., et al., *RANKL and Vascular Endothelial Growth Factor (VEGF) Induce Osteoclast Chemotaxis through an ERK1/2-dependent Mechanism.* Journal of Biological Chemistry, 2003. 278(49): p. 48745-48753.

[224] Gabrilovich, D.I., et al., *Production of vascular endothelial growth factor by human tumors inhibits the functional maturation of dendritic cells (vol 2, pg 1096, 1996).* Nature Medicine, 1996. 2(11): p. 1267-1267.

[225] Dankbar, B., et al., *Vascular endothelial growth factor and interleukin-6 in paracrine tumor-stromal cell interactions in multiple myeloma.* Blood, 2000. 95(8): p. 2630-2636.

[226] Neufeld, G., et al., *Vascular endothelial growth factor (VEGF) and its receptors.* The FASEB Journal, 1999. 13(1): p. 9-22.

[227] Li, J., et al., *Induction of Vascular Endothelial Growth Factor Gene Expression by Interleukin-1 in Rat Aortic Smooth Muscle Cells.* Journal of Biological Chemistry, 1995. 270(1): p. 308-312.

[228] Matsumoto, K., H. Ohi, and K. Kanmatsuse, *Interleukin 10 and interleukin 13 synergize to inhibit vascular permeability factor release by peripheral blood mononuclear cells from patients with lipoid nephrosis.* Nephron, 1997. 77(2): p. 212-218.

[229] Gupta, D., et al., *Adherence of multiple myeloma cells to bone marrow stromal cells upregulates vascular endothelial growth factor secretion: therapeutic applications.* Leukemia, 2001. 15(12): p. 1950-1961.

[230] Goad, D.L., et al., *Enhanced expression of vascular endothelial growth factor in human SaOS-2 osteoblast-like cells and murine osteoblasts induced by insulin-like growth factor I.* Endocrinology, 1996. 137(6): p. 2262-8.

[231] Deroanne, C.F., et al., *Angiogenesis by Fibroblast Growth Factor 4 Is Mediated through an Autocrine Up-Regulation of Vascular Endothelial Growth Factor Expression.* Cancer Research, 1997. 57(24): p. 5590-5597.

[232] Finkenzeller, G., et al., *Sp1 recognition sites in the proximal promoter of the human vascular endothelial growth factor gene are essential for platelet-derived growth factor-induced gene expression.* Oncogene, 1997. 15(6): p. 669-76.

[233] Pertovaara, L., et al., *Vascular endothelial growth factor is induced in response to transforming growth factor-beta in fibroblastic and epithelial cells.* Journal of Biological Chemistry, 1994. 269(9): p. 6271-6274.

[234] Ryuto, M., et al., *Induction of Vascular Endothelial Growth Factor by Tumor Necrosis Factor a in Human Glioma Cells.* Journal of Biological Chemistry, 1996. 271(45): p. 28220-28228.

[235] Wang, T.-H., et al., *Human Chorionic Gonadotropin-Induced Ovarian Hyperstimulation Syndrome Is Associated with Up-Regulation of Vascular Endothelial Growth Factor.* Journal of Clinical Endocrinology & Metabolism, 2002. 87(7): p. 3300-3308.

[236] Hurt, E.M., et al., *Overexpression of c-maf is a frequent oncogenic event in multiple myeloma that promotes proliferation and pathological interactions with bone marrow stroma.* Cancer cell, 2004. 5(2): p. 191-199.

[237] Gerber, H.P., et al., *Vascular endothelial growth factor regulates endothelial cell survival through the phosphatidylinositol 3'-kinase/Akt signal transduction pathway: Requirement for Flk-1/KDR activation.* Journal of Biological Chemistry, 1998. 273(46): p. 30336-30343.

[238] Podar, K., et al., *Vascular Endothelial Growth Factor-induced Migration of Multiple Myeloma Cells Is Associated with β1 Integrin- and Phosphatidylinositol 3-Kinase-dependent PKCa Activation.* Journal of Biological Chemistry, 2002. 277(10): p. 7875-7881.

[239] Qi, J.H. and L. Claesson-Welsh, *VEGF-induced activation of phosphoinositide 3-kinase is dependent on focal adhesion kinase.* Experimental Cell Research, 2001. 263(1): p. 173-182.

[240] Waltenberger, J., et al., *DIFFERENT SIGNAL-TRANSDUCTION PROPERTIES OF KDR AND FLT1, 2 RECEPTORS FOR VASCULAR ENDOTHELIAL GROWTH-FACTOR.* Journal of Biological Chemistry, 1994. 269(43): p. 26988-26995.

[241] Le Gouill, S., et al., *VEGF induces Mcl-1 up-regulation and protects multiple myeloma cells against apoptosis.* Blood, 2004. 104(9): p. 2886-2892.

[242] Meyer, R.D., et al., *The presence of a single tyrosine residue at the carboxyl domain of vascular endothelial growth factor receptor-2/FLK-1 regulates its autophosphorylation and activation of signaling molecules.* Journal of Biological Chemistry, 2002. 277(30): p. 27081-27087.

[243] Rousseau, S., et al., *Vascular Endothelial Growth Factor (VEGF)-driven Actin-based Motility Is Mediated by VEGFR2 and Requires Concerted Activation of Stress-activated Protein Kinase 2 (SAPK2/p38) and Geldanamycin-sensitive Phosphorylation of Focal Adhesion Kinase.* Journal of Biological Chemistry, 2000. 275(14): p. 10661-10672.

[244] Kim, K.J., et al., *Inhibition of vascular endothelial growth factor-induced angiogenesis suppresses tumour growth in vivo.* Nature, 1993. 362(6423): p. 841-844.

[245] Ferrara, N., et al., *Discovery and development of bevacizumab, an anti-VEGF antibody for treating cancer.* Nat Rev Drug Discov, 2004. 3(5): p. 391-400.

[246] Lin, B., et al., *The Vascular Endothelial Growth Factor Receptor Tyrosine Kinase Inhibitor PTK787/ZK222584 Inhibits Growth and Migration of Multiple Myeloma Cells in the Bone Marrow Microenvironment.* Cancer Research, 2002. 62(17): p. 5019-5026.

[247] Wood, J.M., et al., *PTK787/ZK 222584, a Novel and Potent Inhibitor of Vascular Endothelial Growth Factor Receptor Tyrosine Kinases, Impairs Vascular Endothelial Growth Factor-induced Responses and Tumor Growth after Oral Administration.* Cancer Research, 2000. 60(8): p. 2178-2189.

[248] Sloan, B. and N.S. Scheinfeld, *Pazopanib, a VEGF receptor tyrosine kinase inhibitor for cancer therapy.* Current Opinion in Investigational Drugs, 2008. 9(12): p. 1324-1335.

[249] Thiery, J.P., *Cell adhesion in cancer.* Comptes Rendus Physique, 2003. 4(2): p. 289-304.

[250] Sanz-Rodríguez, F. and J. Teixidó, *VLA-4-dependent myeloma cell adhesion.* Leukemia and Lymphoma, 2001. 41(3-4): p. 239-245.

[251] Sanz-Rodríguez, F., et al., *Characterization of VLA-4-dependent myeloma cell adhesion to fibronectin and VCAM-1.* British Journal of Haematology, 1999. 107(4): p. 825-834.

[252] Uchiyama, H., et al., *Characterization of adhesion molecules on human myeloma cell lines.* Blood, 1992. 80(9): p. 2306-2314.

[253] Sanz-Rodríguez, F., A. Hidalgo, and J. Teixidó, *Chemokine stromal cell-derived factor-1a modulates VLA-4 integrin-mediated multiple myeloma cell adhesion to CS-1/fibronectin and VCAM-1.* Blood, 2001. 97(2): p. 346-351.

[254] Damiano, J.S., et al., *Cell adhesion mediated drug resistance (CAM-DR): Role of integrins and resistance to apoptosis in human myeloma cell lines.* Blood, 1999. 93(5): p. 1658-1667.

[255] Landowski, T.H., et al., *Cell adhesion-mediated drug resistance (CAM-DR) is associated with activation of NF-κB (RelB/p50) in myeloma cells.* Oncogene, 2003. 22(16): p. 2417-2421.

[256] Shain, K.H., et al., *β1 integrin adhesion enhances IL-6-mediated STAT3 signaling in myeloma cells: Implications for microenvironment influence on tumor survival and proliferation.* Cancer research, 2009. 69(3): p. 1009-1015.

[257] Fulciniti, M., et al., *A high-affinity fully human anti-IL-6 mAb, 1339, for the treatment of multiple myeloma.* Clinical Cancer Research, 2009. 15(23): p. 7144-7152.

[258] Hideshima, T., et al., *Proteasome inhibitor PS-341 abrogates IL-6 triggered signaling cascades via caspase-dependent downregulation of gp130 in multiple myeloma.* Oncogene, 2003. 22(52): p. 8386-8393.

[259] Tai, Y.T., et al., *Human anti-CD40 antagonist antibody triggers significant antitumor activity against human multiple myeloma.* Cancer research, 2005. 65(13): p. 5898-5906.

[260] Voorhees, P.M., et al., *Inhibition of interleukin-6 signaling with CNTO 328 enhances the activity of bortezomib in preclinical models of multiple myeloma.* Clinical Cancer Research, 2007. 13(21): p. 6469-6478.

[261] Hunsucker, S.A., et al., *Blockade of interleukin-6 signalling with siltuximab enhances melphalan cytotoxicity in preclinical models of multiple myeloma.* British Journal of Haematology, 2011. 152(5): p. 579-592.

[262] Voorhees, P.M., et al., *Targeted inhibition of interleukin-6 with CNTO 328 sensitizes pre-clinical models of multiple myeloma to dexamethasone-mediated cell death.* British Journal of Haematology, 2009. 145(4): p. 481-490.

[263] Todoerti, K., et al., *Pleiotropic anti-myeloma activity of ITF2357: Inhibition of interleukin-6 receptor signaling and repression of miR-19a and miR-19b.* Haematologica, 2010. 95(2): p. 260-269.

[264] Bisping, G., et al., *Targeting receptor kinases by a novel indolinone derivative in multiple myeloma: Abrogation of stroma-derived interleukin-6 secretion and induction of apoptosis in cytogenetically defined subgroups.* Blood, 2006. 107(5): p. 2079-2089.

[265] Tassone, P., et al., *Combination therapy with interleukin-6 receptor superantagonist Sant7 and dexamethasone induces antitumor effects in a novel SCID-hu in vivo model of human multiple myeloma.* Clinical Cancer Research, 2005. 11(11): p. 4251-4258.

[266] Lamm, W., et al., *Bortezomib combined with rituximab and dexamethasone is an active regimen for patients with relapsed and chemotherapy-refractory mantle cell lymphoma.* Haematologica, 2011. 96(7): p. 1008-1014.

[267] Wemeau, M., S. Balkaran, and X. Leleu, *Increased sensitivity to bortezomib after mobilization of multiple myeloma cells with the CXCR4 antagonist AMD3100.* Majoration de la sensibilité au bortézomib dans le myélome multiple en favorisant la migration des cellules tumorales dans le sang par un inhibiteur de CXCR4, l'AMD3100, 2009. 15(3): p. 194-196.

[268] Rossi, J.F., et al., *Atacicept in relapsed/refractory multiple myeloma or active Waldenstrom's macroglobulinemia: a phase I study.* Br J Cancer, 0000. 101(7): p. 1051-1058.

[269] Presta, L.G., et al., *Humanization of an Anti-Vascular Endothelial Growth Factor Monoclonal Antibody for the Therapy of Solid Tumors and Other Disorders.* Cancer Research, 1997. 57(20): p. 4593-4599.

[270] Lin, B., et al., *The vascular endothelial growth factor receptor tyrosine kinase inhibitor PTK787/ZK222584 inhibits growth and migration of multiple myeloma cells in the bone marrow microenvironment.* Cancer research, 2002. 62(17): p. 5019-5026.

[271] Hagedorn, M. and A. Bikfalvi, *Target molecules for anti-angiogenic therapy: from basic research to clinical trials.* Critical reviews in oncology/hematology, 2000. 34(2): p. 89-110.

[272] *Development of SU5416, a selective small molecule inhibitor of VEGF receptor tyrosine kinase activity, as an anti-angiogenesis agent.* Anti-Cancer Drug Design, 2000. 15: p. 29-41.

[273] Ramakrishnan, V., et al., *Sorafenib, a dual Raf kinase/vascular endothelial growth factor receptor inhibitor has significant anti-myeloma activity and synergizes with common anti-myeloma drugs.* Oncogene, 2010. 29(8): p. 1190-1202.

[274] Flier, J.S., P. Usher, and A.C. Moses, *Monoclonal antibody to the type I insulin-like growth factor (IGF-I) receptor blocks IGF-I receptor-mediated DNA synthesis: clarification of the*

mitogenic mechanisms of IGF-I and insulin in human skin fibroblasts. Proceedings of the National Academy of Sciences, 1986. 83(3): p. 664-668.

[275] Hayry, P., et al., *Stabile D-peptide analog of insulin-like growth factor-1 inhibits smooth muscle cell proliferation after carotid ballooning injury in the rat.* The FASEB Journal, 1995. 9(13): p. 1336-1344.

[276] Pietrzkowski, Z., et al., *Inhibition of Growth of Prostatic Cancer Cell Lines by Peptide Analogues of Insulin-like Growth Factor 1.* Cancer Research, 1993. 53(5): p. 1102-1106.

[277] *Insulin-Like Growth Factor 1 Receptor Targeted Therapeutics: Novel Compounds and Novel Treatment Strategies for Cancer Medicine.* Recent Patents on Anti-Cancer Drug Discovery, 2009. 4: p. 54-72.

[278] Hayashi, T., et al., *Transforming growth factor β receptor I kinase inhibitor down-regulates cytokine secretion and multiple myeloma cell growth in the bone marrow microenvironment.* Clinical Cancer Research, 2004. 10(22): p. 7540-7546.

[279] Beider, K., et al., *CXCR4 antagonist 4F-benzoyl-TN14003 inhibits leukemia and multiple myeloma tumor growth.* Experimental Hematology, 2011. 39(3): p. 282-292.

[280] Azab, A.K., et al., *CXCR4 inhibitor AMD3100 disrupts the interaction of multiple myeloma cells with the bone marrow microenvironment and enhances their sensitivity to therapy.* Blood, 2009. 113(18): p. 4341-4351.

[281] Oliveira, A.M., et al., *Thalidomide treatment down-regulates SDF-1a and CXCR4 expression in multiple myeloma patients.* Leukemia Research, 2009. 33(7): p. 970-973.

[282] Haridas, V., et al., *Avicin D: A protein reactive plant isoprenoid dephosphorylates Stat3 by regulating both kinase and phosphatase activities.* PLoS ONE, 2009. 4(5).

[283] Hamasaki, M., et al., *Azaspirane (N-N-diethyl-8,8-dipropyl-2-azaspiro [4.5] decane-2-propanamine) inhibits human multiple myeloma cell growth in the bone marrow milieu in vitro and in vivo.* Blood, 2005. 105(11): p. 4470-4476.

[284] Kannaiyan, R., et al., *Celastrol Inhibits Proliferation and Induces Chemosensitization through downregulation of NF-kappaB and STAT3 Regulated Gene Products in Multiple Myeloma Cells.* Br J Pharmacol, 2011.

[285] Burger, R., et al., *Janus kinase inhibitor INCB20 has antiproliferative and apoptotic effects on human myeloma cells in vitro and in vivo.* Molecular cancer therapeutics, 2009. 8(1): p. 26-35.

[286] Sandur, S.K., et al., *5-Hydroxy-2-methyl-1,4-naphthoquinone, a vitamin K3 analogue, suppresses STAT3 activation pathway through induction of protein tyrosine phosphatase, SHP-1: Potential role in chemosensitization.* Molecular Cancer Research, 2010. 8(1): p. 107-118.

[287] Bhardwaj, A., et al., *Resveratrol inhibits proliferation, induces apoptosis, and overcomes chemoresistance through down-regulation of STAT3 and nuclear factor-κB-regulated antiapoptotic and cell survival gene products in human multiple myeloma cells.* Blood, 2007. 109(6): p. 2293-2302.

[288] Khong, T., J. Sharkey, and A. Spencer, *The effect of azacitidine on interleukin-6 signaling and nuclear factor-κB activation and its in vitro and in vivo activity against multiple myeloma.* Haematologica, 2008. 93(6): p. 860-869.

[289] Dai, Y., et al., *Interruption of the NF-κB pathway by Bay 11-7082 promotes UCN-01-mediated mitochondrial dysfunction and apoptosis in human multiple myeloma cells.* Blood, 2004. 103(7): p. 2761-2770.

[290] He, H., et al., *Genistein down-regulates the constitutive activation of nuclear factor-κB of bone marrow stromal cells in multiple myeloma, leading to suppression of gene expression and proliferation.* Drug Development Research, 2008. 69(4): p. 219-225.

[291] Hideshima, T., et al., *MLN120B, a novel IκB kinase β inhibitor, blocks multiple myeloma cell growth in vitro and in vivo.* Clinical Cancer Research, 2006. 12(19): p. 5887-5894.

[292] Kong, F., et al., *Inhibitory effects of parthenolide on the angiogenesis induced by human multiple myeloma cells and the mechanism.* Journal of Huazhong University of Science and Technology - Medical Science, 2008. 28(5): p. 525-530.

[293] Hossain, Z., et al., *Chitosan and marine phospholipids reduce matrix metalloproteinase activity in myeloma SP2 tumor-bearing mice.* European Journal of Lipid Science and Technology, 2009. 111(9): p. 877-883.

[294] Ritchie, J.P., et al., *SST0001, a chemically modified heparin, inhibits myeloma growth and angiogenesis via disruption of the heparanase/syndecan-1 axis.* Clinical Cancer Research, 2011. 17(6): p. 1382-1393.

[295] Mori, Y., et al., *Anti-a4 integrin antibody suppresses the development of multiple myeloma and associated osteoclastic osteolysis.* Blood, 2004. 104(7): p. 2149-2154.

[296] Olson, D.L., et al., *Anti-a4 integrin monoclonal antibody inhibits multiple myeloma growth in a murine model.* Molecular cancer therapeutics, 2005. 4(1): p. 91-99.

[297] Wang, X., Z. Zhang, and C. Yao, *Targeting integrin-linked kinase increases apoptosis and decreases invasion of myeloma cell lines and inhibits IL-6 and VEGF secretion from BMSCs.* Medical Oncology, 2010: p. 1-5.

6

The SUMOylation Pathway as a Potential Therapeutic Target in Multiple Myeloma

James J. Driscoll
Division of Hematology and Oncology, Department of Internal Medicine
University of Cincinnati Medical Center and Barrett Cancer Center
Cincinnati, OH
Medical Oncology Branch, National Cancer Institute, National Institutes of Health
Bethesda, MD
USA

1. Introduction

The Ubiquitin+Proteasome System (UPS) represents a successful anti-cancer strategy that has translated from preclinical studies to clinical development and significantly improved the survival of Multiple Myeloma (MM) patients (1). The proteasome is high molecular weight structure that contains multiple proteolytic sites and functions as the catalytic core of the UPS to degrade Ub~conjugated proteins (2-4). Inhibition of the proteasome's chymotryptic-like peptidase activity blocks the entire UPS and leads to selective tumor cell death. Bortezomib is the first proteasome inhibitor used in human clinical trials and treatment leads to a reduction in tumor burden in MM patients (5,6). However, cellular resistance to proteasome-based therapy generally results and reduces the efficacy. Resistance to proteasome inhibitors may result from altered expression of either proteasome or non-proteasome encoding genes. SUMOylation is a post-translational modification that attaches a **S**mall **U**biquitin-like **MO**difier to target proteins and, similar to Ub, may target proteins for proteasomal degradation. Gene expression profiling of MM patient samples indicated that bortezomib resistance may be achieved through induction of non-proteasome components. Importantly, certain effectors of the SUMOylation pathway were induced in the samples of MM patients that did not respond to bortezomib. A molecular-based, biologically-relevant supervised approach was used to identify a compendium of genes within the SUMO+UPS that were induced in MM patients and correlated with a decreased response to bortezomib. This molecular approach is relevant to a heterogeneous disease like MM where patients with similar clinical and pathologic features have vastly different genetic mutations responsible for disease and varying responses to therapies and clinical outcomes. The potential role of the SUMOylation pathway is only beginning to emerge, however, evidence indicates that SUMOylation is induced in myelomagenesis and also in bortezomib-resistant cells.

An aggresome is a proteinaceous inclusion body that forms when the cellular protein degradation machinery is impaired or overwhelmed and leads to an accumulation of proteins for disposal (7,8). Aggresome formation is thought to represent a cellular protective response to the presence of abnormal, misfolded or damaged proteins within the cytoplasm that cannot be eliminated by the UPS. Aggresomes form adjacent to the microtubule-organizing center (MTOC) and neighboring the centrosome. The microtubule-based motor protein dynein, heat shock proteins and the histone deacetylase 6 (HDAC6) have been reported as aggresome components (9). HDAC6 specifically functions as an adaptor protein between the dynein motor protein and accumulating polyubiquitinated substrate proteins. The protein aggregates that reside in an aggresome are sequestered in a cage that consists largely of intermediate filaments. Aggresome formation may serve as an alternative mechanism to eliminate the cytotoxic effect of accumulated Ub~protein conjugates. Recent evidence indicates that SUMOylation effectors and SUMO-modified proteins are related to aggresome formation. Inhibition of SUMOylation could preclude aggresome formation and consequently overcome bortezomib resistance.

The formation of the aggresome functions as a mechanism not only to sequester potentially cytotoxic aggregates but also to serve as a platform for the eventual autophagic clearance of these aggregates (10, 11). Autophagy is a catabolic process that involves the degradation of the cell's own constituents through the lysosomal machinery (12, 13). It is a tightly-regulated process that plays a normal part in cell growth, development, and homeostasis and maintains the balance between the synthesis, degradation and subsequent recycling of cellular products. It is a major mechanism by which a starving cell reallocates nutrients from unnecessary processes to more-essential processes. A variety of autophagic processes exist, all having in common the degradation of intracellular components through the lysosome. The most well-known mechanism of autophagy involves the formation of a membrane around a targeted region of the cell, separating the contents from the rest of the cytoplasm. The resultant vesicle then fuses with a lysosome and subsequently degrades the contents.

Importantly, new evidence indicates upon proteasome inhibition, the accumulated Ub~protein conjugates are bound by autophagy cargo receptors for clearance (14, 15). Thus, it appears that aggresome formation is a prerequisite for autophagic clearance of Ub~protein conjugates (16). In addition, selective autophagy may serve to eliminate these aggregates and overcome proteasome inhibition and yield drug resistance. It remains to be determined whether SUMOylated proteins are also cleared by autophagic clearance. However, inhibition of the SUMOylation pathwya may prevent aggresome formation, impede their autophagic clearance of Ub~protein conjugates and overcome bortezomib resistance. Future studies will address these questions and may yield new therapeutic targets, novel anti-cancer agents and lead to improved strategies for the treatment of MM and other malignancies.

2. Clinical success of proteasome inhibitor-based therapy in multiple myeloma

Multiple myeloma (MM) is a hematologic neoplasm of B-cell origin characterized by the clonal proliferation and progressive accumulation of malignant plasma cells within the bone marrow. MM accounts for greater than 10% of all hematologic cancers and in spite of conventional high-dose chemotherapies, remains uniformly fatal, in part, because of either intrinsic (primary) or acquired (secondary) drug resistance. Recent advances in translational medicine have led to the development of molecularly-based targeted therapies as well as highly effective synergistic drug combinations that have the potential to achieve a higher frequency of durable responses in a greater number of MM patients. Molecular, genomic and proteomic studies have further increased understanding of the biology of myelomagenesis, provided the basis for better prognostic classification in the context of uniform therapies and generated a sound rationale for combining targeted therapies in current and emerging clinical development.

The 26S proteasome is a high-molecular weight, multi-subunit complex that consists of a 20S catalytic core and a 19S regulatory particle. Proteasomes are found in eukaryotes, archaebacteria and some bacteria. The 20S proteasome functions as the catalytic core of the ubiquitin-proteasome system to hydrolyze proteins into short polypeptide and is capable of hydrolyzing peptides C-terminal to chymotryptic, tryptic or acidic residues. 20S proteasomes are cylindrical structures composed of four stacked rings with each ring composed of seven individual subunits. The two inner rings are made of seven *β subunits* that contain the various active sites and the two outer rings are each composed of seven *a subunits*. The two outer rings comprised of α subunits are then bound at either pole by the 19S regulatory particles.

Proteasome inhibition is a promising therapeutic strategy for the treatment of an increasing number of B cell malignancies, especially MM. Bortezomib is a low molecular weight boron-based agent that inhibits the chymotryptic-like activity of the proteasome. Inhibition of the chymotryptic-like activity inhibits all proteasome activity and acts as a blockade of the entire ubiquitin+proteasome pathway. The result is the intracellular accumulation of Ub~protein conjugates, activation of cellular stress sensors and eventually cell death. The selective cytotoxic effect of proteasome inhibition on tumor cells further validated protein degradation as a therapeutic target in oncology and has been translated in the treatment of certain malignancies. Bortezomib was US Food and Drug Administration (FDA) approved for the treatment of newly diagnosed, relapsed and refractory MM. The introduction of bortezomib into the treatment of MM resulted in a paradigm shift and significantly improved patient survival. The concurrent targeting of both the tumor cell as well as the surrounding bone marrow microenvironment may promote tumor cell death and efficacy. The FDA has recently approved a more effective three drug combination of bortezomib, lenalidomide and dexamethasone for the treatment of MM that may act on the malignant plasma cell and also to counteract the protective effect of the bone marrow milieu.

Many MM patients, however, exhibit an intrinsic (primary) resistance and do not initially respond to bortezomib. Furthermore, in those patients that do respond, clinical efficacy is dampened by the inevitable emergence of acquired drug-resistance that eventually develops through unidentified mechanisms. While bortezomib has significantly transformed the management of MM, the mechanism(s) of action and bases of individual patient susceptibility remain unclear. These recent advances in mechanistic understanding and treatment modalities have extended median survival to >6 years and 10% of patients now survive >10 years. However, the vast majority of MM remains incurable even with these strategies.

Though the catabolism of ubiquitinated substrates has been targeted therapeutically with significantly improved prognosis, patient response to bortezomib remains highly variable and cannot be predicted accurately. E3 Ub ligases are the specific components of the UPS that recognize substrates for degradation and confer specificity on target selection for the UPS. Therefore, the expression of individual E3's was analyzed using a microarray dataset obtained from MM patient tumor samples and found a striking variability in the expression level of individual E3 Ub ligases between normal plasma cells and patients MM cells. Specifically, RNF4, an E3 specific for poly-sumoylated proteins, was induced in MM patients and correlated with decreased patient response to the proteasome inhibitor bortezomib. Expression profiling of pretreatment tumor samples obtained from MM patients in independent clinical trials were used to generate a signature that correlated expression of SUMO+Ub+Proteasome pathway components with clinical outcome to predict patient response to bortezomib.

3. The Ub+Proteasome System (UPS) and the Ub-like SUMOylation pathway

The UPS regulates numerous critical cellular processes by maintaining the appropriate intracellular level of key proteins. Whereas *de novo* protein synthesis is a comparatively slow process, proteins are rapidly degraded at a rate compatible with the control of cell cycle transitions and cell death induction. The critical role played by Ub-mediated protein turnover in cell cycle regulation makes this process a high-value target for oncogenic mutations. SUMO proteins are similar to ubiquitin, and SUMOylation is directed by an three-step enzymatic cascade analogous to that involved in ubiquitination. SUMOylation is a highly dynamic, reversible, post-translational protein modification, similar to ubiquitination that attaches a family of polypeptides to target proteins to modify their function, subcellular localization or stability. A role for SUMOylation in the UPS has been established since SUMO attachment signals the recruitment of specific E3 Ub ligases to target proteins, e.g., PML, PEA, PARP-1 and HIF1-alpha, for ubiquitination and proteasomal degradation. Induction of individual SUMOylation and UPS effectors has been demonstrated in MM cell lines and patient samples and SUMO pathway induction has been correlated with resistance to bortezomib-based therapy. Similarly, proteasome components are induced in bortezomib-resistant cells ad ndecrease the toxic accumulation of Ub~conjugates. The mechanistic link of SUMOylation to proteasomal resistance is uncertain. An important unresolved issue is the clinical significance of sumoylation during proteasomal degradation and proteasome inhibitor-based therapy. SUMOylation was recently shown to have a role in proteasomal degradation since SUMO-2/3 attachment can signal Ub-dependent degradation. Novel RING family Ub ligases, e.g., RNF4, bear SUMO interaction motifs and have been implicated in the proteasomal degradation of SUMO-modified target protein PML. Similarly, the E3 Ub ligase von Hippel–Lindau (VHL) has been reported to control the levels of sumoylated HIF-1α while VHL and RNF4 control the levels of HIF-2□ to indicate that sumoylated HIF-2α is degraded through SUMO-targeted ubiquitination. SUMO modification as a signal for degradation is conserved in eukaryotes and Ub ligases that specifically recognize SUMO-modified proteins have been discovered from yeasts to humans. proteasome components to further link the pathways. Individual components of the sumoylation pathway serve as biomarkers to predict clinical response to bortezomib and provide evidence for targeting SUMO pathway to improve therapeutic outcome in myeloma in general and specifically in combination with proteasome inhibitors.

SUMO modification as a signal for degradation is conserved in eukaryotes and Ub ligases that specifically recognize SUMO-modified proteins have been discovered from yeasts to humans. E3 Ub ligases are engaged in the recognition of biologically relevant proteins that are degraded by the proteasome. While proteasome inhibition generates the accumulation of Ub~conjugated proteins and ultimately cell death, the selectivity of this process and the role of individual E3 ligases has not been previously addressed. We investigated whether UPS effectors and specifically, E3 ligases were differentially expressed in MM patients and whether expression correlated with resistance to bortezomib-based therapy. Recently, we demonstrated that genes encoding SUMOylation pathway effectors were induced during myelomagenesis and correlated with decreased patient survival.

4. Aggresomes and proteasome-based therapy

Aggresomes are novel cellular structures that employ HDAC6 to sequester and transport protein aggregates to the autophagy-lysosome system for efficient disposal. These poorly defined structures have been shown to consist of HDAC6, microtubules, heat shock proteins and ubiquitin. Aggresome formation is induced by a number of cellular and genotoxic stressors, including proteasomal inhibition. These structures may represent a potential compensatory mechanism to for cells to eliminate Ub~protein conjugates that accumulate upon proteasomal inhibiton. The result may be resistance to proteasome inhibitors and promote tumor survival. Similar to Ub, the small Ub-like MOdifier (SUMO) is attached to target certain proteins for proteasomal degradation but an association with aggresomes has not been established. The proteasome is limited in its capacity to degrade certain proteins, such as membrane-associated, oligomeric and protein aggregates. SUMOylation, like ubiquitination, may be mechanistically and biologically linked to aggresomes to promote the removal of toxic proteins that accumulate upon proteasomal inhibition. SUMOylation may also be required for the formation of aggresomes. Genetic or pharmacologic targeting of SUMOylation pathway effectors may impair functioning and formation of aggresomes to overcome drug resistance and enhance the cytotoxicity of proteasome inhibitors.

5. Autophagy

Removal of harmful protein aggregates is mediated by autophagy, a mechanism that sequesters cytosolic cargo and delivers it to the lysosome (17-20). Autophagy is of great importance for cellular homeostasis and survival, while its deregulation has been linked to pathological conditions, e.g., certain neurodegenerative diseases and cancer (21-23). The process of autophagy for many years has been thought of as a random degradative process to eliminate long-lived cell constituents. However, recent evidence indicates that autophagy can be selective and mediated through specialized Ub-binding cargo receptors.

The involvement of Ub as a specificity factor for selective autophagy has resulted in a rapid emergence of studies that have demonstrated active communication between the UPS and the aggresome-autophagy-lysosomal system (25). The identification and characterization of autophagy receptors, such as p62/SQSTM1, NBR1, p97/ VCP which can simultaneously bind both Ub and autophagy-specific Ub-like modifiers, e.g., LC3/GABARAP, and possible SUMO has provided a molecular link between the UPS and autophagy (26-28). Since the UPS regulates the selective degradation of certain short-lived, mutant and misfolded proteins, autophagy may remove not only aggregates which are comprised of long-lived proteins but also UPS substrates. Selective autophagy may protect cells from oxidative and genotoxic stresses. In addition, this process may remove Ub~ and SUMO~protein conjugates that accumulate upon proteasome inhibition and overcome the cytotoxic effect of bortezomib. Induction of selective autophagy may be induced in tumor cells to provide a mechanism of cell survival and drug resistance (29, 30). Selective autophagy represents a promising new pathway to investigate as means to overcome resistance to proteasome inhibitors and further advance the treatment of MM.

6. Conclusions

Multiple myeloma accounts for a substantial amount of all hematologic malignancies seen worldwide. In the US and Europe, the incidence of MM exceeds 40,000 cases annual. MM has assumed a position of prominence as a model system for preclinical studies, drug development and clinical trials. Unlike other malignancies, in which surgery and radiation are important treatment modalities, MM is nearly exclusively treated with stem cell transplantation (SCT) or synergistic chemotherapeutic combinations. SCT has produced statistically significant survival benefit for MM patients. However, a number of MM patients are not eligible for SCT either because of age, toxicities and many patients can relapse. Novel therapeutic agents such as the immunomodulatory agents and bortezomib have revolutionized therapy and improved overall survival. However, despite these advances, MM remains largely incurable as disease relapse is inevitable. Therefore, there is an urgent need for new, tolerable agents that demonstrate the ability to either overcome or prevent drug resistance. The role of the SUMOylation pathway in Multiple Myeloma is only beginning to be understood and appears to be a novel therapeutic target that can be used not only to treat MM but also to overcome drug resistance. Future studies will address the role of this emerging pathway in myelomagenesis.

7. References

[1] Hideshima T, Bradner JE, Chauhan D, Anderson KC. Intracellular protein degradation and its therapeutic implications. Clin Cancer Res 2005;11:8530-8533.

[2] Hershko, A. and Ciechanover, A. The ubiquitin system. Annu. Rev. Biochem. 1998; 67, 425-479.

[3] Kirkin V, Dikic I. Ubiquitin networks in cancer. Curr Opin Genet Dev. 2011, 21:21-28.

[4] Kerscher O, Felberbaum R, Hochstrasser M. Modification of proteins by ubiquitin and ubiquitin-like proteins. Annu Rev Cell Dev Biol. 2006;22:159–180.

[5] Hideshima T, Bradner JE, Wong J, et al. Small-molecule inhibition of proteasome and aggresome function induces synergistic antitumor activity in multiple myeloma. Proc Natl Acad Sci U S A 2005;102(24):8567-8572.

[6] Mitsiades CS, Davies FE, Laubach JP, et al. Future directions of next-generation novel therapies, combination approaches, and the development of personalized medicine in myeloma. J Clin Oncol 2011 29:1916–1923.

[7] Kopito, R R. Aggresomes, inclusion bodies and protein aggregation. Trends Cell Biol. 2000; 10:524-30.

[8] Pang, T. The Role of Ubiquitin in Autophagy-Dependent Protein Aggregate Processing Genes and Cancer 2010; 779- 786.

[9] Kawaguchi, Y., Kovacs, J. J., McLaurin, A., Vance, J. M., Ito, A., and Yao, T.-P. The deacetylase HDAC6 regulates aggresome formation and cell viability in response to misfolded protein stress. Cell. 115. 727-738 (2003).
[10] Kirkin V, McEwan DG, Novak I, Dikic I., A Role for Ubiquitin in Selective Autophagy. Mol Cell 2010; 34:259-269.
[11] Kondo Y, Kanzawa T, Sawaya R, Kondo S. The role of autophagy in cancer development and response to therapy. Nat Rev Cancer 2005; 5: 726–34.
[12] White E., DiPaola R. S. The Double-Edged Sword of Autophagy Modulation in Cancer. *Clin. Cancer Res.* 2009 15, 5308–5316.
[13] 50. Mathew R, et al. Role of autophagy in cancer. *Nat Rev Cancer.* 2007;7:961–967.
[14] I. Dikic, T. Johansen, V. Kirkin, Selective autophagy in cancer development and therapy. Cancer Res. 70, 3431–3434 (2010).
[15] Amaravadi, R.K., Thompson, C.B. 2007. The roles of therapy-induced autophagy and necrosis in cancer treatment. Clin. Cancer Res. 13:7271-7279.
[16] Hoeller D, Dikic I. Targeting the ubiquitin system in cancer therapy. Nature; 2009; 458 (7237): 438-44.
[17] Dikic I, Johansen T, Kirkin V. Selective autophagy in cancer development and therapy. Cancer Res. 2010, 70(9):3431-4.
[18] Kraft C, Peter M, Hofmann K. Selective autophagy: ubiquitin-mediated recognition and beyond. Nat Cell Biol. 2010;12:836–841.
[19] Amaravadi RK, Lippincott-Schwartz J, Yin XM, Weiss WA, Takebe N, Timmer W, DiPaola RS, Lotze MT, White E. (2011) Principles and current strategies for targeting autophagy for cancer treatment. Clin Cancer Res. Feb 15;17(4):654-66.
[20] White, E., and DiPaola, R. S. (2009). The double-edged sword of autophagy modulation in cancer. Clinical Cancer Res. 15(17):5308-16.
[21] Levine B. and Kroemer G. Autophagy in the pathogenesis of disease. Cell 2008; 132:27–42.
[22] Shintani T, Klionsky DJ. Autophagy in health and disease: a double-edged sword. Science 2004; 306: 990–5.
[23] Rubinsztein DC: The roles of intracellular protein-degradation pathways in neurodegeneration. Nature 2006, 443:780-786.
[24] Korolchuk VI, Menzies FM, Rubinsztein DC. Mechanisms of cross-talk between the ubiquitin-proteasome and autophagy-lysosome systems. FEBS Lett 584: 1393–1398, 2010.
[25] Lee, J.-Y. and T.-P. Yao (2010). "Quality control autophagy: A joint effort of ubiquitin, protein deacetylase and actin cytoskeleton." Autophagy 6(4): 555-557.
[26] Xie Z, Klionsky DJ. Autophagosome formation: core machinery and adaptations. Nat Cell Biol. 2007;9:1102–1109.
[27] Komatsu M, Waguri S, Koike M, et al. Homeostatic levels of p62 control cytoplasmic inclusion body formation in autophagy-deficient mice. Cell 2007;131:1149–63.
[28] 35. Kirkin V, Lamark T, Sou Y, Bjorkoy G, Nunn J, Bruun J, Shvets E, Mc Ewan D, Clausen T, Wild P, Bilusic I, Theurillat JP, Overvatn A, Ishii T, Elazar Z, Komatsu M, Dikic I, Johansen T (2009) A role for NBR1 in autophagosomal degradation of ubiquitinated substrates. Mol Cell 33:505-516
[29] Hoang B, Benavides A, Shi Y, Frost P, Lichtenstein A. Effect of autophagy on multiple myeloma cell viability. Mol Cancer Ther2009;8:1974–84.

[30] Catley L, Weisberg E, Kiziltepe T, et al.(2006) Aggresome induction by proteasome inhibitor bortezomib and alpha-tubulin hyperacetylation by tubulin deacetylase (TDAC) inhibitor LBH589 are synergistic in myeloma cells. Blood 2006, 108:3441-3449.

7

Therapeutic Approaches for Targeting Hypoxia-Inducible Factor in Multiple Myeloma

Keita Kirito
University of Yamanashi
Japan

1. Introduction

1.1 Regulation of HIF function

Hypoxia-inducible factor (HIF) is a transcription factor that is a master regulator of cellular responses to hypoxia and regulates many genes that are required for adaptation to hypoxia. [1]HIF is composed of two subunits, HIFα and HIFβ. HIFα is composed of three family members, HIF-1α, HIF-2α and HIF-3α. [2]Among these family members, HIF-1α and HIF-2α play crucial roles in hypoxic responses. HIF activity is regulated via two mechanisms in response to hypoxia. First, HIFα expression is dependent on oxygen levels. [1] Under normoxic conditions, HIFα is hydroxylated at specific proline residues via prolyl-hydroxylase domain proteins (PHDs). The enzymatic activities of PHDs are dependent on oxygen levels. Hydroxylation of the proline residues of HIFs increases the interaction of HIFα with the von Hippel-Lindau (VHL) proteins, which recruit an E3 ubiquitin-protein ligase. In turn, HIFα is ubiquitinated and subsequently degraded by the proteasome. In hypoxic conditions, PHD activity is suppressed and HIFα degradation is reduced. In addition to protein levels, oxygen levels control the transcriptional activities of HIFs. [2]The factors that inhibit HIF (FIHs) play central roles in the process. At normoxic conditions, FIHs catalyze hydroxylation of asparagine residues of HIFα, which represses the interaction of HIF with the transcriptional coactivator CBP/P300. Using these mechanisms, HIF is activated during hypoxia under normal physiological conditions.

2. Abnormal activation of HIFs in multiple myeloma

Under physiological conditions, HIFs are active during hypoxia. However, HIFs can be activated in many types of cancer cells, even under normoxic conditions, by oncogene products, impaired activities of tumor suppressor genes,[3] or the accumulation of metabolic glucose intermediates. [4] HIFs are known to be activated in multiple myeloma cells. The hypoxic microenvironment of multiple myeloma bone marrow and oxygen-independent mechanisms contribute to abnormal activation of HIFs in myeloma cells. Asosingh and colleagues reported HIF-1α expression in 5T2 MM cells in the mouse myeloma model. [5]These researchers showed that the hypoxic microenvironment of the bone marrow contributed to HIF-1 activation, especially in the initial stages of the disease. [5] Hypoxia-induced HIF-1α expression in myeloma cells in multiple myeloma bone marrow was reported by Hu et al, who used the murine 5T3MM myeloma model to demonstrate that the majority of myeloma cells localize in an extensively hypoxic region and show strong expression of HIF-1α. [6]The correlation between bone marrow hypoxia and HIF-1 activation in multiple myeloma cells was detected in human clinical samples. [7] Colla and colleagues analyzed the expression of HIF-1α in bone marrow biopsies and demonstrated HIF-1α immunostaining in the nuclei of myeloma cells in all multiple myeloma patients. [7] Additionally, Colla and colleagues analyzed oxygen levels of bone marrow samples from multiple myeloma patients and found that the bone marrow of the myeloma patients was hypoxic. The researchers speculated that this hypoxia may cause the accumulation of HIF-1α. However, the oxygen levels in the bone marrow of healthy volunteers were equivalent to those of myeloma patients. Therefore, it is not clear whether a reduced oxygen level in the bone marrow is the only inducer of HIF-1α expression. Colla and colleagues detected HIF-1α protein in isolated CD138-positive myeloma cells in approximately 28% of myeloma patients in normoxic conditions. [7] These observations suggest that the hypoxia-independent mechanisms regulate HIF-1α in multiple myeloma cells. Our group detected constitutive expression of HIF-1α in several multiple myeloma cell lines and in CD138-positive primary myeloma cells even in normoxic conditions. [8] We found that growth factors for myeloma cells, including insulin-like growth factor-1 (IGF-1) and IL-6, enhanced the expression of HIF-1α in myeloma cells through activation of AKT. LY294002, which is an inhibitor of PI3-kinase and AKT, inhibited IGF-1-induced HIF-1α elevation. [8] The oncogene product c-Myc is also involved in aberrant activation of HIF-1 under normoxia. [9] [10]Downregulation of c-Myc by chemical inhibitors or siRNA diminished HIF-1α expression levels in myeloma cells. [9] Increased DNA methylation was detected in the promoter region of VHL[11] and PHD[12] genes in myeloma cells and may contribute to abnormal HIF activation. In addition to protein levels, transcriptional activity of HIFs is modulated in multiple myeloma cells. The inhibitor of growth family member 4 (ING4) is a tumor suppressor gene that is involved in the process. Colla et al. found that myeloma cells showed reduced ING4 expression, which inversely correlated with the expression of pro-angiogenic factors such as IL-8 and osteopontin. [13] Colla et al. concluded that ING4 suppressed HIF-1 function via PHD interactions.[13]

Abnormal activation of HIF-2 is found in multiple myeloma cells. Martin et al. examined the expression of HIF-1α and HIF-2α with bone marrow trephine specimens from patients with multiple myeloma. [14] They detected weak HIF-1α expression in numerous types of bone marrow cells, whereas HIF-2α expression was strong and restricted to CD138-positive cells. [14] Abnormal activation of HIF-2 was reported by another group. [15] In their study, the expression of HIF-1α and HIF-2α was assessed in the bone marrow of 106 multiple myeloma patients. Among the patients, HIF-1α and HIF-2α were expressed in 33% and 13.2%, respectively. [15]The aforementioned findings indicate that HIF-1α and HIF-2 are activated in multiple myeloma cells using multiple mechanisms, including the hypoxic environment of the myeloma bone marrow, growth factors for myeloma cells and oncogene products (Fig.1).

3. Role of abnormal HIF activation in the pathophysiology of MM

HIFα forms a complex with the beta-subunit of HIF and binds conserved DNA sequences that are known as hypoxia-response elements (5′-RCGTG-3′) to regulate mRNA expression of target genes. [1]HIFs regulate many genes that are required for adaptation to hypoxic conditions. Among the first group of genes regulated by HIF are pro-angiogenetic factors

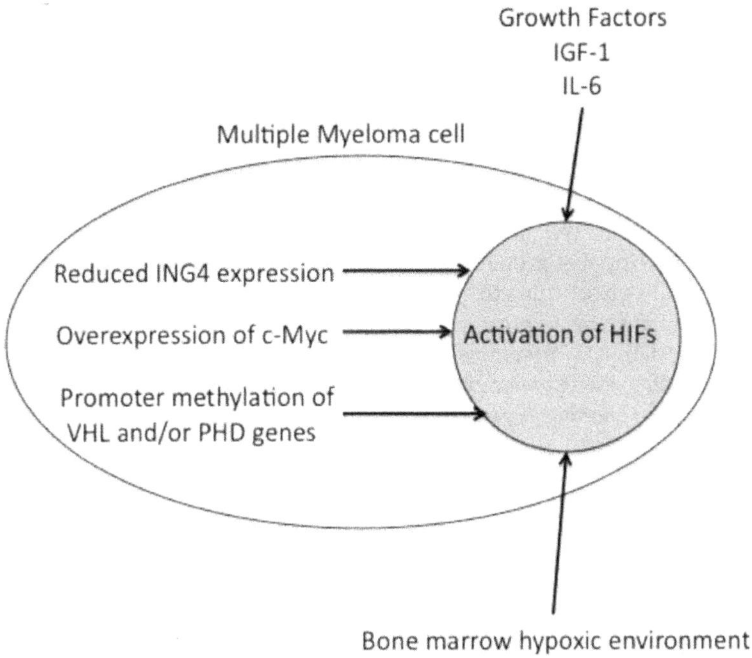

Fig. 1. Abnormal activation of HIFs in multiple myeloma cells
The bone marrow of multiple myeloma patients is hypoxic, which induces HIF activation in multiple myeloma cells. Growth factors activate HIFs via increased protein synthesis in myeloma cells. Overexpression of c-Myc and decreased ING4 enhance HIF activity. DNA methylation of the promoter regions of VHL and PDHs, which are required for HIF α degradation, may enhance HIFα levels.

including vascular endothelial growth factor (VEGF), IL-8 and osteopontin. [13] HIFs regulate several chemokines and their receptors SDF-1[16] (also known as CXCL12) and CXCR4. [17] Several anti-apoptotic proteins are also HIF targets. HIF-1 regulates the Bcl-2 family of anti-apoptotic proteins: Bcl-xL[18] and Mcl-1. [19] Furthermore, HIF-1 controls the expression of survivin, which is a member of the inhibitor for apoptosis family of proteins (IAPs). [20] Under hypoxic conditions, glucose metabolism is shifted from oxidative phosphorylation, which requires oxygen, to glycolysis. HIFs contribute to this metabolic shift[21] via up-regulation of glycolytic enzymes including glucose transporters, hexokinase and pyruvate dehydrogenase kinase (PDK). [22-24]In addition, HIFs suppress mitochondrial function to reduce oxidative phosphorylation. [21]

Aberrant HIF activation in multiple myeloma cells enhances the expression of these genes and contributes to the pathophysiology of multiple myeloma. HIFs enhance VEGF production in myeloma cells. [9]In addition, HIF-1 may contribute to increased angiogenesis via up-regulation of IL-8 and osteopontin. [13] Osteopontin stimulates the survival and migration of endothelial cells to enhance angiogenesis. [25] HIF-2 activation induces CXCL12 expression, which contributes to aberrant angiogenesis. [14] The promoter of CXCL12 has several hypoxia responsive elements (HREs). Treatment of myeloma cell lines with hypoxia increases the binding of HIF-2 to HRE on the CXCL12 promoter and enhances transcriptional activity. Ectopic expression of HIF-2 in myeloma cells increases production of CXCL2. The role of CXCL12 in angiogenesis was revealed by a study using a mouse xenograft model. In this model, the addition of an agonist for CXCR4, which is a receptor for CXCL12, inhibited angiogenesis. [14] In addition to pathological angiogenesis, HIFs induce survival molecules in multiple myeloma cells. We found that activation of HIF-1 by IGF-1 enhanced the expression of the anti-apoptotic protein survivin. [8] Recently, target genes of HIFs in multiple myeloma cells were analyzed using high-throughput methods. [7] Colla et al. compared the transcriptional profile of CD138-positive myeloma cells under normoxia and treated with the hypoxic mimetic drug $CoCl_2$. They detected 714 genes that were significantly modulated by hypoxia including heme oxygenase-1, heat shock protein 90 (Hsp90), VEGF and IL-8. [7] In summary, HIFs contribute to the pathogenesis of multiple myeloma by inducing the expression of their target genes to enhance angiogenesis in the bone marrow and suppressing apoptosis in myeloma cells (Fig. 2).

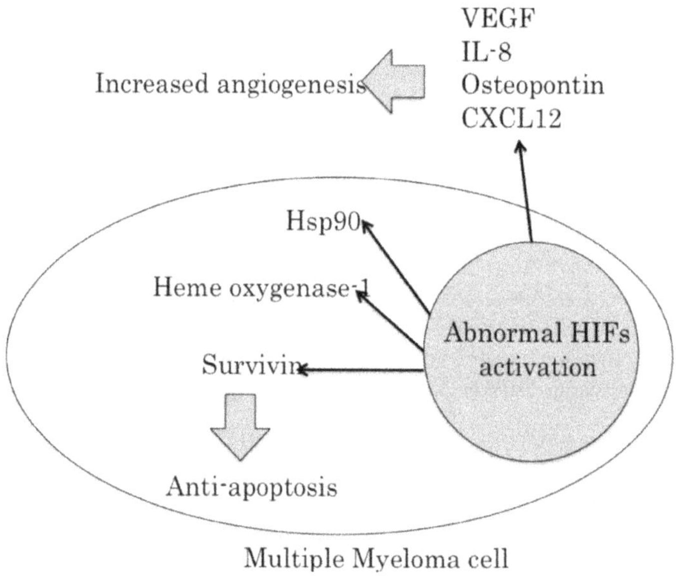

Fig. 2. Pathological role of HIFs in multiple myeloma
HIF activation induces the production of several pro-angiogenetic factors and enhances angiogenesis in the bone marrow. HIFs suppress apoptosis in myeloma cells by inducing anti-apoptotic factors.

4. HIFs as therapeutic targets for multiple myeloma

As described above, evidence has accumulated that implicates the important role of HIFs in the pathophysiology of multiple myeloma. These findings suggest the possibility for new therapeutic approaches that target hypoxic bone marrow microenvironments and HIFs. Our group showed that inhibition of HIF-1 function via the chemical inhibitor echinomycin[26], which disrupts HIF binding to DNA, or siRNA against HIF-1α disrupted the anti-apoptotic effects of IGF-1. [8] Importantly, echinomycin enhanced melphalan-induced apoptosis in primary CD138-positive myeloma cells. [8] Zhang et al. found that adaphostin, which is a tyrphostin kinase inhibitor, [27] [28]blocked expression of c-Myc and HIF-1α in several multiple myeloma cells. [9] They reported that adaphostin down-regulated c-Myc and HIF-1α in the xenograft mouse myeloma model. In this model, the compound suppressed VEGF secretion, tumor angiogenesis and tumor progression and increased the survival of the animals. [9] Known anti-myeloma drugs inhibit function of HIFs. Bortezomib suppresses transcriptional activity of HIF-1. [29]Lenalidomide inhibits the synthesis of HIF-1α in endothelial cells and suppresses the expression of HIF-1α in multiple myeloma cells. [30]Recent studies also revealed that HIFs were molecular targets of a new generation of agents against multiple myeloma. A molecular chaperone, heat shock protein 90 (Hsp90), stabilizes a series of proteins that are required for cell cycle progression and survival. [31] In multiple myeloma cells, Hsp90 is known to enhance survival, and several inhibitors for HSp90 show anti-myeloma effects. [31] Interestingly, HIF-1α is a target protein for Hsp90. [32] Treatment of myeloma cells with Hsp90 inhibitor blocked expression of HIF-1α expression. [32]Together with these observations, there is evidence that Hsp90 inhibitor may exert anti-myeloma effects through the suppression of HIFs. Histone deacetylase (HDAC) inhibitors are attractive new-generation agents against multiple myeloma. [33] HDAC inhibitors suppress the growth and survival of myeloma cells in vitro. [34] Furthermore, several HDAC inhibitors are currently being used in clinical trials. [35]Although the main target of HDAC inhibitors is histone deacetylase, the inhibitors modify the function of numerous proteins including HIFs. The HDAC inhibitor induces the degradation of HIF-1α independent of VHL function. [36] [37]Taken together, HIFs may be a molecular target of HDAC inhibitors in multiple myeloma. Finally, TH-302, which is a hypoxia-activated prodrug, [38] shows significant anti-myeloma effects in the murine myeloma model. [6] These results suggest that the hypoxic environment of multiple myeloma bone marrow might be an attractive therapeutic target.

5. Conclusions

The microenvironment of bone marrow is hypoxic in multiple myeloma and supports the survival and growth of myeloma cells, especially during the initial stage of the disease. Hypoxia enhances HIF activity and induces the production of pro-angiogenetic factors. Subsequently, angiogenesis in the bone marrow is enhanced and supports further growth of myeloma cells. [39] Growth factors for myeloma cells and intrinsic cellular changes (i.e., increased c-Myc expression and reduced ING4 levels) modify HIF activity and may contribute to increased angiogenesis. Furthermore, HIFs are survival factors for myeloma cells that induce the production of anti-apoptotic proteins and may be involved in the acquisition of drug-resistance. Treatments targeting both HIFs and hypoxic microenvironments represent novel strategies to improve treatment outcomes for multiple myeloma.

6. References

[1] Semenza GL. Oxygen sensing, homeostasis, and disease. N Engl J Med. 2011;365:537-547.

[2] Lisy K, Peet DJ. Turn me on: regulating HIF transcriptional activity. Cell Death Differ. 2008;15:642-649.

[3] Zundel W, Schindler C, Haas-Kogan D, et al. Loss of PTEN facilitates HIF-1-mediated gene expression. Genes Dev. 2000;14:391-396.

[4] Semenza GL. Defining the role of hypoxia-inducible factor 1 in cancer biology and therapeutics. Oncogene. 2010;29:625-634.

[5] Asosingh K, De Raeve H, de Ridder M, et al. Role of the hypoxic bone marrow microenvironment in 5T2MM murine myeloma tumor progression. Haematologica. 2005;90:810-817.

[6] Hu J, Handisides DR, Van Valckenborgh E, et al. Targeting the multiple myeloma hypoxic niche with TH-302, a hypoxia-activated prodrug. Blood. 2010;116:1524-1527.

[7] Colla S, Storti P, Donofrio G, et al. Low bone marrow oxygen tension and hypoxia-inducible factor-1alpha overexpression characterize patients with multiple myeloma: role on the transcriptional and proangiogenic profiles of CD138(+) cells. Leukemia. 2010;24:1967-1970.

[8] Hu Y, Kirito K, Yoshida K, et al. Inhibition of hypoxia-inducible factor-1 function enhances the sensitivity of multiple myeloma cells to melphalan. Mol Cancer Ther. 2009;8:2329-2338.

[9] Zhang J, Sattler M, Tonon G, et al. Targeting angiogenesis via a c-Myc/hypoxia-inducible factor-1alpha-dependent pathway in multiple myeloma. Cancer Res. 2009;69:5082-5090.

[10] Podar K, Anderson KC. A therapeutic role for targeting c-Myc/Hif-1-dependent signaling pathways. Cell Cycle. 2010;9:1722-1728.

[11] Hatzimichael E, Dranitsaris G, Dasoula A, et al. Von Hippel-Lindau methylation status in patients with multiple myeloma: a potential predictive factor for the development of bone disease. Clin Lymphoma Myeloma. 2009;9:239-242.

[12] Hatzimichael E, Dasoula A, Shah R, et al. The prolyl-hydroxylase EGLN3 and not EGLN1 is inactivated by methylation in plasma cell neoplasia. Eur J Haematol. 2010;84:47-51.

[13] Colla S, Tagliaferri S, Morandi F, et al. The new tumor-suppressor gene inhibitor of growth family member 4 (ING4) regulates the production of proangiogenic molecules by myeloma cells and suppresses hypoxia-inducible factor-1 alpha (HIF-1alpha) activity: involvement in myeloma-induced angiogenesis. Blood. 2007;110:4464-4475.

[14] Martin SK, Diamond P, Williams SA, et al. Hypoxia-inducible factor-2 is a novel regulator of aberrant CXCL12 expression in multiple myeloma plasma cells. Haematologica. 2010;95:776-784.

[15] Giatromanolaki A, Bai M, Margaritis D, et al. Hypoxia and activated VEGF/receptor pathway in multiple myeloma. Anticancer Res. 2010;30:2831-2836.

[16] Ceradini DJ, Kulkarni AR, Callaghan MJ, et al. Progenitor cell trafficking is regulated by hypoxic gradients through HIF-1 induction of SDF-1. Nat Med. 2004;10:858-864.

[17] Staller P, Sulitkova J, Lisztwan J, Moch H, Oakeley EJ, Krek W. Chemokine receptor CXCR4 downregulated by von Hippel-Lindau tumour suppressor pVHL. Nature. 2003;425:307-311.

[18] Chen N, Chen X, Huang R, et al. BCL-xL Is a Target Gene Regulated by Hypoxia-inducible Factor-1Œ±. Journal of Biological Chemistry. 2009;284:10004-10012.

[19] Piret J-P, Minet E, Cosse J-P, et al. Hypoxia-inducible Factor-1-dependent Overexpression of Myeloid Cell Factor-1 Protects Hypoxic Cells against tert-Butyl Hydroperoxide-induced Apoptosis. Journal of Biological Chemistry. 2005;280:9336-9344.

[20] Peng X-H, Karna P, Cao Z, Jiang B-H, Zhou M, Yang L. Cross-talk between Epidermal Growth Factor Receptor and Hypoxia-inducible Factor-1{alpha} Signal Pathways Increases Resistance to Apoptosis by Up-regulating Survivin Gene Expression. J Biol Chem. 2006;281:25903-25914.

[21] Semenza GL. Hypoxia-inducible factor 1: regulator of mitochondrial metabolism and mediator of ischemic preconditioning. Biochim Biophys Acta. 2010;1813:1263-1268.

[22] Kim JW, Tchernyshyov I, Semenza GL, Dang CV. HIF-1-mediated expression of pyruvate dehydrogenase kinase: a metabolic switch required for cellular adaptation to hypoxia. Cell Metab. 2006;3:177-185.

[23] Papandreou I, Cairns RA, Fontana L, Lim AL, Denko NC. HIF-1 mediates adaptation to hypoxia by actively downregulating mitochondrial oxygen consumption. Cell Metab. 2006;3:187-197.

[24] Kirito K, Hu Y, Komatsu N. HIF-1 prevents the overproduction of mitochondrial ROS after cytokine stimulation through induction of PDK-1. Cell Cycle. 2009;8:2844-2849.

[25] Takahashi F, Akutagawa S, Fukumoto H, et al. Osteopontin induces angiogenesis of murine neuroblastoma cells in mice. Int J Cancer. 2002;98:707-712.

[26] Kong D, Park EJ, Stephen AG, et al. Echinomycin, a small-molecule inhibitor of hypoxia-inducible factor-1 DNA-binding activity. Cancer Res. 2005;65:9047-9055.

[27] Avramis IA, Christodoulopoulos G, Suzuki A, et al. In vitro and in vivo evaluations of the tyrosine kinase inhibitor NSC 680410 against human leukemia and glioblastoma cell lines. Cancer Chemother Pharmacol. 2002;50:479-489.

[28] Chandra J, Tracy J, Loegering D, et al. Adaphostin-induced oxidative stress overcomes BCR/ABL mutation-dependent and -independent imatinib resistance. Blood. 2006;107:2501-2506.

[29] Shin DH, Chun YS, Lee DS, Huang LE, Park JW. Bortezomib inhibits tumor adaptation to hypoxia by stimulating the FIH-mediated repression of hypoxia-inducible factor-1. Blood. 2008;111:3131-3136.

[30] Lu L, Payvandi F, Wu L, et al. The anti-cancer drug lenalidomide inhibits angiogenesis and metastasis via multiple inhibitory effects on endothelial cell function in normoxic and hypoxic conditions. Microvasc Res. 2009;77:78-86.

[31] Richardson PG, Mitsiades CS, Laubach JP, Lonial S, Chanan-Khan AA, Anderson KC. Inhibition of heat shock protein 90 (HSP90) as a therapeutic strategy for the treatment of myeloma and other cancers. Br J Haematol. 2010;152:367-379.

[32] Mabjeesh NJ, Post DE, Willard MT, et al. Geldanamycin induces degradation of hypoxia-inducible factor 1alpha protein via the proteosome pathway in prostate cancer cells. Cancer Res. 2002;62:2478-2482.

[33] Dimopoulos MA, San-Miguel JF, Anderson KC. Emerging therapies for the treatment of relapsed or refractory multiple myeloma. Eur J Haematol. 2011;86:1-15.

[34] Mandl-Weber S, Meinel FG, Jankowsky R, Oduncu F, Schmidmaier R, Baumann P. The novel inhibitor of histone deacetylase resminostat (RAS2410) inhibits proliferation

and induces apoptosis in multiple myeloma (MM) cells. Br J Haematol. 2010;149:518-528.

[35] Niesvizky R, Ely S, Mark T, et al. Phase 2 trial of the histone deacetylase inhibitor romidepsin for the treatment of refractory multiple myeloma. Cancer. 2011;117:336-342.

[36] Kong X, Lin Z, Liang D, Fath D, Sang N, Caro J. Histone deacetylase inhibitors induce VHL and ubiquitin-independent proteasomal degradation of hypoxia-inducible factor 1alpha. Mol Cell Biol. 2006;26:2019-2028.

[37] Fath DM, Kong X, Liang D, et al. Histone deacetylase inhibitors repress the transactivation potential of hypoxia-inducible factors independently of direct acetylation of HIF-alpha. J Biol Chem. 2006;281:13612-13619.

[38] Duan JX, Jiao H, Kaizerman J, et al. Potent and highly selective hypoxia-activated achiral phosphoramidate mustards as anticancer drugs. J Med Chem. 2008;51:2412-2420.

[39] Martin SK, Diamond P, Gronthos S, Peet DJ, Zannettino AC. The emerging role of hypoxia, HIF-1 and HIF-2 in multiple myeloma. Leukemia. 2011.

8

The Contribution of Prognostic Factors to the Better Management of Multiple Myeloma Patients

Marie-Christine Kyrtsonis, Dimitrios Maltezas, Efstathios Koulieris, Katerina Bitsani, Ilias Pessach, Anna Efthymiou, Vassiliki Bartzis, Tatiana Tzenou and Panayiotis Panayiotidis
Hematology Section – First Department of Propedeutic Internal Medicine
Athens Medical School
Greece

1. Introduction

Multiple myeloma (MM) is an heterogeneous plasma cell disorder of unknown etiology, with a wide range of clinical manifestations and a highly variable disease course. Survival varies from a few months to more than ten years. The disease is characterized by bone marrow (BM) infiltration by malignant plasma cells usually secreting a serum or urine monoclonal immunoglobulin (Ig) component. Progress has been made in the understanding of its pathogenesis including knowledge of BM microenvironment and of cellular and genetic factors implicated in disease mechanisms that are not uniform in all patients, thus partly explaining disease variability. Furthermore, based on these, new very performing biology-based treatment modalities have been developed and are either already available for patients or under evaluation.

Prognostic factors (PFs) are needed to predict disease behavior and chemosensitivity to a given regimen in order to schedule the most efficient therapeutic approach. They are useful both at diagnosis and during disease course, because ongoing biologic transformations are taking place, related to further disease manifestations after response or resistance to treatment.

Existing PFs can be divided into those expressing host characteristics, reflecting tumor load and associated with malignant plasma cell or BM microenvironment peculiarities.

In the present context, existing knowledge regarding PFs and risk stratification-systems in MM, as well as their contribution in clinical practice, will be summarised. The need for re-evaluation of some established concepts or guidelines as a consequence of the recent therapeutic advances, will be discussed. Focus will be made on symptomatic MM only, because this is the field where PFs and risk-stratification systems can contribute the most to a better disease management.

2. Prognostic factors evaluated before treatment

Routine clinical and laboratory data assessed upon initial evaluation of newly diagnosed symptomatic MM patients include an important number of prognostic factors (Figure 1). Their ability to predict disease outcome has usually been established by retrospective clinical observations. Other important markers of disease behavior emerged more recently and resulted from a better knowledge of disease biology and from advances in laboratory technology. Because of the clinical importance of the information they provide, their evaluation became strongly recommended (Dimopoulos et al, 2011; Munshi et al, 2011).

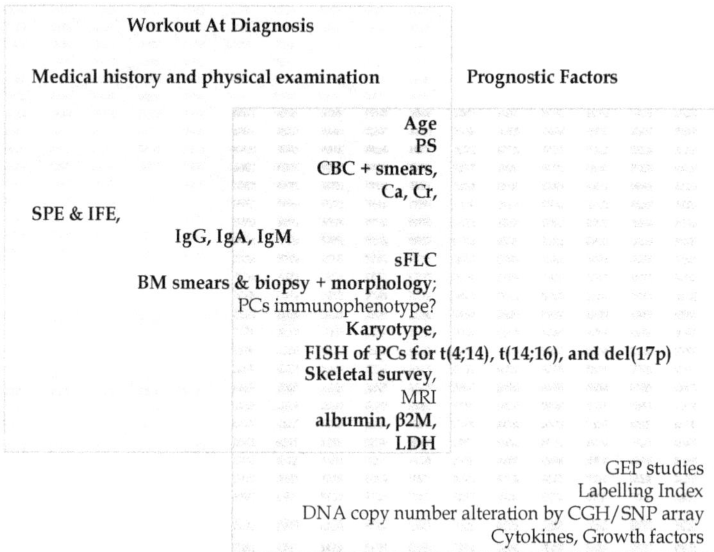

PS: performance status, CBC: complete blood count, Ca: calcium, Cr: creatinine, Ig: immunoglobulin, PC: plasma cell, β2M: beta2-microglobulin, LDH: lactate dehydrogenase, sFLC: serum free light chain, MRI: magnetic resonance imaging, PET: positron emission tomography. FISH: fluorescence in situ hybridization, GEP: gene expression profiling, SNP: single nucleotide polymorphism

Fig. 1. Recommended Workout And Prognostic Factors for MM Patients at Diagnosis.

2.1 Prognostic factors expressing host characteristics

2.1.1 Age

The median age at the time of disease diagnosis is approximately 70 years and about 37% of patients are younger than 65 years (Durie et al, 2004; Durie et al, 2006). In several studies, younger age was associated with longer survival, both after conventional therapy and high-dose treatment (Kyle R, 1995; Ludwig et al, 2008; Lenhoff et al, 2006). Indeed age is closely related to performance status and the presence of co-morbidities and consequently affects treatment choice. Elderly patients are weaker and present frequently other chronic diseases such as diabetes mellitus, increased blood pressure or cardiac diseases, thus eventually compromising the administration of simple drugs like corticosteroids that are an indispensable component of MM chemotherapy. They also develop more frequently than younger ones, post-therapy cytopenias and are more prone to infections.

2.1.2 Performance status

Performance status (PS), assessed by the Eastern Cooperative Oncology Group (ECOG) or Karnofsky scale, has a considerable impact on patients' outcome (Rajkumar & Buady, 2007). It was shown in a large unselected observational study that the adverse effect of PS on outcome was greater than any other single prognostic variable (Kyle et al, 2003). In addition, patients with a bad PS are not eligible for high dose treatment with autologous stem cell transplantation, independently of age.

2.2 Prognostic factors derived from initial laboratory tests

As already mentioned, during initial MM patients' workout, routine haematology, biochemistry, immunology, histopathology, nuclear medicine and radiology tests are undertaken, both for diagnostic and prognostic purposes. Many of them are included in the Durie-Salmon staging system (Durie & Salmon, 1975) that has been for 30 years the standard risk-stratification model for MM patients and is still in use. It is a disease specific staging system that combines haemoglobin, calcium, paraprotein concentration and skeletal status by x-rays to separate MM patients into 3 distinct prognostic groups, further subdivided according to creatinine value. In addition, "disease mass" corresponding to each stage, was evaluated with complex mathematic calculations, thus suggesting that the aforementioned factors reflect to some extend tumour load, while renal status and extend of BM infiltration at aspiration's site, do not. The major limitations of the Durie-Salmon staging were that evaluation of bone disease by x-rays is observer-dependent and that paraprotein quantification in light chain MM was evaluated by the amount of 24 hours proteinuria.

2.2.1 Complete Blood Count (CBC)

With regard to CBC assessed at diagnosis, anaemia is the most common finding. It confers an adverse prognosis without being an independent factor; it may reflect in part tumor burden although anaemia is mostly due to cytokines' inhibitory activity and to impaired erythropoietin secretion or function. The other blood counts are usually normal. However, all kind of cytopenias (anemia, thrombocytopenia, neutropenia, lymphocytopenia), when observed, present a significant correlation with early death (Augustson et al, 2005). Thrombocytopenia in particular (Cavo et al, 1989) is a rare but powerful independent PF.

2.2.2 Serum creatinine

Renal impairment, due to excessive free light chain (FLC) secretion in urine, is associated with an adverse prognosis (Kyle et al, 2003; Drayson et al, 2005). Until 2001 FLC secretion was estimated by the amount of protein in the urine collected during 24 hours. During the past decade, a new assay was developed which allows precise quantification of serum free light chains (Bradwell, 2001). This method was shown useful for both diagnostic and prognostic purposes (see below in the current chapter).

About 20% of patients have increased serum creatinine at the time of diagnosis, while 10% present acute renal failure and need haemodialysis. Their long term prognosis depends on renal recovery (Wirk et al, 2011), meaning that the correlation between increased creatinine and early death is mostly due to short term complications. Thus, the survival of patients with recovered kidney function is equivalent to those without renal failure.

2.2.3 Serum albumin

Serum albumin, produced in the liver, regulates blood volume by maintaining blood compartment's osmotic pressure and carries several molecules. The first reports of albumin being an important prognostic factor in MM patients came in the late 80s. (Simonsson et al, 1988; Blade et al, 1989). These results were further validated later on (Kyle et al, 2003), leading to the incorporation of albumin into two staging systems, the SWOG (Jacobson et al, 2003) and the currently widely used ISS (Greipp et al, 2005).

2.2.4 Serum calcium

Hypercalcemia is the most common metabolic disorder in MM patients. The main cause is bone destruction, which is induced by mediator proteins (RANKL, MIP-1a, DKK-1 and proinflammatory cytokines) produced by plasmacytes and stromal cells. Elevated serum calcium levels have a toxic effect on the kidneys, enhancing the damage caused by paraprotein. Inappropriate parathyroid hormone-like secretion may also contribute to increased calcium levels.

The importance of elevated serum calcium as an adverse prognostic factor was recognized early and was incorporated into the Durie-Salmon staging system. In addition, calcium levels were shown to constitute an independent predictor of life quality (Wisløff et al., 2007).

2.2.5 Imaging for the evaluation of bone disease

X-rays of the spine, skull, chest, pelvis, humeri, and femora remain the standard to identify MM related bone lesions. Magnetic resonance imaging (MRI) is recommended to evaluate symptoms in patients with normal x-rays results and in all patients with findings suggesting the presence of solitary bone plasmacytoma. In Durie - Salmon staging, the presence of spontaneous fractures (bone scale 3) leads by itself to stage III disease, independently of any other factor. Accordingly, in a series of 158 consecutive MM patients from our department, those (24%) presenting spontaneous fractures at diagnosis had a worse outcome than the others (Figure 2), with a median disease specific survival of 38 versus 90 months (p=0.012).

On the contrary, a recent study on the impact of bone lesions as evaluated by conventional radiography compared survival of patients with bone scale 0 and 1 (no lesions and diffuse osteoporosis) to the others, and failed to prove any difference (Li et al, 2010).

Indeed, the evaluation of Durie-Salmon bone scale 0, 1 and 2 is much more subjective and depends on x-rays quality than scale 3 which involves the presence of fractures. In addition plain radiographs are relatively insensitive and can only demonstrate lytic bone disease when 30% or more of trabecular bone has been lost (Snapper I, 1971; Lecouvet et al, 1999). For all these reasons, Durie proposed in 2006, the incorporation into the system he had developed in the 70s, of MRI and positron emission tomography (PET) scan findings for the precise evaluation of lytic and other bone lesions (Durie BGM, 2006). The new staging was named Durie-Salmon Plus but was not widely adopted.

MRI showed utility as a prognostic factor (Moulopoulos et al, 2005). The Hellenic MM working group evaluated 142 symptomatic MM patients with MRI. Focal marrow lesions were identified in 50% of patients, diffuse marrow replacement in 28%, a variegated pattern in 14%, and normal pattern in 8% of patients. Patients with diffuse pattern had a median survival of 24 months, while it was longer than 50 months for the remaining patterns. It was shown in addition that patients with more than 7 focal lesions detected by MRI, had a worse outcome, while in contrast, the number of lesions on plain radiography did not contribute to prognosis (Walker et al, 2007).

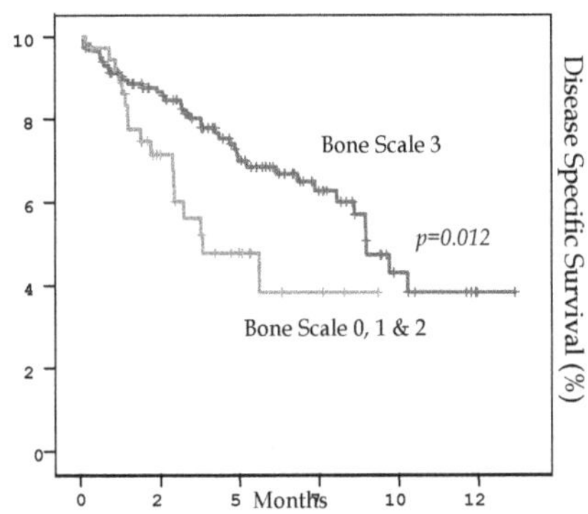

Fig. 2. Survival According to the Presence or Absence of Spontaneous Fractures.

2.3 Prognostic factors related to tumor burden and growth fraction

2.3.1 Beta-2-Microglobulin (β_2M)

Beta2-Microglobulin (β_2-M) is a subunit of the MHC class I molecule, associated with the outer membrane of almost all nucleated cells. High serum β_2-M levels are detected in patients with renal impairment, lymphoid malignancies and autoimmune disorders. In MM, β_2-M emerged as a predictor of survival in the late 1970s (Cassuto et al, 1978; Norfolk et al, 1979). Its role in the initial staging and subsequent monitoring of monoclonal plasma cell disorders was studied (Garewal et al, 1984). However, it was not found helpful for monitoring MM disease course, since there are patients that relapse without a previous raise in β_2-M levels, while others show increases without any evidence of disease progression (Cuzick et al, 1990). Several stratification systems of β_2-M in combination with other disease parameters were afterwards proposed (Bataille et al, 1992). In 2005 the International Staging System (ISS) (Greip et al, 2005), based on clinical and laboratory data gathered on 11171 MM patients showed that the combination of β_2-M and albumin separated very efficiently prognostic subgroups. Median overall survival was 62, 44, and 29 months, for patients with ISS stages 1, 2, and 3 respectively. That system was simple and potent and replaced the Durie–Salmon staging system. ISS has important pitfalls; it is not disease specific and cannot separate the small subgroup of patients with a very limited survival, who will benefit from a different therapeutic approach (Rajkumar & Buadi, 2007). Attempts were therefore made to improve ISS prognostication by adding other variables (Table 1), namely LDH (Terpos et al, 2010), serum free light chain ratio (Kyrtsonis et al, 2007b; Snozek et al, 2008) or cytogenetic abnormalities (Avet-Loiseau et al, 2009; Neben et al, 2010).

Study	Model	Results			
Terpos et al, 2010	LDH ≥ or <300 U/L within ISS groups	ISS 1: 27,7%	High LDH 7%	Median OS (months)	22
			Normal LDH 93%		76
		ISS 2: 38%	High LDH 10%		11
			Normal LDH 90%		40
		ISS 3: 34,3%	High LDH 12%		17
			Normal LDH 88%		27
Neben et al, 2010	Low risk: ISS 1 and absence of t(4;14) or del17p13 High Risk: ISS 2/3 and t(4;14) or del17p13 Int risk: All others	Low: 42%	5 years OS (%)		72
		Intermediate: 44%			62
		High: 14%			41
Snozek et al, 2008	Presence of 0,1,2,3 of sFLC abnormal, β_2M≥ 3,5 g/dl, albumin 3,5<g/dl	0 factors: 12,6%	5 years OS (%)		41,5
		1 factor: 29,9%			32
		2 factors: 34,5%			24.5
		3 factors: 23,5%			13.4
Kyrtsonis et al, 2007	Low risk: sFLCR <median and ISS <3 Int risk: Either sFLCR> median or ISS=3 High risk: sFLCR> median and ISS=3	Low: 29%	5 years OS (%)		90
		Intermediate: 46%			56
		High: 24%			24

ISS: International Staging System, OS = overall survival, sFLCR = serum free light chain ratio, β_2 *M: B2-microglobulin.*

Table 1. Risk-Stratification Models Attempting ISS Prognostication Improvement

2.3.2 Lactate Dehydrogenase (LDH)

Since the late 70s, the relationship between hematological malignancies and elevated LDH has been intensively studied (Talageri et al, 1977). In aggressive lymphoma patients, increased LDH was found linked to high tumor burden and turnover (Vezzoni MA et al, 1983). Later on several investigators reported its prognostic value in MM patients (Simonsson et al, 1987; Barlogie et al, 1989), it was however not incorporated in any widely used staging system, although its ability to identify patients with an especially adverse outcome was shown (Dimopoulos et al, 1991; Kyrtsonis et al, 2007b).

2.3.3 Plasma cell proliferation

Increased plasma cell proliferating potential determined by either labeling index, Ki-67 immunostaining or flow cytometry predicts shorter survival.

Plasma cell labeling index (PCLI) detects the percentage of cells in S-phase, by assessing bromodeoxyuridine uptake (Greipp et al, 1993). High PCLI was associated with both poor overall survival and progression-free survival (Boccadoro et al, 1989).

Ki-67, a nuclear protein expressed in proliferating cells and absent from resting cells, constitutes an excellent marker of the neoplastic growth fraction. Increased Ki-67 immunostaining on BM trephine biopsy specimens was found associated with shorter survival, hypodiploidy and identified an adverse prognostic group within ISS stage 1 patients (Gastinne et al, 2010).

Plasma cell proliferation can also be evaluated by flow cytometry using fluorescent dye which stains nucleic acids to detect the proportion of cells that actively double their DNA (Trendle et al, 1999). Actively proliferating cells' immunophenotype was characterized and is $CD45^{bright}CD11a^{pos}$ (Robillard et al, 2005).

2.4 Prognostic factors reflecting cell and microenvironment characteristics

In this part, prognostic factors related to plasma cell appearance, secretion, expression, genetic lesions and interaction with the BM microenvironment will be presented.

2.4.1 Plasma cell morphology

In older studies, special attention was given to PCs morphology on BM smears (Fritz et al, 1984). The presence of 2% or more plasmablasts in the plasma-cell population, was associated with a shorter survival (Greipp et al, 1998; Rajkumar et al, 1999). Plasmablasts were characterized as follows: fine reticular chromatin pattern in the nucleus; large nucleus less-abundant cytoplasm (Figure 3). In addition plasmablastic morphology was associated with increased presence of cytogenetic abnormalities.

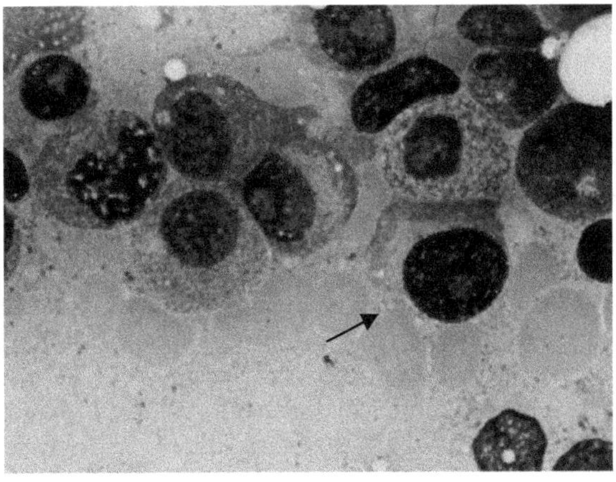

Fig. 3. Presence of Plasma Cells With Plasmablastic Morphology on BM Smears

2.4.2 Immunoglobulin heavy and light chain secretion

The hallmark of MM is the secretion of monoclonal Ig by BM infiltrating PCs. Paraprotein can be detected by serum protein electrophoresis (SPEP) and immunofixation (IFE) and quantified nephelometrically or by SPEP densitometry. About 20% of patients secrete light chains only (LCO) that can be assessed by serum/urine IFE and precisely quantified by the serum free-light-chain (FLC) assay. Although serum monoclonal Ig quantification was one of Durie and Salmon staging system's risk factors and was included in older prognostic algorithms (Bettini R, 1983), it was shown that MM aggressiveness or tumor load is not necessarily related to the amount of serum Ig heavy chain and subsequent stratification models did not retain it as a risk parameter (Kyrtsonis et al, 2009). However, paraprotein type was shown to influence survival; IgG patients enjoy the longest one, followed by IgA while LCO patients have the shortest (Drayson et al, 2006)

With regard to the amount of Ig light chains secreted by malignant plasma cells, they were traditionally grossly evaluated by 24h proteinuria. In 2001, a new assay was introduced which allows precise quantification of serum free light chains (Bradwell et al, 2001; Bradwell et al, 2003). This highly sensitive method offered significant improvement in identifying and monitoring patients with oligo-secretory and LCO disease. In the next years, serum free light chain ratio (sFLCR) was shown a powerful and independent prognostic factor in newly diagnosed MM patients (Kyrtsonis et al, 2007; Snozek et al, 2008). Furthermore, the addition of sFLCR to factors of disease activity (LDH, β2M, genetic abnormalities) provided powerful prognostic models (Kyrtsonis et al, 2007b; Kumar et al, 2010).

Immunoassays using antibodies that target junctional epitopes between the heavy and light chains of each Ig molecule were recently manufactured for the analysis of Ig heavy chain/light chain (HLC) pairs (Hevylite™). These assays allow the precise quantification of the absolute value of the monoclonal IgGκ, IgGλ, IgAκ and IgAλ separately and of their deriving ratios (Keren 2009; Bradwell 2010). Preliminary results suggest that HLC and their ratios are prognostic with regard to time to treatment (Avet-Loiseau et al, 2009b) and overall survival (Koulieris et al, 2010; Ludwig et al, 2010).

2.4.3 Plasma cell genetic abnormalities

Chromosomal abnormalities may be evaluated by conventional karyotype, fluorescence in situ hybridization (FISH), comparative genomic hybridization, or by single nucleotide polymorphism (SNP). Classical cytogenetic analysis is rarely successful because of the low plasma cell proliferation rate; however, any chromosomal abnormality that is detected on standard cytogenetic analysis is associated with a worse outcome. Monosomy or partial deletion of chromosome 13 (del13q14) is a recurrent chromosomal aberration of adverse prognosis, observed in approximatively 50% of patients with abnormal karyotypes. The frequency of the aforementioned finding is much higher when evaluated by FISH that is more sensitive and significantly increases the proportion of patients with chromosomal aberrations. However, It seems that the adverse prognostic effect of 13q deletions, as detected by FISH, is related to other associated abnormalities, such as t(4;14) translocation and partial deletion on chromosome 17p and that patients who have only a chromosome 13 deletion have the same prognosis as those who do not have this abnormality (Avet-Loiseau et al, 2007; Kyrtsonis et al, 2010b). Specific translocations in the Ig heavy chain region that are detected by FISH, such as t(4;14), deletion 17p13, and chromosome 1 abnormalities, are associated with a poor prognosis and high risk, while standard-risk disease is defined by the presence of hyperdiploidy or t(11;14) (Fonseca et al, 2009; Avet-Loiseau, 2010b). The reported adverse impact of other rarer translocations such as t(14;16) is still under investigation due to the absence of large testing series. Prognostic information provided by GEP and SNP studies recognizes abnormalities throughout the whole genome, but they require plasma cell purification and highly specified centers; they are not routinely available for clinical prognostic evaluation.

2.4.4 plasma cell immunophenotype

Multiparameter flow cytometry (MFC) immunophenotyping can recognize normal plasma cell (N-PC) from malignant ones (MPC) according to cell surface markers (CD19, CD38, CD45, CD56). It was shown that symptomatic MM patients who have more than 5% N-PC/MPC at diagnosis present unique clinical, biological, and cytogenetic signature characterized by higher haemoglobin levels, less extended BM PC infiltration, lower paraprotein levels, and absence of high-risk cytogenetic abnormalities[t(4;14), t(14;16), del17p] (Paiva et al, 2009).

The presence or absence of combined specific cell surface markers predicts outcome. Thus, positive staining for CD19 and CD28, as well as absence of CD117 detected on clonal PC were associated with significantly shorter survival (Bahlis et al, 2007; Paiva et al, 2011).

Ploidy status evaluation, determination of the percentage of S-phase PC and stringent complete remission (sCR) categorization (Durie et al, 2006) are additional prognostic tools provided by MFC immunophenotype.

2.4.5 Prognostic factors derived from plasma cells and microenvironment cells interactions

The contribution of the medullary milieu to MM pathogenesis, was extensively studied during the past 30 years (Mitsiadis et al, 2006). Numerous cytokines and growth factors that sustain myeloma cell survival and proliferation are secreted upon plasma cells' adhesion to stromal cells. The serum concentrations of some of these, namely soluble interleukin-6 receptor (Pulki et al, 2006; Kyrtsonis et al, 2006) and soluble syndecan-1 (Seidel et al 2001, Kyrtsonis et al, 2004), are strongly prognostic for adverse survival.

The formation of new vessels and interactions between plasma cells and osteoclasts (OCs) are other important microenvironment processes accompanied by the secretion of cytokines and soluble factors that may also constitute prognostic factors. Bone marrow neo-vascularization is required to support neoplastic cells' metabolic requirements. The microvessel density correlates with disease stage and prognosis (Vacca et al, 1994; Kumar et al, 2004). Evolution from monoclonal gammopathy of unknown significance to MM, has been found associated with loss of marrow angiogenesis inhibitory activity (Kumar et al, 2004b). Myeloma and stromal cells produce angiogenic growth factors such as vascular endothelial growth factor (VEGF) and basic fibroblast growth factor (bFGF) that may account, in part, for the increased microvessel density observed in the BM. Both factors are specific endothelial cell mitogens and their serum levels were found in correlation with disease activity markers in MM patients (Sezer et al, 2001). VEGF also induces proliferation and triggers migration of MM cells by increasing vascular permeability (Podar et al, 2001). In addition, hepatocyte growth factor (HGF) stimulates epithelial cells' growth, further induces blood vessel formation and promotes osteoclasts formation and activation; high serum HGF levels predicted poor response to therapy and survival (Di Raimondo et al, 2000). The process of angiogenesis in MM is not yet fully elucidated; it is thought that imbalance of angiogenic regulators including angiopoietins along with other known and unknown factors are additionally involved. Increased serum Angiopoietin-2 or low Angiopoietin-1/Angiopoietin-2 ratio were recently found correlated with markers of disease activity and overall survival (Joshi et al, 2011; Terpos et al, 2011). Moreover, inhibition of neovascularization offers promising therapeutical implications and such mechanisms account in part for the improved anti-myeloma activity of new drugs.

Osteolyses in MM is caused by OCs proliferating in bony areas adjacent to myeloma cells. This promiscuity favours both cell types to secrete soluble factors sustaining one each other's activity. The main stimulator of OC formation is a member of the TNF family, namely the receptor activator of NF-kappaB ligand (RANKL). RANKL binds to the RANK receptor, on osteoclast progenitors, inducing OC differentiation and maturation while on the contrary, osteoprotegerin (OPG), a natural decoy receptor, blocks RANKL/RANK ligation. In addition, OCs are further regulated by other factors, including TNF, IL-1, IL-6, MIP-1a, while at the same time osteoblast inactivation is induced by IL-3, IL-7 and DKK1. RANKL/OPG ratio, MIP-1a, and DKK1 serum levels were all found of prognostic significance (Terpos et al, 2003a & b; Gavriatopoulou et al, 2009).

3. Prognostic factors of response to treatment

Treatment options for patients with MM at diagnosis and in relapse have dramatically increased. High dose treatment (HDT) with autologous stem cell transplantation (ASCT), thalidomide, lenalidomide, and bortezomib, introduced in the past 2 decades, resulted in improved outcomes and duration of response (Kumar et al, 2008; Lonial S, 2010). In addition, the depth of response seen with these modalities was never observed before, opening horizons for eventual cure. The aforementioned treatments are able to overcome the impact of well-known adverse prognostic factors and risk-stratification models, rendering the establishment of newer, more appropriate ones, mandatory.

3.1 Quality of response and response duration

Achieving complete response (CR) is an important goal based on the general principle that focuses in reaching the lowest tumor burden possible, in an intend to cure. In numerous studies, it was shown that the "quality" of response positively influenced both event free survival (EFS) and overall survival (OS). As "qualitative" responses, very good partial responses (VGPR), near complete responses (nCR) and CR (Blade et al, 1998), were included.

In an attempt to better define deeper CR, stringent CR was introduced as a new category in the recent "uniform international response criteria", concerning patients that, in addition to the previous criteria for CR (Blade et al, 1998), also presented normalization of free light chain ratio (FLCR) and absence of clonal cells as determined either by bone marrow immunfluoresence or immunohistochemistry (Durie et al, 2006). However the importance of FLCR in this context remains controversial. An important limitation of the definition is that "abnormal" FLCR has not been well defined. FLCR assesses both eventual increase of involved FLC (iFLC) and suppression of the polyclonal one of the same class (pFLC); in addition normal values for kappa and lambda FLCs are not exactly the same. Setting the appropriate normal range for FLCR in general or cutoff for the "high FLCR" group has been proven a challenging task. The mostly widely accepted reference range for FLCR is 0.26-1.65. In our experience, the use of "high" and "low" FLCR with different cutoff values for kappa and lambda patients was more appropriate; we therefore used the median value of each group separately as cut - off (Kyrtsonis et al, 2007; Kyrtsonis et al 2008). Indeed, the median value changes from a patients' series to another. An international consensus agreement defining appropriate normal values is urgently needed. We also believe that the choice of a "high" and "low" cutoff will resolve to some extend, the problem of the so called "discordant" presence of abnormal FLCR with normal IFE (de Larrea CF et al, 2009; Singal et al, 2009), given that absence of minimal residual disease (MRD) does not necessarily mean absence of polyclonal Ig depression involving pFLC and resulting in an abnormal FLCR when using the proposed "lower than 0.26 or higher than 1.65" range, while it would have been "low" FLCR if our system was used. Eventually because of this limitation, although it has been four years since the introduction of the sCR entity, the impact of its achievement has not been yet evaluated in large clinical trials.

Multiparameter flow cytometry (MFC) and polymerase chain reaction (PCR) are very sensitive methods for MRD evaluation (Liu H et al, 2008; Paiva et al, 2011; Corradini et al, 2003; Martínez-Sanchez et al, 2008). A recent study showed that achievement of immunophenotypic response leads to better response duration and OS than CR and sCR. The inclusion of these methods for response evaluation was thus proposed. They are however less widely available.

3.2 Prognostic factors for high dose treatment and autologous transplant

With conventional treatment CR did not exceed 5% while few patients were primary resistant, the median overall survival (OS) being 3 years. The addition of HDT with autologous bone marrow or stem cell rescue increased the CR rate up to 30-40% (Attal et al, 1992; Lenhoff et al, 2000; Barlogie et al, 2004) and median OS to 4-5 years. However, although HDT with ASCT may overcome the adverse prognosis of a significant number of classical adverse PFs, unsatisfactory response duration was observed after high dose treatment and bone marrow transplantation or stem cell rescue in patients with partial or complete deletions of chromosome 13 by conventional cytogenetics (Tricot et al, 1995), t(4;14)(p16;q32), t(14;16)(q32;q23) and 17p13 deletions (Gertz et al, 2005; Avet-Loiseau, 2007), deletions and gains of chromosome 1p21 (Chang et al, 2005) or its associated gene *CKS1B* amplification (Chang et al, 2006). However, a recent retrospective study showed that only HDT with ASCT overcome the adverse prognosis conferred by high FLCR, while the same was not true for novel agents (Maltezas et al, 2011).

An interesting observation was that, symptomatic MM patients with more than 5% normal BM PCs displayed a greater response rate to HDT/ASCT; The CR rate was 64% versus 33% in the rest with significantly longer progression free and overall survival rates (Paiva et al, 2010).

3.3 Prognostic factors for new agents

Over the last years, new therapeutic agents, such as thalidomide, lenalidomide and bortezomib have become approved and available for the treatment of MM (Engelhardt et al, 2006; Pangalis et al, 2006). When they are given alone or in combination with corticosteroids or other agents, they produce high response rates including a considerable percentage of complete remissions (CR) or near CR (nCR). The latter is probably due to their capacity to overcome some markers of adverse prognosis (Table 2).

Marker	ASCT	New Agent			Comments
		Thalidomide	Lenalidomide	Bortezomib	
Age	S	S	O	O	
PS	Ineligible	S	S	S	
LC MM	O	O	O	O	
↓ Hb	O	S	O	O	
↑ Cr	O	S	O	O	
↑ Ca	U	S	O	O	
↑ LDH	S	S	S	S	
FLC/FLCR	O	S	S	S	
sIL-6R	U	U	U	U	
s-syndecan-1	U	U	U	U	
VEGF	U	S	U	U	
HGF	U	S	U	U	
PCLI	S	S	S	U	
Hypodiploidy	U	U	S	U	
Del13q/Δ13[c]	S	S	S	O	
t(4;14)	S	S	S	O	
del 17p13	S	S	S	O	Conflicting data for bortezomib
1p21 lesions	S	S	S	O	
CKS1B amp	S	U	U	O	

S: sustained, O: overcome, U: unknown, [c]: By conventional cytogenetics,

Table 2. Ability of Novel Agents To Overcome Some Markers Of Adverse Prognosis.

3.3.1 Thalidomide

The introduction of thalidomide in MM therapeutics was revolutionary because it constituted the first treatment able to act both on myeloma and microenvironmental cells. Its mechanism of action includes direct inhibition of malignant plasmacytes via immunomodulation of T-cells and enhancement of NK-cells (Davies et al, 2009). It also affects BM stromal cells, creating a hostile microenvironment (Mitsiades et al, 2002). The last is mediated through reduction of expression of angiogenic factors (IL-6, TNF-a, bFGF, VEGF) via gene downregulation in BM endothelial cells (Vacca et al, 2005).

The first important study on thalidomide as a single agent (Singal et al, 1999), showed a response rate of 32% in relapsed-refractory MM patients. Subsequently other investigators confirmed thalidomide efficacy as a single agent or in combination with dexamethasone, chemotherapy or other new agents (Rajkumar et al, 2000; Juliusson et al, 2000; Blade et al, 2001). However, thalidomide does not seem able to overcome established adverse prognostic factors such as advanced stage, age ≥ 65 years, abnormal karyotype, increased LDH and β2M, del q13/Δ13, hypodiploidy, t(4;14), t(14;16), 17p13 deletions, chromosome 1 abnormalities, nor that of increased VEGF and HGF levels (Mileshkin et al, 2007); however it was shown able to reverse the poor prognosis associated with cyclin-D1 negativity and fibroblast growth factor-3 positivity (Kelly et al, 2009). The adverse impact of PCLI was not overcome by Thalidomide (Kapoor et al, 2009).

3.3.2 Lenalidomide

Lenalidomide is an immunomodulatory drug. In combination with dexamethasone it constitutes an effective treatment option for most patients with relapse/refractory MM. In myeloma cells, lenalidomide inhibits cell growth, promotes apoptosis and blocks their adhesion to stromal cells in the BM milieu (Richardson et al, 2002). In stromal cells, lenalidomide reduces the expression of angiogenic factors and several additional factors that support plasma cell growth (Dredge et al, 2002). In addition, lenalidomide stimulates T cells and natural killer cells (Marriot et al, 2002).It may be beneficial regardless of patient age, disease stage and renal function, although the starting dose of lenalidomide should be adjusted for renal impairment and cytopenias (Dimopoulos et al, 2011). It was relatively recently (early 2008) approved in Europe for the treatment of relapse/refractory patients and there are at present only few studies on its effectiveness in the presence of cytogenetic findings conferring adverse prognosis. A study on 100 newly diagnosed patients that received front-line lenalidomide/dexamethasone showed that patients with high risk MM defined by the presence of hypodiploidy, del(13q) by metaphase cytogenetics, del(17p), t(4;14), or t(14;16) and high plasma cell labeling index, had a shorter progression-free survival compared to standard-risk patients (Kapoor et al, 2009). In addition it was shown unable to overcome the adverse prognosis of chromosome 1 abnormalities (Chang et al, 2010).

3.3.3 Bortezomib

Bortezomib (Velcade®) is a reversible inhibitor of the chymotryptic component of the 26S proteasome. Thus, by inhibiting the proteasome, it inactivates key proteins implicated in cell growth and function such as nuclear factor kappa B (NF-κB), leading to the inhibition of cytokines and growth factors, immunoreceptors, adhesion molecules, transcription factors and to the induction of apoptosis. In addition, angiogenesis is downregulated through inhibition of VEGF and IL-6, which are produced by vascular endothelial cells. In addition, normalization of the angiopoietin-1/angiopoietin-2 ratio was shown a surrogate marker of response to bortezomib in relapsed/refractory MM patients (Anargyrou et al, 2008). Furthermore, indirect anti-tumor effects resulting from gene silencing of RANKL have been reported. The drug has an osteoblast activating effect by reducing serum dickkopf-1, resulting in an increase of bone-type alkaline phosphatase (Terpos et al, 2006).

In Europe, it has been licensed only for the treatment of relapsed/refractory MM patients or those with previously untreated MM, who are not eligible for high-dose chemotherapy with ASCT, in combination with melphalan and prednisone, while in the US there are no restrictions.

It was shown able to overcome the adverse effect of deleterious genetic aberrations (13q deletions, t(4;14), amplification *CKS1B* (Chang et al, 2007; Jannagath, 2007; Sagaster, 2007). Drug effectiveness in patients with del(17p) is controversial (Avet-Loiseau et al, 2010b); patients may respond but rapidly relapse. Some subanalyses and prospective studies suggest that up-front bortezomib-based treatment followed by HDT/ASCT and reinductions with bortezomib-lenalidomide-dexamethasone combinations may benefit high-risk patients with t(4;14) or del(17p). Nevertheless a subset of patients will still present early death (Avet-Loiseau, 2010).

4. Prognostic factors related to specific disease manifestations

The prediction of particularly morbid MM manifestations in order to avoid them, if possible, would have been of special interest. Unfortunately, although there are a number of markers that reflect specific manifestations, almost none predict their acute onset. For example, bone disease is more extended when increased concentrations of cytokines and soluble factors involved in bone metabolism are observed, but this is not enough to predict spontaneous fractures. In the same way, patients with polyclonal hypogammaglobulinaemia are more prone to infections but the presence of depressed polyclonal antibodies is not a strong enough predictor of infection in order to administer antibiotics. The most "predictable" disease manifestation is renal failure and evidences of genetic predisposition for peripheral neuropathy are emerging (Corthals et al, 2011).

4.1 Renal failure

Rapidly increasing sFLCs, observed while monitoring patients, predict imminent renal failure. Approximately 40% of MM patients have renal impairment at clinical presentation and 5-10% will require haemodialysis because of acute renal failure from cast nephropathy. Since the pre-renal load of sFLCs is the direct cause of renal damage, it is logical to monitor for rising concentrations on a regular basis, so that acute renal failure during disease relapse can be avoided by early treatment initiation (Hutchison et al, 2007).

5. Conclusion

In current clinical practice, MM patients' workout at diagnosis, automatically include prognostic factors such as CBC, creatinine, albumin, β_2M, LDH, 24 hours proteinuria, SPE, IFE and quantitative Ig and FLC measurements (with FLCR calculation), bone survey, bone marrow aspiration and biopsy with conventional karyotype. Information provided allows staging as well as additional prognostication based on LDH and FLC/FLCR values, thus helping treatment choices. However, if the decision to make is between thalidomide- and Bortezomib- containing regimens, FISH studies, eventually revealing high risk translocations, are useful. Therefore, they should also be routinely performed. Indeed, other more sensitive and patients' specific prognostic information can possibly be provided by

GEP and SNP studies but, for the time being these highly specified techniques concern research and are not available for clinical purposes.

After treatment, best response depth estimation is important. The introduction of stringent CR improves response evaluation but a more rigorous definition is needed and results of large clinical trials on the impact of sCR achievement are awaited. Possible additional information provided by multiparameter flow cytometry should be explored, if available. The question raised at that time is weather some kind of maintenance would make remission last longer.

During follow-up of MM patients in remission and plateau phase, FLC monitoring allows prevention of renal damage and early recognition of relapse.

At the time of relapse, PFs are once again needed to predict outcome; practically, the same that were determined at diagnosis, should be tested.

In conclusion, prognostic factors and systems have evolved during the past years. They allow a better disease management and contribute to the improvement observed with regard to survival. Unfortunately, there is still a proportion of patients with suboptimal outcomes and disease remains incurable at present.

6. Acknowledgment

We warmly thank Irini Rissakis for technical support.

7. References

Anargyrou, K., Terpos, E., Vassilakopoulos, T.P., Pouli, A., Sachanas, S., Tzenou, T., Masouridis, S., Christoulas, D., Angelopoulou, MK., Dimitriadou, E.M., Kalpadakis, C., Tsionos, K., Panayiotidis, P., Dimopoulos, M.A., Pangalis, G.A. & Kyrtsonis, M-C. (2008). Normalization of the serum angiopoietin-1 to angiopoietin-2 ratio reflects response in refractory/resistant multiple myeloma patients treated with bortezomib. Haematologica, Vol. 93, No.3, (Mars 2008), pp. 451-454, Print ISSN: 0390-6078 Online ISSN: 1592-8721.

Attal, M., Huguet, F., Schlaifer, D., Payen, C., Laroche, M., Fournie, B., Mazieres, B., Pris, J., & Laurent, G. (1992). Intensive combined therapy for previously untreated aggressive myeloma. *Blood*, Vol.79, No.5, (March 1992), pp. 1130-6, Print ISSN: 0006-4971 Online ISSN: 1528-0020

Augustson, B.M., Begum, G., Dunn, J.A., Barth, N., Davies, F., Morgan, G., Behrens, J., Smith, A., Child, J.A., & Drayson, M.T. (2005). Early mortality after diagnosis of multiple myeloma: analysis of patients entered onto the United kingdom Medical Research Council trials between 1980 and 2002--Medical Research Council Adult Leukaemia Working Party. *J Clin Oncol*, Vol.23, No.36, (December 2005), pp. 9219-26, Print ISSN: 0732-183X Online ISSN: 1527-7755

Avet-Loiseau, H., Attal, M., Moreau, P., Charbonnel, C., Garban, F., Hulin, C., Leyvraz, S., Michalle, M., Yakoub-Agha, I., Garderet, L., Marit, G., Michaux, L., Voillat, L., Renaud, M., Grosbois, B., Guillerm, G., Benboubker, L., Monconduit, M., Thieblemont, C., Casassus, P., Caillot, D., Stoppa, A.M., Sotto, J.J., Wetterwald, M.,

Dumontet, C., Fuzibet, J.G., Azais, I., Dorvaux, V., Zandecki, M., Bataille, R., Minvielle, S., Harousseau, J.L., Facon, T., & Mathiot, C. (2007). Genetic abnormalities and survival in multiple myeloma: the experience of the Intergroupe Francophone du Myelome. *Blood*, Vol.109, No.8, (April 2007), pp. 3489-95, Print ISSN: 0006-4971 Online ISSN: 1528-0020

Avet-Loiseau, H., Durie, B., Haessler, J., Crowley, J., Hoering, A., Barlogie, B., Shaughnessy, J.D. Jr., Sezer, O., Shustik, C., Hajek, R., Goldschmidt, H., Sonneveld, P., Moreau, P., Attal, M., Palumbo, A., Boccadoro, M., Lee, J.H., Westin, J., Turesson, I., San Miguel, J.F., Blade, J., Lahuerta, J.J., Pavlovsky, S., Fantl, D.B., Rajkumar, S.V., & Fonseca, R. (2009). Impact of FISH and Cytogenetics On Overall and Event Free Survival in Myeloma: An IMWG Analysis of 9,897 Patients. *Blood (ASH Annual Meeting Abstracts)*, Vol.114, No.22, (November 2009), abstr 743, ISSN: 0006-4971 Online ISSN: 1528-0020

Avet-Loiseau, H., Harousseau, J.L., Moreau, P., Mathiot, C., Facon, T., Attal, M., Bradwell, A. & Harding, S. (2009). Heavy/Light Chain Specific Immunoglobulin Ratios at Presentation Are Prognostic for Progression Free Survival in the IFM 2005-01 Myeloma Trial. *Blood (ASH Annual Meeting Abstracts)*, Vol 114, 1818, (November 2009), ISSN: 0006-4971 Online ISSN: 1528-0020

Avet-Loiseau, H. (2010). Ultra High-Risk Myeloma. In: *Hematology 2010*, Gewirtz A, Mikhael J, Schwartz B, &Crowther M, pp. 489-93, American Society of Hematology , Print ISSN: 1520-4391 Online ISSN 1520-4383, Washington

Avet-Loiseau H, Leleu X, Roussel M, Moreau P, Guerin-Charbonnel C, Caillot D, Marit G, Benboubker L, Voillat L, Mathiot C, Kolb B, Macro M, Campion L, Wetterwald M, Stoppa AM, Hulin C, Facon T, Attal M, Minvielle S, Harousseau JL. (2010). Bortezomib plus dexamethasone induction improves outcome of patients with t(4;14) myeloma but not outcome of patients with del(17p). *J Clin Oncol*. Vol.28, No. 30, (October 2010), pp. 4630-4, Print ISSN: 0732-183X Online ISSN: 1527-7755

Bahlis, N.J., King, A.M., Kolonias, D., Carlson, L.M., Liu, H.Y., Hussein, M.A., Terebelo, H.R., Byrne, G.E.Jr., Levine, B.L., Boise, L.H., & Lee, K.P. (2007). CD28-mediated regulation of multiple myeloma cell proliferation and survival. *Blood*, Vol.109, No.11, (June 2007), pp. 5002-10, Print ISSN: 0006-4971 Online ISSN: 1528-0020

Barlogie, B., Smallwood, L., Smith, T., & Alexanian, R. (1989). High serum levels of lactic dehydrogenase identify a high-grade lymphoma-like myeloma. *Ann Intern Med*, Vol.110, No.7, (April 1989), pp. 521-5, Print ISSN: 0003-4819 Online ISSN: 1539-3704

Barlogie, B., Shaughnessy, J., Tricot, G., Jacobson, J., Zangari, M., Anaissie, E., Walker, R., & Crowley, J. (2004) Treatment of multiple myeloma. *Blood*, Vol.103, No.1, (January 2004), pp. 20-32, Print ISSN: 0006-4971 Online ISSN: 1528-0020

Bataille, R., Boccadoro, M., Klein, B., Durie, B., & Pileri, A. (1992). C-reactive protein and beta-2 microglobulin produce a simple and powerful myeloma staging system. *Blood*, Vol.80, No.3, (August 1992), pp. 733–737, Print ISSN: 0006-4971 Online ISSN: 1528-0020

Bettini, R., Steidl, L., Rapazzini, P., & Giardina, G. (1983) Prognostic value of the staging system proposed by Merlini, Waldenström and Jayakar for multiple myeloma. *Acta Haematol*, Vol.70, No.6, pp. 379-85, Print ISSN: 0001-5792 Online ISSN: 1421-9662

Bladé, J., Rozman, C., Cervantes, F., Reverter, J.C., & Montserrat, E. (1989). A new prognostic system for multiple myeloma based on easily available parameters. *Br J Haematol*, Vol.72, No.4, (August 1989), pp. 507-11, Print ISSN: 0007-1048 Online ISSN: 1365-2141

Blade, J., Samson, D., Reece, D., Apperley, J., Björkstrand, B., Gahrton, G., Gertz, M., Giralt, S., Jagannath, S., & Vesole, D. (1998). Criteria for evaluating disease response and progression in patients with multiple myeloma treated by high-dose therapy and hemopoietic stem cell transplantation. Myeloma Subcommittee of the EBMT. European Group for Blood and Marrow Transplant. *Br J Haematol*, Vol.102, No.5, (September 1998), pp. 1115–23, Print ISSN: 0007-1048 Online ISSN: 1365-2141

Blade, J., Esteve, J., Rosiño,l L., Perales, M., Montoto, S., Tuset, M., & Montserrat, E. Thalidomide in refractory and relapsing multiple myeloma. *Semin Oncol*, Vol.28, No.6, (December 2001), pp. 588-92, Print ISSN: 0093-7754

Boccadoro, M., Marmont, F., Tribalto, M., Fossati, M.G., Redoglia, V., Battaglio, S., Massaia, M., Gallamini, A., Comotti, B., Barbui, T., Campobasso, N., Dammacco, F., Cantonetti, M., Petrucci, M.T., Mandelli, F., Resegotti, L., & Pileriet, A. (1989). Early responder myeloma: kinetic studies identify a patient subgroup characterized by very poor prognosis. *J Clin Oncol*, Vol.7, No.1, (January 1989), pp. 119–25, , Print ISSN: 0732-183X Online ISSN: 1527-7755

Bradwell, A.R., Carr-Smith, H.D., Mead, G.P., Tang, L.X., Showell, P.J., Drayson, M.T., & Drew, R. (2001) Highly sensitive, automated immunoassay for immunoglobulin free light chains in serum and urine. *Clin Chem*, Vol 47, No 4, (April 2001), pp 673-680, Print ISSN: 0009-9147 Online ISSN: 1530-8561

Bradwell, A.R.,Carr-Smith H.D., Mead, G.P., Harvey, T.C., & Drayson, M.T. (2003). Serum test for assessment of patients with Bence Jones myeloma. *The Lancet*, Vol.361, No.9356, (February 2003), pp. 489-91, Print ISSN: 0140-6736 Online ISSN: 1474-547X

Bradwell AR. (2010). *Serum Free Light Chain Analysis (Plus Hevylite)* (6th edition) The Binding Site Ltd, Birmingham, UK

Cassuto, J.P., Krebs, B.P., Viot, G., Dujardin, P., & Masseyeff, R. (1978). Beta 2microglobulin, a tumor marker of lymphoproliferative disorders. *The Lancet*, Vol.312, No.8096, (October 1978), pp. 950, Print ISSN: 0140-6736 Online ISSN: 1474-547X

Cavo, M., Galieni, P., Zuffa, E., Baccarani, M., Gobbi, M., & Tura, S. (1989). Prognostic variables and clinical staging in multiple myeloma. *Blood*, Vol.74, No.5, (October 1989), pp. 1774-1780, Print ISSN: 0006-4971 Online ISSN: 1528-0020

Chang, H., Trieu, Y., Qi. X., Xu, W., Stewart, K.A., & Reece, D. (2007). Bortezomib therapy response is independent of cytogenetic abnormalities in relapsed/refractory multiple myeloma. *Leuk Res*, Vol.31, No.6, (June 2007), pp. 779-82, Print ISSN: 0145-2126 Online ISSN: 1873-5835

Chang, H., Qi, X., Trieu, Y., Xu, W., Reader, J.C., Ning, Y., & Reece, D. (2006) Multiple myeloma patients with CKS1B gene amplification have a shorter progression-free survival post-autologous stem cell transplantation. *Br J Haematol*, Vol.135, No.4, (November 2006), pp. 486-91, Print ISSN: 0007-1048 Online ISSN: 1365-2141

Chang, H., Qi, X., Jiang, A., Xu, W., Young, T., & Reece, D. (2010). 1p21 deletions are strongly associated with 1q21 gains and are an independent adverse prognostic factor for the outcome of high-dose chemotherapy in patients with multiple myeloma. *Bone Marrow Transplant*, Vol 45, No 1, (January 2010), pp 117-21, Print ISSN: 0268-3369 Online ISSN: 1476-5365

Chang, H., Jiang A., Qi, C., Trieu, Y., Chen, C., & Reece, D. (2010). Impact of genomic aberrations including chromosome 1 abnormalities on the outcome of patients with relapsed or refractory multiple myeloma treated with lenalidomide and dexamethasone. *Leuk Lymphoma,* Vol.51, No.11, (November 2010), 2084-9, Print ISSN: 1042-8194 Online ISSN: 1029-2403.

Corradini, P., Cavo, M., Lokhorst, H., Martinelli, G., Terragna, C., Majolino, I., Valagussa, P., Boccadoro, M., Samson, D., Bacigalupo, A., Russell, N., Montefusco, V., Voena, C., & Gahrton, G.; Chronic Leukemia Working Party of the European Group for Blood and Marrow Transplantation (EBMT). (2003). Molecular remission after myeloablative allogeneic stem cell transplantation predicts a better relapse-free survival in patients with multiple myeloma. *Blood*, Vol.102, No.5, (September 2003), pp. 1927-9, Print ISSN: 0006-4971 Online ISSN: 1528-0020

Corthals, S.L., Kuiper, R., Johnson, D.C., Sonneveld, P., Hajek, R., van der Holt, B., Magrangeas, F., Goldschmidt, H., Morgan, G.J., & Avet-Loiseau H. (2011). Genetic factors underlying the risk of bortezomib induced peripheral neuropathy in multiple myeloma patients. *Haematologica,* (Epub ahead of print, July 2011), Print ISSN: 0390-6078 Online ISSN: 1592-8721

Cuzick, J., De Stavola, B.L., Cooper, E.H., Chapman, C., & MacLennan, I.C. (1990). Long-term prognostic value of serum beta 2 microglobulin in myelomatosis. *Br J Haematol*, Vol.75, No.4, (August 1990), pp. 506–510, Print ISSN: 0007-1048 Online ISSN: 1365-2141

de Larrea, C.F., Cibeira, M.T., Elena, M., Arostegui, .JI., Rosiñol, L., Rovira, M., Filella, X., Yagüe, J., & Bladé, J. (2009). Abnormal serum free light chain ratio in patients with multiple myeloma in complete remission has strong association with the presence of oligoclonal bands: Implications for stringent complete remission definition. *Blood*, Vol.114, No.24, (December 2009), pp. 4954-6, Print ISSN: 0006-4971 Online ISSN: 1528-0020

Davies, F.E., Raje, N., Hideshima, T., Lentzsch, S., Young, G., Tai, Y.T., Lin, B., Poda, K., Gupta, D., Chauhan, D., Treon, S.P., Richardson, P.G., Schlossman, R.L., Morgan, G.J., Muller, G.W., Stirling, D.I., Anderson, K.C. (2001). Thalidomide and immunomodulatory derivatives augment natural killer cell cytotoxicity in multiple myeloma. *Blood*, Vol.98, No.1, (July 2001), pp. 210-6, Print ISSN 0006-4971 Online ISSN 1528-0020

Dimopoulos, M.A., Barlogie, B., Smith T.L., & Alexanian, R. (1991). High serum lactate dehydrogenase level as a marker for drug resistance and short survival in multiple myeloma. *Ann Intern Med*, Vol.115, No.12, (December 1991), pp. 931-5 Print ISSN: 0003-4819 Online ISSN: 1539-3704

Dimopoulos, M., Kyle, R., Fermand, J.P., Rajkumar, SV., San Miguel, J., Chanan-Khan, A., Ludwig, H., Joshua, D., Mehta, J., Gertz, M., Avet-Loiseau, H., Beksaç, M., Anderson, K.C., Moreau, P., Singhal, S., Goldschmidt, H., Boccadoro, M., Kumar, S., Giralt, S., Munshi, N.C., & Jagannath, S. (2011). Consensus recommendations for standard investigative workup: report of the International Myeloma Workshop Consensus Panel 3. *Blood*, Vol.117, No.18, (May 2011), pp. 4701-5, Print ISSN: 0006-4971 Online ISSN: 1528-0020

Dimopoulos, M.A., Palumbo, A., Attal, M., Beksaç, M., Davies, F.E., Delforge, M., Einsele, H., Hajek, R., Harousseau, J.L., da Costa, F.L., Ludwig, H., Mellqvist, U.H., Morgan, G.J., San-Miguel, J.F., Zweegman, S., & Sonneveld, P.; European Myeloma Network. (2011). optimizing the use of lenalidomide in relapsed or refractory multiple myeloma: consensus statement. *Leukemia*, Vol.25, No.5, (May 2011), pp. 749-60, Print ISSN: 0887-6924, Online ISSN: 1476-5551

Di Raimondo, F., Azzaro, M.P., Palumbo, G., Bagnato, S., Giustolisi, G., Floridia, P., Sortino, G. & Giustolisi, R. (2000). Angiogenic factors in multiple myeloma: high levels in bone marrow than in peripheral blood. *Haematologica*, Vol.85, No.8, (August 2000), pp. 800–805,Print ISSN: 0390-6078 Online ISSN: 1592-8721

Drayson, M., Begum, G., Basu, S., Makkuni, S., Dunn, J., Barth, N., & Child, J.A. (2006). Effects of paraprotein heavy and light chain types and free light chain load on survival in myeloma: an analysis of patients receiving conventional-dose chemotherapy in Medical Research Council UK multiple myeloma trials. *Blood*, Vol.108, No.6, (September 2006), pp. 2013-19, Print ISSN: 0006-4971 Online ISSN: 1528-0020

Dredge, K., Marriott, J.B., Macdonald, C.D., Man, H.W., Chen, R., Muller, G.W., Stirling, D., & Dalgleish, A.G.. (2002). Novel thalidomide analogues display anti-angiogenic activity independently of immunomodulatory effects. *Br J Cancer*, Vol.87, No.4, (November 2002), pp. 1166–72, Print ISSN: 0007-0920 Online ISSN: 1532-1827

Durie, B.G., & Salmon, S.E. (1975). A clinical staging system for multiple myeloma. Correlation of measured myeloma cell mass with presenting clinical features, response to treatment, and survival. *Cancer*, Vol.36, No.3, (May 1975), pp. 842–54, Online ISSN: 1097-0142

Durie, B.G., Kyle, R.A., Belch, A., Bensinger, W., Blade, J., Boccadoro, M., Child, J.A., Comenzo, R., Djulbegovic, B., Fantl, D., Gahrton, G., Harousseau, J-L., Hungria, V., Joshua, D., Ludwig, H., Mehta, J., Morales, A.R., Morgan, G., Nouel, A., Oken, M., Powles, R., Roodman, D., San Miguel, J., Shimizu, K., Singhal, S., Sirohi, B., Sonneveld, P., Tricot, G., & Van Ness, B. Myeloma management guidelines: a consensus report from the Scientific Advisors of the International Myeloma Foundation. (2003). *Hematol J*, Vol.4 No.6, pp. 379-98 [Erratum in: *Hematol J* 2004;5:285], Print ISSN: 1466-4860

Durie, B.G. M. (2006). The role of anatomic and functional staging in myeloma: Description of Durie/Salmon plus staging system. *Eur J Cancer*, Vol.42, No.11, (July 2006), pp. 1539-43, Print ISSN:0959-8049 Online 1879-0852

Durie, B.G., Harousseau, J-L., Miguel, J.S., Bladé, J., Barlogie, B., Anderson, K., Gertz, M., Dimopoulos, M., Westin, J., Sonneveld, P., Ludwig, H., Gahrton, G., Beksac, M., Crowley, J., Belch, A., Boccadaro, M., Cavo, M., Turesson, I., Joshua, D., Vesole, D., Kyle, R., Alexanian, R., Tricot, G., Atta,l M., Merlini, G., Powles, R., Richardson, P., Shimizu, K., Tosi, P., Morgan, G., & Rajkumar, S.V. (2006). International uniform response criteria for multiple myeloma. *Leukemia*, Vol.20, No.9, (September 2006) pp. 1467-73, [Errata, Leukemia 2006; 20:2220, 2007;21:1134], Print ISSN: 0887-6924 Online ISSN: 1476-5551

Drayson, M., Begum, G., Basu, S., Makkuni, S., Dunn, J., Barth, N., & Child, J.A. (2006). Effects of paraprotein heavy and light chain type and free light chain load on survival in myeloma: An analysis of patients receiving conventional dose chemotherapy in Medical Research Council UK Multiple Myeloma trials. *Blood*, Vol.108, No.6, (September 2006), pp. 2013-9, Print ISSN: 0006-4971, Online ISSN: 1528-0020

Engelhardt, M., & Mertelsmann R. (2006). 160 years of multiple myeloma Progress and challenges. *Eur J Cancer*, Vol.42, No.42, (July 2006), pp. 1507-9, Print ISSN: 0959-8049

Fonseca, R., Bergsagel, P.L., Drach, J., Shaughnessy, J., Gutierrez, N., Stewart, A.K., Morgan, G., Van Ness, B., Chesi, M., Minvielle, S., Neri, A., Barlogie, B., Kuehl, W.M., Liebisch, P., Davies, F., Chen-Kiang, S., Durie, B.G., Carrasco, R., Sezer, O., Reiman, T., Pilarski, L., & Avet-Loiseau, H.; International Myeloma Working Group. (2009). International Myeloma Working Group molecular classification of multiple myeloma: spotlight review. Leukemia, Vol.23, No.12, (December 2009), pp 2210-21, Print ISSN: 0887-6924 Online ISSN: 1476-5551

Garewal, H., Durie, B.G., Kyle, R.A., Finley, P., Bower, B., & Serokman, R. (1984). Serum beta 2-microglobulin in the initial staging and subsequent monitoring of monoclonal plasma cell disorders. *J Clin Oncol*, Vol.2, No.1, (January 1984), pp. 51-7, Print ISSN: 0732-183X Online ISSN: 1527-7755

Gastinne, T., Leleu, X., Duhamel, A., Moreau, A.S., Frank, G., Andrieux, J., Lai, J.L., Coiteux V., Yakoub-Agha, I., Bauters, F., Harousseau, J.L., Zandecki, M., & Facon, T., On behalf of the Intergroupe Francophone du Myelome (IFM).[1]On behalf of the Intergroupe Francophone du Myelome. (2010). Plasma cell growth fraction using Ki-67 antigen expression identifies a subgroup of Multiple Myeloma patients displaying short survival within the ISS stage I. *Eur J Haematol.*, (August 5 2010), (Epub ahead of print doi: 10.1111/j.1600-0609.2007.0915), Print ISSN: 0902-4441 Online ISSN: 1600-0609

Gertz, M.A., Lacy, M.Q., Dispenzieri, A., Greipp, P.R., Litzow, M.R., Henderson, K.J., Van Wier, S.A., Ahmann, G.J., & Fonseca, R. (2005). Clinical implications of t(11;14)(q13;q32), t(4;14)(p16.3;q32), and -17p13 in myeloma patients treated with high-dose therapy. *Blood*, Vol.106, No.8, (October 2005), pp. 2837-40, Print ISSN: 0006-4971 Online ISSN: 1528-0020

Greipp, P.R., Lus, J.A., O'Fallon, W.M. Katzmann, J.A., Witzig, T.E., & Kyle, R.A. (1993). Plasma cell labeling index and beta 2-microglobulin predict survival independent of thymidine kinase and C-reactive protein in multiple myeloma. *Blood*, Vol.81, No.12, (June 1993), pp. 3382-7, Print ISSN: 0006-4971 Online ISSN: 1528-0020

Greipp, P.R., Leong, T., Bennett, J.M., Gaillard, J.P., Klein, B., Stewart, J.A., Oken, M.M., Kay, N.E., Van Ness, B., & Kyle, R.A. (1998). Plasmablastic Morphology—An Independent Prognostic Factor With Clinical and Laboratory Correlates: Eastern Cooperative Oncology Group (ECOG) Myeloma Trial E9486 Report by the ECOG

Myeloma Laboratory Group. *Blood*, Vol.91, No.7 (April 1998), pp. 2501-7, Print ISSN: 0006-4971, Online ISSN: 1528-0020

Greipp, P.R., San Miguel, J., Durie, B.G., Crowley, J.J., Barlogie, B., Bladé, J., Boccadoro, M., Child, J.A., Avet-Loiseau, H., Kyle, R.A., Lahuerta, J.J., Ludwig, H., Morgan, G., Powles, R., Shimizu, K., Shustik, C., Sonneveld, P., Tosi, P., Turesson, I., & Westin, J. (2005). International Staging System for Multiple Myeloma. *J Clin Oncol*, Vol.23, No.15, (May 2005), pp. 3412-20, Print ISSN: 0732-183X Online ISSN: 1527-7755

Fritz, E., Ludwig, H., & Kundi, M. (1984). Prognostic Relevance of Cellular Morphology in Multiple Myeloma. *Blood*, Vol.63, No.5, (May 1984), pp. 1072-9, Print ISSN: 0006-4971, Online ISSN: 1528-0020

Gavriatopoulou, M., Dimopoulos, M.A., Christoulas, D., Migkou, M., Iakovaki, M., Gkotzamanidou, & M., Terpos, E. (2009). Dickkopf-1: a suitable target for the management of myeloma bone disease. Expert Opin Ther Targets, Vol.13, No.7, (July 2009), pp. 839-48, Print ISSN: 1472-8222 Online ISSN : 1744-7631

Hutchison, C.A., Cockwell, P., Reid, S., Chandler, K., Mead, G.P., Harrison, J., Hattersley, J., Evans, N.D., Chappell, M.J., Cook, M., Goehl, H., Storr, M., & Bradwell, A.R. (2007). Efficient removal of immunoglobulin free light chains by hemodialysis for multiple myeloma: in vitro and in vivo studies. *J Am Soc Nephrol*, Vol.18, No.3, (March 2007), pp. 886-95, Print ISSN: 1046-6673 Online ISSN: 1533-3450

Jacobson, J.L., Hussein, M.A., Barlogie, B., Durie, B.G., & Crowley, J.J. (2003). Southwest Oncology Group: A new staging system for multiple myeloma patients based on the Southwest Oncology Group (SWOG) experience. *Br J Haematol*, Vol.122, No.3, (August 2003), pp. 441-50, Print ISSN: 0007-1048 Online ISSN: 1365-2141

Jagannath, S., Richardson, P.G., Sonneveld, P., Schuster, M.W., Irwin, D., Stadtmauer, E.A., Facon, T., Harousseau, J.L., Cowan, J.M., & Anderson, K.C. (2007). Bortezomib appears to overcome the poor prognosis conferred by chromosome 13 deletion in phase 2 and 3 trials. *Leukemia*, Vol.21, No.1, (January 2007), pp. 151-7, Print ISSN: 0887-6924 Online ISSN: 1476-5551

Joshi, S., Khan, R., Sharma, M., Kumar, L., & Sharma, A. (2011). Angiopoietin-2: a potential novel diagnostic marker in multiple myeloma. *Clin Biochem*, Vol.44, No.8-9, (June 2011), pp. 590-5, Print ISSN: 0009-9120

Juliusson, G., Celsing, F., Turesson, I., Lenhoff, S., Adriansson, M.;, & Malm, C. (2000). Frequent good partial remissions from thalidomide including best response ever in patients with advanced refractory and relapsed myeloma. *British Journal of Haematology*, Vol.109, No.1, (April 2000), pp. 89-96, Print ISSN: 0007-1048 Online ISSN: 1365-2141

Kapoor, P., Kumar, S., Fonseca, R., Lacy, M.Q., Witzig, T.E., Hayman, S.R., Dispenzieri, A., Buadi, F., Bergsagel, P.L., Gertz, M.A., Dalton, R.J., Mikhael, J.R., Dingli, D., Reeder, C.B., Lust, J.A., Russell, S.J., Roy, V., Zeldenrust, S.R., Stewart, A.K., Kyle, R.A., Greipp, P.R., & Rajkumar, S.V.(2009). Impact of risk stratification on outcome among patients with multiple myeloma receiving initial therapy with lenalidomide and dexamethasone. *Blood*, Vol.114, No.3, (July 2009), pp. 518-21, Print ISSN: 0006-4971, Online ISSN: 1528-0020

Kelley, T.W., Baz, R., Hussein, M., Karafa, M., & Cook, J.R. (2009). Clinical significance of cyclin D1, fibroblast growth factor receptor-3 and p53 immunohistochemistry in plasma cell myeloma treated with a thalidomide-based regimen. *Human Pathology* , Vol.40, No.3, (May 2009), pp. 405-12, Print ISSN: 0046-8177 Online ISSN: 1532-8392

Keren D.F.(2009). Heavy/Light-Chain analysis of monoclonal gammopathies. *Clin Chem,* Vol.55, No.9, (September 2009), pp. 1606-8, Print ISSN: 0009-9147 Online ISSN: 1530-8561

Koulieris, E., Kyrtsonis, M.C., Kafassi, N., Maltezas D., Bartzis., Tzenou, T., Dimou, M., Georgiou, G., Mirbahai, L., Panayiotidimm P., Bradwell, A., & Harding, S. (2010). Heavy Chain Ratio (HLCR) IgG{kappa}/IgG{lambda} or IgA{kappa}/IgA{lambda}: Experience and Clinical Implications In Multiple Myeloma at Diagnosis and During Disease Course. *Blood (ASH Annual Meeting Abstracts),* Vol.116, No.21, (November 2010), abstr 5019, ISSN: 0006-4971 Online ISSN: 1528-0020

Kumar, S., Gertz, M.A., Dispenzieri, A.,Lacy, M,Q., Wellik, L.A., Fonseca, R., Lust, J.A., Witzig, T.E., Kyle, R.A., Greipp, P.R. & Rajkumar, S.V. (2004). Prognostic value of bone marrow angiogenesis in patients with multiple myeloma undergoing high-dose therapy. *Bone Marrow Transplant,* Vol.34, No.3, (August 2004), pp. 235–239, Print ISSN: 0268-3369 Online ISSN: 1476-5365

Kumar, S., Witzig, T., Timm, M., Haug, J., Wellik, L., Kimlinger, T., Greipp, P., & Rajkumar, V. (2004). Bone marrow angiogenic ability and expression of angiogenic cytokines in myeloma: evidence favoring loss of marrow angiogenesis inhibitory activity with disease progression. *Blood,* Vol.104, No.4, (August 2004), pp. 1159-65, Print ISSN: 0006-4971 Online ISSN: 1528-0020

Kumar, S.K., Rajkumar, S.V., Dispenzieri. A., Lacy, M.Q., Hayman, S.R., Buadi, F.K., Zeldenrust, S.R., Dingli, D., Russell, S.J., Lust, J.A., Greipp, P.R., Kyle, R.A., & Gertz, M.A. (2008). Improved survival in multiple myeloma and the impact of novel therapies. *Blood,* Vol.111, No.5, (Mar 2008), pp. 2516–20, Print ISSN: 0006-4971, Online ISSN: 1528-0020

Kumar, S., Dispenzieri, A., van Wier, S., Katzmann, J.A., Snyder, M., Blood, E., DeGoey, R., Henderson, K., Kyle, R.A., Bradwell, A.R., Greipp, P.R., Rajkumar, S.V.,& Fonseca, R. (2010). Relationship between elevated immunoglobulin free light chain and the presence of IgH translocations in multiple myeloma. *Leukemia,* Vol.24, No.8, (August 2010), pp. 1498-1505, Print ISSN: 0887-6924 Online ISSN: 1476-5551

Kyle, R.A. (1995). Prognostic factors in multiple myeloma. *Stem Cells,* Suppl 2, (August 1995), pp. 56-63, Print ISSN: 1066-5099 Online ISSN: 1549-4918

Kyle, R.A., Gertz, M.A., Witzig, T.E., Lust, J.A., Lacy, M.Q., Dispenzieri, A., Fonseca, R., Rajkumar, S.V., Offord, J.R., Larson, D.R., Plevak, M.E., Therneau, T.M., & Greipp, P.R. (2003). Review of 1,027 patients with newly diagnosed multiple myeloma. *Mayo Clinic Proceedings,* Vol.78, No.1, (January 2003), pp. 21–33, Print ISSN: 0025-6196

Kyrtsonis, M.C., Dedoussis, G., Baxevanis, C., Stamatelou, M., & Maniatis, A. (1996). Serum interleukin-6 (IL-6) and interleukin-4 (IL-4) in patients with multiple myeloma (MM). *Br J Haematol,* Vol.92, No.2, (February 1996), pp. 420-22, Print ISSN: 0007-1048 Online ISSN: 1365-2141

Kyrtsonis, M.C., Dedoussis, G., Zervas, C., Perifanis, V., Baxevanis, C., Stamatelou, M., & Maniatis A.M-C. (1996). Soluble interleukin-6 receptor (sIL-6R), a new prognostic factor in multiple myeloma. *Br J Haematol*, Vol.93, No.2, (May 1996), pp. 398-400, Print ISSN: 0007-1048 Online ISSN: 1365-2141

Kyrtsonis, M.C.,Vassilakopoulos, T.P., Siakantaris, M.P., Kokoris, S.I., Gribabis, D.A., Dimopoulou, M.N., Angelopoulou, M.K., & Pangalis G.A. (2004). Serum syndecan-1, basic fibroblast growth factor and osteoprotegerin in myeloma patients at diagnosis and during the course of the disease. *Eur J Haematol*, Vol.72, No.4, (April 2004), pp. 252-8, Print ISSN: 0902-4441 Online ISSN: 1600-0609

Kyrtsonis, M-C., Vassilakopoulos, T.P., Kafasi, N., Sachanas, S., Tzenou, T., Papadogiannis, A., Galanis, Z., Kalpadakis, C., Dimou, M., Kyriakou, E., Angelopoulou, M.K., Dimopoulou, M.N., Siakantaris, M.P., Dimitriadou, E.M., Kokoris, S.I., Panayiotidis, P., & Pangalis, G.A. (2007). Prognostic value of serum free light chain ratio at diagnosis in multiple myeloma. *Br J of Haematol*, Vol.137, No.3, (May 2007), pp 240-3, Print ISSN: 0007-1048 Online ISSN: 1365-2141

Kyrtsonis, M.C., Vassilakopoulos, T.P., Kafasi, N., Maltezas, D., Anagnostopoulos, A., Terpos, E., Elefterakis-Papaiakovou, E., Pouli, A., Repousis, P., Delimpasi, S., Anargyrou, A., Stefanoudaki, C., Michalis, E., Sachanas, S., Tzenou, T., Masouridis, S., Dimou, M., Angelopoulou, M.K., Dimopoulou, M.N., Siakantaris, M., MD1,Dimitriadou, E., Kokoris, S.I., Kalpadakis, C., Panayiotidis, P., Dimopoulos, M.A., & Pangalis, G.A. (2007). The addition of sFLCR improves ISS prognostication in multiple myeloma. *Blood (ASH Annual Meeting Abstracts)*, Vol.110, Abstr 1490, Print ISSN 0006-4971 online ISSN 1528-0020

Kyrtsonis M.C., Vassilakopoulos T.P., Maltezas, D., Kafasi, N., Terpos, E., Eleftherakis-Papaiakovou, E., Repousis, P., Pouli, A., Delimpasi, S., Anargyrou, K., Stefanoudaki, A., Michalis, E., Sachanas, S., Tzenou, T., Dimou, M., Gavrieletopoulou, M., Panayiotidis, P., Dimopoulos, M.A., & Pangalis G.A. Hellenic Myeloma, Study Group. (2008). Suggested risk-stratification models including serum free light chain ratio for improved prognistication in multiple myeloma. *Hematology Meeting Reports* , Vol.2, No.2, (September 2008), pp. 32, ISSN 1970-7339

Kyrtsonis, M.C., Maltezas, D., Tzenou, T., Koulieris, E., & Bradwell, A.R. (2009). Staging Systems and Prognostic factors as a Guide to Therapeutic Decisions in Multiple Myeloma. *Semin Hematol* Vol.46, No.2, (April 2009), pp. 110–7, Print ISSN: 0037-1963 On line ISSN: 1532-8686

Kyrtsonis, M-C., Maltezas, D., Koulieris, E., Zaroulis, C., Tzenou, T., Sachanas, S., Bartzis, V., Georgiou, G., Dimou, M., Siakavellas, S., Vassilakopoulos, T.P., Angelopoulou, M.K., Koutra, E., Mouzaki, A., Pangalis, G.A., & Panayiotidis, P. (2010) Response to Bortezomib in Refractory/Relapsed Multiple Myeloma Patients: A Single Center Experience with Discussion on Specific Issues. *The Asia-Pacific Journal of Oncology & Hematology*, Vol.2, No.1, (February 2010), pp. 1-11, Print ISSN 1759-6637

Kyrtsonis, M-C., Bartzis, V., Papanikolaou, X., Koulieris, E., Georgiou, G., Dimou, M., Tzenou, T., & Panayiotidis, P. (2010) Genetic and Molecular Advances in Multiple

Myeloma: A Route to Better Understand Disease Heterogeneity. *The Application Of Clinical Genetics*, Vol.3, (July 2010), pp. 41-51, ISSN: 1178-704X

Lecouvet, F.E., Malghem, J., Michaux, L., Maldague, B., Ferrant, A., Michaux, J.L., & Vande Berg, B.C. (1999). Skeletal survey in advanced multiple myeloma: radiographic versus MR imaging survey. *Br J Haematol*, Vol.106, No.1, (July 1999), pp. 35–9, Print ISSN: 0007-1048 Online ISSN: 1365-2141

Lenhoff, S., Hjorth, M., Holmberg, E., Turesson, I., Westin, J., Nielsen, J.L., Wislöff, F., Brinch, L., Carlson, K., Carlsson, M., Dahl, I.M., Gimsing, P., Hippe, E., Johnsen, H.E., Lamvik, J., Löfvenberg, E., Nesthus, I., & Rödjer, S. (2000). Impact on survival of high-dose therapy with autologous stem cell support in patients younger than 60 years with newly diagnosed multiple myeloma: a population-based study. Nordic Myeloma Study Group. *Blood*, Vol 95, No 1, (January 2000), pp7-11 {Erratum in: *Blood*, Vol.116, No.13, (September 30, 2010), pp. 2402. Johnsen, H [corrected to Johnsen, H E]}, Print ISSN: 0006-4971 Online ISSN: 1528-0020

Lenhoff, S., Hjorth, M., Westin, J., Brinch, L., Bäckström, B., Carlson, K., Christiansen, I., Dahl, I.M., Gimsing, P., Hammerström, J., Johnsen, H.E., Juliusson, G., Linder, O., Mellqvist, U.H., Nesthus, I., Nielsen, J.L., Tangen, J.M., & Turesson, I. (2006). Impact of age on survival after intensive therapy for multiple myeloma: a population-based study by the Nordic Myeloma Study Group. *Br J Haematol*, Vol.133, No.4, (May 2006), pp. 389-96, Print ISSN: 0007-1048 Online ISSN: 1365-2141

Li, Si-dan., Wang,Ya-fei., Qi, Jun-yuan., & Qiu, Lu-gui. (2010). Clinical Features of Bone Complications and Prognostic Value of Bone Lesions Detected by X-ray Skeletal Survey in Previously Untreated Patients with Multiple Myeloma. *Indian J Hematol Blood Transfus*, Vol.26, No.3, (July-Sept 2010), pp. 83–88, Print ISSN: 0971-4502 Online ISSN: 0974-0449

Liu, H., Yuan, C., Heinerich, J., Braylan, R., Chang, M., Wingard, J., & Moreb, J. (2008). Flow cytometric minimal residual disease monitoring in patients with multiple myeloma undergoing autologous stem cell transplantation: A retrospective study. *Leuk Lymphoma*, Vol.49, No.2, (February 2008), pp. 306-14, Print ISSN: 1042-8194 Online ISSN: 1029-2403

Lonial, S. (2010). Presentation and risk stratification – improving prognosis for patients with multiple myeloma. *Cancer Treatment Reviews*, Vol.36, Suppl 2, (May 2010), pp. S12–7, ISSN: 0305-7372

Ludwig, H., Nachbaur, D.M., Fritz, E., Krainer, M., & Huber, H. (1991). Interleukin-6 is a prognostic factor in multiple myeloma. *Blood*, Vol .77, No.12, (June 1991), pp. 2794-5, Print ISSN: 0006-4971 Online ISSN: 1528-0020

Ludwig, H., Durie, B.G., Bolejack, V., Turesson, I., Kyle, R.A., Blade, J., Fonseca, R., Dimopoulos, M., Shimizu, K., San Miguel, J., Westin, J., Harousseau, J.L., Beksac, M., Boccadoro, M., Palumbo, A., Barlogie, B., Shustik, C., Cavo, M., Greipp, P.R., Joshua, D., Attal, M., Sonneveld, & P., Crowley, J. (2008). Myeloma in patients younger than age 50 years presents with more favorable features and shows better survival: an analysis of 10 549 patients from the International Myeloma Working Group. *Blood*, Vol.111, No.8, (April 2008), pp. 4039-47, Print ISSN: 0006-4971 Online ISSN: 1528-0020

Ludwig, H., Mirbahai, L., Zojer, N., Bradwell, A., & Harding, S. (2010). The Ratio of Monoclonal to Polyclonal Immunoglobulins Assessed with the Hevylite Test Predicts Prognosis, Is Superior for Monitoring the Course of the Disease and Allows Detection of Monoclonal Immunoglobulin In Patients with Normal or Subnormal Involved Immunoglobulin Isotype. *Blood (ASH Annual Meeting Abstracts)*, Vol 116, No 21, (November 2010), Abstr 4038, Print ISSN: 0006-4971 Online ISSN: 1528-0020

Maltezas, D., Dimopoulos, M.A., Katodritou, I., Repoussis, P., Pouli, A., Terpos, E., Panayoitidis, P., Delimpasi, S., Michalis, E., Anargyrou, K., Gavriatopoulou, M., Stefanoudaki, A., Kafassi, N., Tzenou, T., Koulieris, E., Bartzis, V., Dimou, M., Vassilakopoulos, T.P., Zervas, K., & Kyrtsonis, M.C. Hellenic Myeloma Study Group. (2011). The prognostic impact of sFLCR-ISS is conserved in MM patients treated withnew agents but not in those that underwent ASCT. *Haematologica*, Vol.96, Suppl.1, (May 2011) , Abstr P199, ISSN 0390-6078

Marriott, J.B., Clarke, I.A., Dredge, K., Muller, G., Stirling, D., & Dalgleish, A.G. (2002). Thalidomide and its analogues have distinct and opposing effects on TNF-α and TNFR2 during co-stimulation of both CD4+ and CD8+ T cells. *Clin Exp Immunol* , Vol.130, No.1, (October 2002), pp. 75-84, Print ISSN: 0009-9104 Online ISSN: 1365-2249

Martínez-Sanchez, P., Montejano, L., Sarasquete, M.E., García-Sanz, R., Fernández-Redondo, E., Ayala, R., Montalbán, M.A., Martínez, R., García Laraña, J., Alegre, A., Hernández, B., Lahuerta, J.J., & Martínez-López J. (2008). Evaluation of minimal residual disease in multiple myeloma patients by fluorescent-polymerase chain reaction: The prognostic impact of achieving molecular response. *Br J Haematol*, Vol.142, No.5, (September 2008), pp. 766-74, Print ISSN: 0007-1048 Online ISSN: 1365-2141

Mileshkin, L.,Honemann, D., Gambell, P., Trivett, M., Hayakawa, Y., Smyth, M., Beshay, V., Ritchie, D., Simmons, P., Milner, A.D., Zeldis, J.B., & Prince, H.M. (2007). Patients with multiple myeloma treated with thalidomide: evaluation of clinical parameters, cytokines,angiogenic markers, mast cells and marrow CD57+ cytotoxic T cells as predictors of outcome. *Hematologica,* Vol.92, No.8, (August 2007), pp.1075-82, Print ISSN: 0390-6078 Online ISSN: 1592-8721

Mitsiades, N., Mitsiades, C.S., Poulaki, V., Chauhan, D., Richardson, P.G., Hideshima, T., Munshi, N.C., Treon, S.P., & Anderson, K.C. Apoptotic signaling induced by immunomodulatory thalidomide analogs in human multiple myeloma cells: Therapeutic implications. *Blood*, Vol.99, No.12, (June 2002), pp. 4525-4530, Print ISSN 0006-4971 Online ISSN 1528-0020

Mitsiades, N., Mitsiades, C., Munshi, N., Richardson, P., & Anderson, K. (2006). The role of the bone microenvironment in the pathophysiology and therapeutic management of multiple myeloma: Interplay of growth factors, their receptors and stromal interactions. *Eur. Jour. Cancer*, Vol.42, No.11, (July 2006), pp. 1564-73, Print ISSN: 0959-8049

Moulopoulos, L.A., Gika, D., Anagnostopoulos, A., Delasalle, K., Weber, D., Alexanian, R., & Dimopoulos, M.A. (2005). Prognostic significance of MRI of bone marrow in previously untreated patients with multiple myeloma. *Ann Oncol*, Vol.16, No.11, (Novenber 2005), pp. 1824-8, Print ISSN 0923-7534 Online ISSN 1569-8041

Munshi, N.C., Anderson, K.C., Bergsagel, P.L., Shaughnessy, J., Palumbo, A., Durie, B., Fonseca, R., Stewart, A.K., Harousseau, J-L., Dimopoulos, M., Jagannath, S., Hajek, R., Sezer, O., Kyle, R., Sonneveld, P., Cavo, M., Rajkumar, S.V., San Miguel, J., Crowley, J. & Avet-Loiseau, H. (2011). Consensus recommendations for risk stratification in multiple myeloma: report of the International Myeloma Workshop Consensus Panel 2. *Blood*, Vol.117, No.18, (May 2011), pp. 4696-4700, Print ISSN: 0006-4971 Online ISSN: 1528-0020

Neben, K., Jauch, A., Bertsch, U., Heiss, C., Hielscher, T., Seckinger, A., Mors, T., Müller, N.Z., Hillengass, J., Raab, M.S., Ho, A.D., Hose, D., & Goldschmidt, H. (2010). Combining information regarding chromosomal aberrations t(4;14) and del(17p13) with the International Staging System classification allows stratification of myeloma patients undergoing autologous stem cell transplantation. *Haematologica*, Vol.95, N. 7, (July 2010), pp. 1150-7, Print ISSN: 0390-6078 Online 1592-8721

Norfolk, D., Child, J.A., Cooper, E.H., Kerruish, S., & Ward, A.M. (1980). Serum beta 2 microglobulin in myelomatosis: Potential value in stratification and monitoring. *Br J Cancer*, Vol.42, No.4, (October 1980), pp. 510-15, Print ISSN 0007-0920 Online 1532-1827

Paiva, B., Vidriales, M.B., Mateo, G., Pérez, J.J., Montalbán, M.A., Sureda, A., Montejano, L., Gutiérrez, N.C., García de Coca, A., de las Heras, N., Mateos, M.V., López-Berges, M.C., García-Boyero, R., Galende, J., Hernández, J., Palomera, L., Carrera, D., Martínez, R., de la Rubia, J., Martín, A., González, Y., Bladé, J., Lahuerta, J.J., Orfao, A., & San-Miguel, J.F.; GEM (Grupo Español de MM)/PETHEMA (Programa para el Estudio de la Terapéutica en Hemopatías Malignas) Cooperative Study Groups.(2009). The persistence of immunophenotypically normal residual bone marrow plasma cells at diagnosis identifies a good prognostic subgroup of symptomatic multiple myeloma patients. *Blood*, Vol.114, No.20, (November 2009), pp. 4369-72, Print ISSN: 0006-4971, Online ISSN: 1528-0020

Paiva, B., Almeida, J., Pérez-Andrés, M., Mateo, G., López, A., Rasillo, A., Vídriales, M.B., López-Berges, M.C., Miguel J.F., & Orfao, A. (2010). Utility of flow cytometry immunophenotyping in multiple myeloma and other clonal plasma cell-related disorders. *Cytometry B Clin Cytom*, Vol.78, Suppl 1, (July 2010), pp. S47-60, Print ISSN: 1552-4949 Online ISSN: 1552-4957

Paiva, B., Martinez-Lopez, J., Vidriales, M.B., Mateos, M.V., Montalban, M.A., Fernandez-Redondo, E., Alonso, L., Oriol, A., Teruel, A.I., de Paz, R., Laraña, J.G., Bengoechea, E., Martin, A., Mediavilla, J.D., Palomera, L., de Arriba, F., Bladé, J., Orfao, A., Lahuerta, J.J., & San Miguel, J.F. (2011). Comparison of Immunofixation, Serum Free Light Chain, and Immunophenotyping for Response Evaluation and Prognostication in Multiple Myeloma. *J Clin Oncol*, Vol.29, No.12, (April 2011), pp. 1627-33, Print ISSN: 0732-183X Online ISSN: 1527-7755

Pangalis, G.A., Kyrtsonis, M.C., Vassilakopoulos, T.P., Dimopoulou, M.N., Siakantaris, M.P., Emmanouilides, C., Doufexis, D., Sahanas, S., Kontopidou, F.N., Kalpadakis, C., Angelopoulou, M.K., Dimitriadou, E.M., Kokoris, S.I., & Panayiotidis, P. (2006).

Immunotherapeutic and immunoregulatory drugs in haematologic malignancies. *Current Topics in Medicinal Chemistry*, Vol.6, No.16, pp. 1657-86, ISSN: 1568-0266

Podar, K., Tai, Y.T., Davies, F.E., Lentzsch, S., Sattler, M., Hideshima, T., Lin, B.K., Gupta, D., Shima, Y., Chauhan, D., Mitsiades, C., Raje, N., Richardson, P., & Anderson, K.C. (2001). Vascular endothelial growth factor triggers signaling cascades mediating multiple myeloma cell growth and migration. *Blood*, Vol.98, No.2, (July 2001), pp. 428-435, Print ISSN: 0006-4971 Online ISSN: 1528-0020

Pulkki, K., Pelliniemi, T.T., Rajamäki, A., Tienhaara, A., Laakso, M., & Lahtinen, R. (1996). Soluble interleukin-6 receptor as a prognostic factor in multiple myeloma. Finnish Leukaemia Group. *Br J Haematol*, Vol.92, No.2, (February 1996), pp. 370-4, Print ISSN: 0007-1048 Online ISSN: 1365-2141

Rajkumar, S.V., Fonseca, R., Lacy, M.Q., Witzig, T.E., Therneau, T.M., Kyle, R.A., Litzow, M.R., Gertz, M.A., & Greipp, PR. (1999). Plasmablastic Morphology Is an Independent Predictor of Poor Survival After Autologous Stem-Cell Transplantation for Multiple Myeloma. *J Clin Oncol*, Vol.17, No.5, (May 1999), pp. 1551-57, Print ISSN: 0732-183X Online ISSN: 1527-7755

Rajkumar, S.V., Fonseca, R., Dispenzieri, A., Lacy, M.Q., Lust, J.A., Witzig, T.E., Kyle, R.A., Gertz, M.A., & Greipp, P.R. (2000). Thalidomide in the treatment of relapsed multiple myeloma. *Mayo Clin Proc*, Vol.75, No.9, (September 2000), pp. 897-901, Print ISSN: 0025-6196 Online ISSN: 1942-5546

Rajkumar, S.V. & Buadi, F. (2007). Multiple myeloma: New staging systems for diagnosis, prognosis and response evaluation. *Best Practice & Research Clinical Haematology*, Vol. 20, No. 4, (December 2007), pp. 665–80, Print ISSN: 1521-6926

Richardson, P.G., Schlossman, R.L., Weller, E., Hideshima, T., Mitsiades, C., Davies, F., LeBlanc, R., Catley, L.P., Doss, D., Kelly, K., McKenney, M., Mechlowicz, J., Freeman, A., Deocampo, R., Rich, R., Ryoo, J.J., Chauhan, D., Balinski, K., Zeldis, J., & Anderson, K.C. (2002). Immunomodulatory drug CC-5013 overcomes drug resistance and is well tolerated in patients with relapsed multiple myeloma. *Blood*, Vol.100, No.1, (November 2002), pp. 3063–7, Print ISSN 0006-4971 Online ISSN 1528-0020

Robillard, N., Pellat-Deceunynck, C., & Bataille, R. (2005). Phenotypic characterization of the human myeloma cell growth fraction. *Blood*, Vol.105, No.12, (June 2005), pp. 4845-8, Print ISSN: 0006-4971 Online ISSN: 1528-0020

Sagaster, V., Ludwig, H., Kaufmann, H., Odelga, V., Zojer, N., Ackermann, J., Küenburg, E., Wieser, R., Zielinski, C., & Drach, J. (2007). Bortezomib in relapsed multiple myeloma: response rates and duration of response are independent of a chromosome 13q-deletion. *Leukemia*, Vol.21, No.1, (January 2007), pp. 164-68, Print ISSN: 0887-6924 Online ISSN: 1476-5551

Seidel, C., Sundan, A., Hjorth, M., Turesson, I., Dahl, I.M., Abildgaard, N., Waage, A., & Borset, M. (2000). Serum syndecan-1: a new independent prognostic marker in multiple myeloma. *Blood*, Vol.95, No.2, (January 2000), pp. 388-92, Print ISSN: 0006-4971, Online ISSN: 1528-0020

Sezer, O., Jakob, C., Eucker, J., Niemöller, K., Gatz, F., Wernecke, K., & Possinger, K. (2001). Serum levels of the angiogenic cytokines basic fibroblast growth factor (bFGF), vascular endothelial growth factor (VEGF) and hepatocyte growth factor (HGF) in multiple myeloma. *Eur J Haematol*, Vol.66, No.2, (February 2001), pp. 83-88, Print ISSN: 0902-4441 Online ISSN: 1600-0609

Simonsson, B., Brenning, G., Källander, C., & Ahre, A. (1987) Prognostic value of serum lactic dehydrogenase (S-LDH) in multiple myeloma. *Eur J Clin Invest*, Vol.17, No.4, (August 1987), pp. 336-9, Print ISSN: 0014-2972 Online ISSN: 1365-2362

Simonsson, B., Källander, C.F., Brenning, G., Killander, A., Gronowitz, J.S., & Bergström, R. (1988). Biochemical markers in multiple myeloma: a multivariate analysis. *Br J Haematol*, Vol.69, No.1, (May 1988), pp. 47-53, Print ISSN: 0007-1048 Online ISSN: 1365-2141

Singhal, S., Mehta, J., Desikan, R., Ayers, D., Roberson, P., Eddlemon, P., Munshi, N., Anaissie, E., Wilson, C., Dhodapkar, M., Zeldis, J., & Barlogie, B. (1999). Antitumor activity of thalidomide in refractory multiple myeloma. *The New England Journal of Medicine*, Vol.341, No.21, (November 1999), pp. 1565-71, Print ISSN 0028-4793 Online ISSN 1533-4406

Singhal, S., Vickrey, E., Krishnamurthy, J., Singh, V., Allen, S., & Mehta, J. (2009). The relationship between the serum free light chain assay and serum immunofixation electrophoresis, and the definition of concordant and discordant free light chain ratios. *Blood*, Vol.114, No.1, (July 2009), pp. 38-9, Print ISSN: 0006-4971, Online ISSN: 1528-0020

Snapper, I., & Khan A. (1971). *Myelomatosis: Fundamentals and Clinical Features*, University Park Press, ISBN 0839105886 9780839105886 Baltimore

Snozek, C.L., Katzmann, J.A., Kyle, R.A., Dispenzieri, A., Larson, D.R., Therneau, T.M., Melton, L.J., Kumar, S., Greipp, P.R., Clark, R.J., & Rajkumar, S.V. (2008). Prognostic value of the serum free light chain ratio in newly diagnosed myeloma: proposed incorporation into the international staging system. *Leukemia*, Vol.22, No.10, (October 2008), pp. 1933-37, Print ISSN: 0887-6924 Online ISSN: 1476-5551

Talageri, V.R., Nadkarni, J.S., & Gollerkeri, M.P. (1977). Evaluation of plasma lactate dehydrogenase (LDH) isoenzymes in cancer patients. *Indian J Cancer*, Vol.14, No.1, (March 1977), pp. 42-9, Print ISSN: 0019-509X

Terpos, E., Szydlo, R., Apperley, J.F., Hatjiharissi, E., Politou, M., Meletis, J., Viniou, N., Yatagana,s X., Goldman, J.M., & Rahemtulla, A. (2003). Soluble receptor activator of nuclear factor kappaB ligand-osteoprotegerin ratio predicts survival in multiple myeloma: proposal for a novel prognostic index. *Blood*, Vol. 102, No.3, (August 2003), pp. 1064-9, Print ISSN: 0006-4971 Online ISSN: 1528-0020

Terpos, E., Politou, M., Szydlo, R., Goldman, J.M., Apperley, J.F., & Rahemtulla, A. (2003). Serum levels of macrophage inflammatory protein-1 alpha (MIP-1alpha) correlate with the extent of bone disease and survival in patients with multiple myeloma. Br J Haematol, Vol.123, No.1, (October 2003), pp.106-9, Print ISSN: 0007-1048 Online ISSN: 1365-2141

Terpos, E., Heath, D. J., Rahemtulla, A., Zervas, K., Chantry, A., Anagnostopoulos, A., Pouli, A., Katodritou, E., Verrou, E., Vervessou, E-C., Dimopoulos, M.A. & Croucher, P.I. (2006). Bortezomib reduces serum dickkopf-1 and receptor activator of nuclear factor-κB ligand concentrations and normalises indices of bone remodelling in patients with relapsed multiple myeloma. *Br J Haematol*, Vol.135, No.5, (December 1996), pp. 688–692, Print ISSN: 0007-1048 Online ISSN: 1365-2141

Terpos, E., Katodritou, E., Roussou, M., Pouli, A., Michalis, E., Delimpasi, S., Parcharidou, A., Kartasis, Z., Zomas, A., Symeonidis, A., Viniou, N.A., Anagnostopoulos, N., Economopoulos, T., Zervas, K., & Dimopoulos, M.A.; Greek Myeloma Study Group, Greece. (2010). High serum lactate dehydrogenase adds prognostic value to the international myeloma staging system even in the era of novel agents. *Eur J Haematol*, Vol.85, No.2, (August 2010), pp. 114-9, Print ISSN: 0902-4441 Online ISSN: 1600-0609

Terpos, E., Anargyrou K., Katodritou E., Kastritis E., Papatheodorou A., Christoulas D., Pouli A., Michalis ., Delimpasi S., Gkotzamanidou M., Nikitas N., Koumoustiotis V., Margaritis D., Tsionos K., Stefanoudaki E., Meletis J., Zervas K., & Dimopoulos, M.A. (2011). Circulating angiopoietin-1 to angiopoietin-2 ratio is an independent prognostic factor for survival in newly diagnosed patients with multiple myeloma who received therapy with novel antimyeloma agents. *Int J Cancer*, (April 2011), (Epub ahead of print), Print ISSN: 0020-7136 Online ISSN: 1097-0215

Trendle, M.C., Leong, T., Kyle, R.A., Katzmann, J.A., Oken, M.M., Kay, N.E., Van Ness, B.G., & Greipp, P.R. (1999). Prognostic Significance of the S-phase Fraction of Light-Chain-Restricted Cytoplasmic Immunoglobulin (cIg) Positive Plasma Cells in Patients with Newly Diagnosed Multiple Myeloma Enrolled on Eastern Cooperative Oncology Group Treatment Trial E9486. *American Journal of Hematology,* Vol.61, No.4, (August 1999), pp. 232–7, Print ISSN: 0361-8609 Online ISSN: 1096-8652.

Tricot, G., Barlogie, B., Jagannath, S., Bracy, D., Mattox, S., Vesole, D.H., Naucke, S., & Sawyer J.R. (1995). Poor prognosis in multiple myeloma is associated only with partial or complete deletions of chromosome 13 or abnormalities involving 11q and not with other karyotype abnormalities. *Blood*, Vol.86, No.11, (December 1995), pp. 4250-56, Print ISSN: 0006-4971, Online ISSN: 1528-0020

Vacca, A., Ribatti, D., Roncali, L., Ranieri, G., Serio, G., Silvestris, F., & Dammacco, F. (1994). Bone marrow angiogenesis and progression in multiple myeloma. *Br J Haematol,* Vol.87, No.3, (July 1994), pp. 503–508, Print ISSN: 0007-1048 Online ISSN: 1365-2141

Vacca, A., Scavelli, C., Montefusco, V., Di Pietro, G., Neri, A., Mattioli, M., Bicciato, S., Nico, B., Ribatti, D., Dammacco, F., Corradini, P. (2005). Thalidomide downregulates angiogenic genes in bone marrow endothelial cells of patients with active multiple myeloma. *J Clin Oncol* , Vol.23, No.23, (August 2005), pp. 5334–46, Print ISSN: 0732-183X Online ISSN: 1527-7755

Vezzoni, M.A., Lucchini, R., Giardini, R., Raineri, M., Murone, M., & Vezzoni, P. (1983). Lactate dehydrogenase levels in cellular extracts of human malignant lymphomas. *Tumori*, Vol.69, No.4, (August 1983), pp. 279-82, Print ISSN: 0300-8916

Walker, R., Barlogie, B., Haessler, J., Tricot, G., Anaissie, E., Shaughnessy, J.D. Jr., Epstein, J., van Hemert, R., Erdem, E., Hoering, A., Crowley, J., Ferris, E., Hollmig, K., van Rhee, F., Zangari, M., Pineda-Roman, M., Mohiuddin, A., Yaccoby, S., Sawyer, J., & Angtuaco, E.J. (2007). Magnetic resonance imaging in multiple myeloma: diagnostic and clinical implications. *J Clin Oncol*, Vol.25, No.9, (March 2007), pp. 1121-28, Print ISSN: 0732-183X Online ISSN: 1527-7755

Wirk, B. (2011). Renal failure in multiple myeloma: a medical emergency. *Bone Marrow Transplant*, Vol.46, No.6, (June 2011), pp. 771-83, Print ISSN: 0268-3369 Online ISSN: 1476-5365

Wisloff, F., Kvam, A.K., Hjorth, M., & Lenhoff, S. (2007). Serum calcium is an independent predictor of quality of life in multiple myeloma. *Eur J Haematol*, Vol.78, No.1, (January 2007), pp. 29-34, Print ISSN: 0902-4441 Online ISSN: 1600-0609.

Part 2

Multiple Myeloma Management: Issues and Considerations

9

Solitary Plasmacytoma of Bone

Jianru Xiao, Wending Huang,
Xinghai Yang and Honglin Teng
The Second Military Medical University
China

1. Introduction

Solitary plasmacytoma (SP), histologically indistinguishable from multiple myeloma (MM), is a kind of malignant tumor characterized by the proliferation of monoclonal plasma cells. SP is an independent subtype of plasmacytoma, including extramedullary plasmacytoma and solitary plasmacytoma of bone (SPB) [1]. Most solitary plasmacytomas progress to MM, and are usually treated in the department of hematology. SPB may involve in any bone, however, it mainly occurs in the axial skeleton, especially in a vertebra. SPB has a high risk of progression to MM, and on magnetic resonance imaging (MRI) examination, at least 25% of patients with an apparent solitary lesion have evidence of disease elsewhere.

In patients with solitary plasmacytoma of bone, the diagnosis can be made in the light of clinical and radiographic manifestations combined pathology. Thereafter, systemic treatment should be performed according to the status of the patients and the evidence of disease progression [2-6].

Although definitive local radiotherapy is a choice for the treatment of SPB, no affirmative conclusion can be drawn due to the lack of randomized trials for this kind of disease. Surgical management is usually non-mandatory; however, patients may require decompression or reconstruction if there are spinal cord compression and pathological fracture.

2. Epidemiology and clinical features

SPB is a primary malignant tumor, mainly affecting axial skeleton, especially the vertebra[2]. These tumors occur in the spine twice as often as other bony sites [7]. The male/female ratio of SPB is about 2 to 1 with a mean age of 55 years [2]. Solitary plasmacytoma is one of the most common malignant primary tumors in spine. Involvement of the base of the skull may present with cranial nerve palsies. The early symptoms of SPB are not typical. The most common presenting symptom is pain. If spine is involved, deformity, motor deficits, sensory deficits, n bowel and bladder dysfunction could be seen as well as pain as result of epidural spinal-cord compression and/or instability of the vertebra. Plain radiography shows expansile, irregular osteolytic lesions with or without vertebra instability [8-9]. CT or MRI can detect the lesions and describe the tumor extent at an earlier stage. Particularly, MRI scanning has an important reference value in description of residual tumor, local relapse and progression to MM after treatment [10]. The presence of M protein has been reported in 24%-72% of patients [2].

3. Radiological and laboratory features

All patients with suspected solitary plasmacytoma should undergo X-ray examination, computed tomography (CT) scan or magnetic resonance imaging (MRI). Plain radiographs showed solitary expansile osteolytic lesion with or without collapse of the vertebral body (Fig.A). However, plain radiographs did not show any abnormality in some patients when the disease was in the early stage, thus CT scan or CT three-dimensional reconstruction examinations were needed. Most CT scan showed osteolytic lesions with or without collapse of the vertebral body or even paravertebral soft tissue masses (Fig.B). As a noninvasive technique for detecting a potential lesion of the bone, MRI has been a routine evaluation. However, there are no definitive guidelines to verify the involvement on an MRI examination. Generally, MRI shows Low or intermediate signal on T1-weighted imaging and hyperintense on T2-weighted imaging, and significant enhancement with gadolinium (Fig.C-E). Whole-body MRI may be an effective technique to detect multiple lesions but costly. MRI patterns of marrow involvement play an important role in assessment myeloma bone disease. They include normal appearance of bone marrow despite minor microscopic plasma cell infiltration, focal involvement, homogeneous diffuse infiltration, combined diffuse and focal infiltration, and variegated or "salt-and-pepper" pattern with inhomogeneous bone marrow with interposition of fat islands. It is essential to have investigations of full skeletal survey to rule out multiple lesions. It is well-known that emission computed tomography (ECT) has a primary value in detecting multiple lesions of bone. Therefore, it is recommended for patients' suspicion of multiple myeloma to undergo ECT scan, but the positive incidence of detecting occult disease is not encouraging. With the advent of positron emission tomography/computed tomography (PET-CT)[11-12], it is proved to be an important method to detect occult lesions.

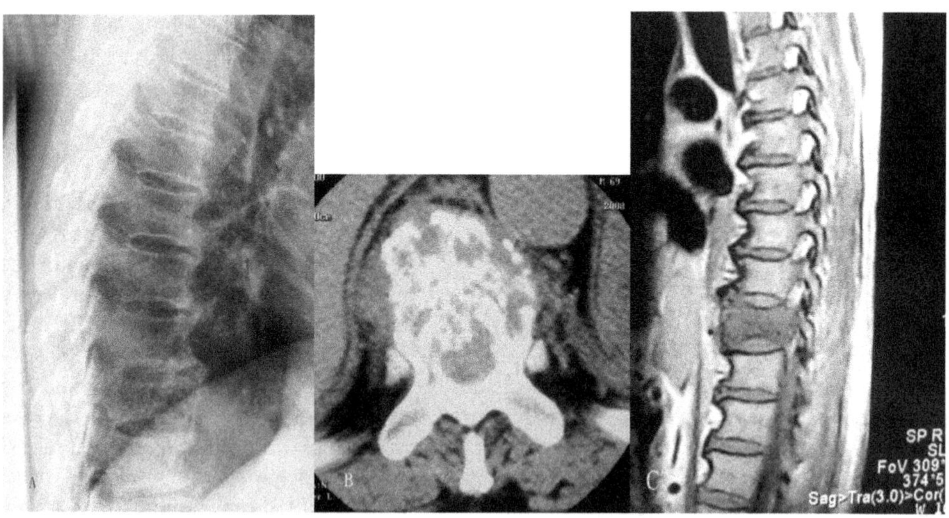

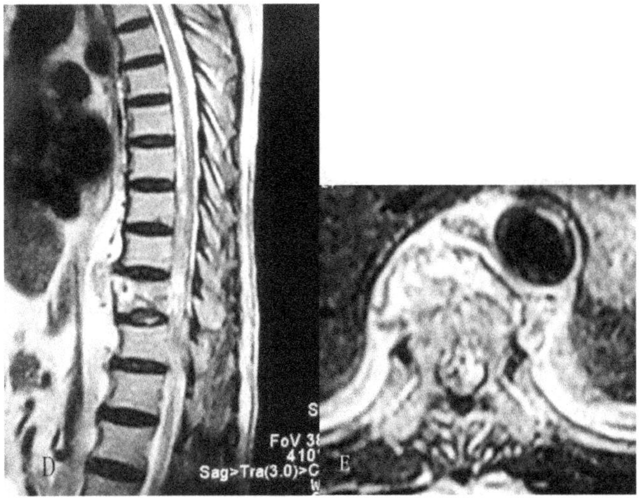

Fig. 1. A 68-year-old man with SBP of T10. Lateral radiograph showing mild collapse of vertebral body height at T10 (A).Computed tomography scan showing lytic bone destruction of the vertebral body (B). Magnetic resonance imaging showing hypointense on T1-weighted imaging(C) and hyperintense on T2-weighted imaging(D), and bright enhancement after administration of gadolinium(E).

If SBP is suspected, the following laboratory investigations should be performed in all patients: complete blood count (CBC), electrolytes, immunoglobulin, serum monoclonal paraprotein (M protein) electrophoresis, urine protein electrophoresis and immune fixation, marrow cell morphology and marrow aspiration biopsy. The prevalence of a monoclonal protein (M protein) in the serum or urine of patients with SBP varies from 24% to 72%, and the levels of the M protein(<3g/dl) are lower than those patients with MM [2]. In our experience, marrow aspiration biopsy is necessary to establish the diagnosis of SBP or MM with certainty.

4. Diagnosis

4.1 Diagnostic criteria

The followings are the recommended diagnostic criteria [3]:

1. A single area of bone damage due to clonal plasma cell hyperplasia.
2. Histologically normal marrow aspirate and trephine.
3. Normal results on skeletal survey, including radiology of long bones.
4. No anemia, hypercalcemia, or renal impairment due to plasma cell dyscrasia.
5. Absent or low serum or urinary level of monoclonal immunoglobulin (level of >20g/L suspicious of MM).
6. No additional lesions on MRI scan of the spine.

4.2 Biopsy and pathology

Biopsy and histopathologic examination play an important role in diagnosing this disease. SPB is generally diagnosed by pathology. Needle biopsy under CT or fluoroscopy guidance can be safe and effective. As this kind of tumor is rare, it is recommended that pathology review should be performed by a senior histopathologist who is skilled in bone tumor or lymphatic system diseases. In our experience, the definitive diagnosis of SPB should be based on clinical, radiologic, and pathologic findings of patients.

5. Treatment of solitary plasmacytoma of bone

5.1 Radiotherapy and recommendations

Radiotherapy is considered the treatment of choice for solitary plasmacytoma of bone. Although high local control rates of 83% to 96% are achieved with moderate doses of radiotherapy, the progression to multiple myeloma is considerably common [6,13-17]. However, the evidence base of radiotherapy is largely consisted of retrospective studies of small series of patients. In addition, data on dose-response relationships are weak in most series of the literatures [3].

On the basis of evidences in the literatures, recommendations were put forward by oncologists [3,5,6]. The recommendation on the dose of radiotherapy is 40Gy in 20 fractions for lesions with a margin of at least 2 centimeters. For lesions of SPB greater than 5 centimeters, a higher dose of up to 50Gy in 25 fractions should be considered. As for the extent of radiation management, the clinical target volume should include the tumor shown on MRI with a margin of at least 2 cm. For a vertebral lesion, the scope of radiotherapy should cover the entire bone involved, together with uninvolved adjacent vertebrae [3,8,18]. For solitary plasmacytoma of spine, considering the anatomical specificity, more exact measurement of radiotherapy dose and target volume is needed to avoid unnecessary irritation or damage of normal tissues and neurological elements. It should include the whole involved vertebra, together with one uninvolved vertebra above and below.

5.2 Surgery and recommendations

Surgery is not the first choice to treat solitary plasmacytoma of bone. However, it remains a reliable option for patients with intractable pain as a result of the vertebral involvement, vertebral instability, neurological compromise, or a combination of these disorders [3,8,9,19]. It is the only method that leads to immediate relief of spinal compression and direct biomechanical stabilization of the involved vertebra. Indications for surgery include [3,8,9,19,20]: any patient with an unstable of spine where surgery is the only way to fix and reconstruct the stabilization of spine; malignant spinal cord compression which can be alleviated by surgery; direct compression by intraspinal bony fragments; existing or impending motor dysfunction for which immediate decompression is required; no response to radiotherapy or radiotherapy tolerance and disease progressing.

The choice of surgical methods depends on the site and extent of the tumor, general condition of each patient, as well as skills and experience of surgeons. It is required that surgical plan should be designed carefully before procedure [21,22]. A gross-total resection is a reasonable choice for cervical spine tumor [23], and total en-bloc resection is feasible but challenging [22,24]. However, total en-bloc spondylectomy or resection is ideal for lesions in thoracic and lumbar spine and extraspinal involvements [22,24-26]. Given to the probability of long-term survival in patients with this disease, it is recommended that reconstruction of the involved spine should be performed [2,8,27]. For extraspinal osseous lesion, definitive local radiotherapy is the main treatment method. However, if pathological fractures of long bones or weight-bearing bones have been detected, surgical resection and fixation may also be required.

If surgery is required, radiotherapy should also be given. However, surgery should be carried out before radiotherapy because surgery may become more difficult in patients with preoperative radiotherapy [2,8,28,29]. Spinal radiation before surgery is associated with a significantly higher rate of major wound complication and may adversely affect the surgical outcome [28].

5.3 Chemotherapy and recommendations

Although there are insufficient data to support and advocate adjuvant chemotherapy for patients with SBP, it may be appropriate to consider to adjuvant radiotherapy in patients at higher risk of treatment failure [2-5]. Aviles et al [30] performed a prospective study which reported a benefit with combined chemotherapy and RT compared to RT alone. This study concluded that combined radiochemotherapy were likely to increase remission and survival duration. A suggested approach is to follow guidelines for the treatment of multiple myeloma [3]. In addition, patients presenting as SBP, but found on MRI to have more extensive disease, should be considered as having MM and treated accordingly [2,3,6]. In addition, bisphosphonate treatment lasting for at least one year may be benefit for patients with SBP. As for patients with MM, the bisphosphonate treatment should be prolonged to 2 years. Such management can be effective in reducing skeletal-related events [3,31-33].

6. Natural history and prognosis

The general prognosis of SP is comparatively better, with a 5-year survival rate about 70% and median overall survival period of 7.5-12 years [2,3,34]. There is no clear factor to predict prognosis of SP. Some researchers consider the following factors as prognosis [3,5,17,18]: old age, tumor size, and persistence of M protein after treatment. Majority of patients probably developed MM in the end with the median time of 2-4 years, especially those with SP of spine [5,15,16-18], and approximately 15%-45% of patients remain disease free at 10 years[4].

However, there is still no effective method to prevent SPB from progressing to MM and there is no consensus in the literature about these adverse prognostic features. Wilder et al[36]performed a multivariate analysis on prognostic factors in a series of 60 patients and considered sustained M protein for over one year after radiotherapy as the adverse prognostic factor, while age, tumor size and paraprotein level were of no special prognostic value. Modalities for monitoring of disease status such as PET/CT, free light chain examination, marrow aspiration biopsy, etc. could identify high risk groups for disease progression [3,5,6,11,12].

For patients with SBP, it is required carefully monitoring to detect progression to MM, possibly 6 weekly for 6 months, with extension of clinic appointments. Assessment of signs and symptoms should be undertaken, together with radiographic and laboratory investigations such as MRI, haematology, biochemistry, serum and urine paraprotein estimation [2-6,14].

7. References

[1] Fletcher CDM, Unni KK, Mertens F. World Health Organization classification of tumours[A]. Pathology and genetics of tumours of soft tissue and bone[M]. Lyon: IARC Press 2002;226-376

[2] Dimopoulos MA, Moulopoulos LA, Maniatis A, et al. Solitary plasmacytoma of bone and asymptomatic multiple myeloma. Blood 2000;96:2037-2044

[3] Soutar R, Lucraft H, Jackson G. Guidelines on the diagnosis and management of solitary plasmacytoma of bone and solitary extramedullary plasmacytoma. Clin Oncol 2004;16:405-413

[4] Weber DM. Solitary Bone and Extramedullary Plasmacytoma. Hematology 2005:373-376.

[5] Ozsahin M, Tsang RW, Poortmans P, et al. Outcomes and patterns of failure in solitary plasmacytoma: a multicenter Rare Cancer Network study of 258 patients. Int J Radiat Oncol Biol Phys 2006;64:210-217

[6] Reed V, Shah J, Medeiros LJ, et al. Solitary plasmacytomas: Outcome and prognostic factors after definitive radiation therapy. Cancer. 2011 117:4468-4474.

[7] Chang MY, Shih LY, Dunn P, Leung WM, Chen WJ. Solitary plasmacytomas of bone. J Formos Med Assoc 1994;93:397-402.

[8] Huang W, Cao D, Ma J, et al. Solitary plasmacytoma of cervical spine: treatment and prognosis in patients with neurological lesions and spinal instability. Spine, 2010;35:E278-284.

[9] Baba1 H, Maezawa1 Y, Furusawa1 N, et al. Solitary plasmacytoma of the spine associated with neurological complications. Spinal Cord 1998; 36, 470 - 475

[10] Moulopoulos LA, Dimopoulos MA, Weber D, et al. Magnetic resonance imaging in the staging of solitary plasmacytoma of bone. J Clin Oncol, 1993; 11:1311-1315

[11] Adam Z, Bolcak K, Stanicek J, et al. Fluorodeoxyglucose positron emission tomography in multiple myeloma, solitary plasmocytoma and monoclonal gammapathy of unknown significance. Neoplasma 2007;54:536-540

[12] Orchard K, Barrington S, Buscombe J, Hilson A, Prentice HG, Mehta A. Fluorodeoxyglucose positron emission tomography imaging for the detection of occult disease in multiple myeloma. Br J Haematol 2002; 117:133-135.

[13] Hu K, Yahalom J. Radiotherapy in the management of plasma cell tumors. Oncology 2000;14:101-108

[14] Holland J, Trenkner DA, Wasserman TH, Fineberg BI. Plasmacytoma. Treatment results and conversion to myeloma. Cancer 1992;69: 1513-1517.

[15] Bolek TW, Marcus RB, Mendenhall NP. Solitary plasmacytoma of bone and soft tissue. Int J Radiat Oncol Biol Phys 1996;36:329-333.

[16] Liebross RH, Ha CS, Cox JD, et al. Solitary bone plasmacytoma: outcome and prognostic factors following radiotherapy. Int J Radiat Oncol Biol Phys 1998; 41:1063-1067

[17] Tsang RW, Gospodarowicz MK, Pintilie M, et al. Solitary plasmacytoma treated with radiotherapy: impact of tumor size on outcome. Int J Radiat Oncol Biol Phys 2001;50:113-120

[18] Mayr NA, Wen BC, Hussey DH, et al. The role of radiation therapy in the treatment of solitary plasmacytomas. Radiother Oncol 1990;17:293-303

[19] Rao G, Ha CS, Chakrabartl I, et al. Multiple myeloma of the cervical spine: treatment strategies for pain and spinal instability. J Neurosurg Spine 2006;5:140–145.

[20] Patchell RA, Tibbs PA, Regine WF, et al. Direct decompressive surgical resection in the treatment of spinal cord compression caused by metastatic cancer: a randomized trial. Lancet 2005;366:643-648.

[21] Boriani S,Weinstein JN,Biagini R. Primary bone tumors of the spine.Terminology and surgical staging. Spine 1997;22:1036-1044.

[22] Yamazaki T, McLoughlin GS, Patel S, Rhines LD, Fourney DR.Feasibility and safety of en bloc resection for primary spine tumors: a systematic review by the Spine Oncology Study Group. Spine 2009; 34:S31-38.

[23] Barrenechea IJ,Perin NI, Triana A,et al.Surgical management of chordomas of the cervical spine. J Neurosurg Spine 2007;6:398-406.

[24] Currier BL, Papagelopoulos PJ, Krauss WE, Unni KK, Yaszemski MJ.Total en bloc spondylectomy of C5 vertebra for chordoma. Spine 2007;32:E294-299.

[25] Tomita K, Kawahara N, Baba H, Tsuchiya H, Fujita T, Toribatake Y. Total en bloc spondylectomy. A new surgical technique for primary malignant vertebral tumors. Spine 1997;22:324-333.

[26] Kawahara N, Tomita K, Murakami H, Demura S. Total en bloc spondylectomy for spinal tumors: surgical techniques and related basic background.Orthop Clin North Am 2009;40:47-63.

[27] McLain RF, Weinstein JN. Solitary plasmacytomas of the spine: a review of 84 cases. J Spinal Disord 1989;2:69-74.

[28] Ghogawala Z,Mansfield FL, Borges LF. Spinal radiation before surgical decompression adversely affects outcomes of surgery for symptomatic metastatic spinal cord compression. Spine 2001;26:818-821.

[29] Chataigner H,Onimus M,Polette A. Surgical treatment of myeloma localized in the spine. Rev Chir Reparatrice Appar Mot 1998;84:31-38.

[30] Aviles A, Huerta-Guzman J, Delgado S, Fernadez A, Diaz-Maqueo JC: Improved outcome in solitary bone plasmacytoma with combined therapy. *Hematol Oncol* 1996, 14:111-117.

[31] Kyle RA, Yee GC, Somerfield MR,et al. American Society of Clinical Oncology 2007 clinical practice guideline update on the role of bisphosphonates in multiple myeloma. J Clin Oncol 2007;25:2464-2472.

[32] Berenson JR, Rosen LS, Howell A, et al. Zoledronic acid reduces skeletal-related events in patients with osteolytic metastastes. Cancer 2001;91:1991-1200.

[33] Terpos E, Moulopoulos LA, Dimopoulos MA. Advances in imaging and the management of myeloma bone disease. J Clin Oncol 2011; 29:1907-1915.

[34] Dimopoulos MA, Hamilos G. Solitary bone plasmacytoma and extramedullary plasmacytoma. Curr Treat Options Oncol 2002;3:255-259.

[35] Wilder RB, Ha CS, Cox JD, et al. Persistence of myeloma protein for more than one year after radiotherapy is an adverse prognostic factor in solitary plasmacytoma of bone. Cancer 2002; 94:1532-1537.

10

Solitary Bone and Extramedullary Plasmacytoma

Galina Salogub, Ekaterina Lokhmatova and Sergey Sozin
Saint Petersburg State Medical University n. a. I.P.Pavlov
Russian Federation

1. Introduction

Plasmacytomas are clonal proliferations of plasma cells that are cytologically and immunophenotypically identical to those of plasma cell myeloma, but manifest a localized osseous or extraosseous growth pattern (Jaffe et al., 2001).

Solitary plasmacytomas are tumors of plasma cell origin that constitute less than 10% of all plasma cell neoplasms (Osserman, 1959) with a slightly lower median age of approximately 63 years (Hernandez et al., 1995).

The World Health Organization classification recognizes solitary plasmacytoma of bone (solitary bone plasmacytoma, SBP) and extramedullary / extraosseous plasmacytoma (EMP) (Jaffe et al., 2001).

The International Myeloma Working Group (IMWG) recognizes solitary plasmacytoma of bone, extramedullary plasmacytoma and multiple solitary plasmacytomas (+/-recurrent) as distinct entities (The International Myeloma Working Group. Criteria for the classification of monoclonal gammopathies, multiple myeloma and related disorders: a report of the International Myeloma Working Group, 2003).

2. Solitary bone plasmacytoma

2.1 Epidemiology and clinically-laboratory features

Solitary bone plasmacytoma has a male:female ratio of 2:1, with a median age of 55 years and primarily affects the axial skeleton especially the vertebrae (Dimopoulos et al, 2000) (Table 1). Osseous lesions constitute approximately 70% of all plasmacytomas. They involve primarily marrow-containing bones, with a predilection for the vertebrae, femurs, and pelvis (Bolek et al., 1996).

Malignant bone tumours of the spine are extremely rare (<0,05% of primary neoplasms). Solitary plasmacytoma is the commonest separate entity within this group, accounting for approximately 30% of the total (McLain & Weinstein, 1989). These tumours occur in the spine twice as often as other bony sites (Chang et al, 1994).

The most common presenting symptom is pain due to bone destruction, but patients with vertebral involvement may also have evidence of spinal cord or nerve root compression.

A few patients with solitary bone plasmacytoma present with symptoms and signs of demyelinating polyneuropathy. In evaluating such patients, the syndrome of polyneuropathy, organomegaly, endocrinopathy, M protein, and skin changes (POEMS) should be considered. Involvement of the base of the skull can present with cranial nerve palsies (Vaicys et al, 1999;Vijaya-Sekaran et al, 1999).

	SBP	SEP
Age (years), median	55	55
M:F	2:1	3:1
Predominant site	Axial skeleton, especially vertebrae	Head and neck
% with M protein	60	<25
% developing MM	>75	<30
% survival at 10 years	40–50	70

Table 1. Clinical features of solitary bone plasmacytoma and extramedullary plasmacytoma (United Kingdom Myeloma Forum, Guidelines on the diagnosis and management of solitary plasmacytoma of bone and solitary extramedullary plasmacytoma, 2004).

The involvement of the nervous system is a common complication of plasma cell neoplasms. Cranial myelomas (osseous, such as skull bones) and intracranial myelomas (other than bones, ie, extramedullary, such as hypothalamus) can be broadly classified into three clinical groups (Moossy et al. 1967) as shown in Table 2.

Group	**Syndrome**	**Involvement**	**Clinical Picture**
I	cranial nerve palsies	base of the skull	single or multiple cranial nerve palsies
II	intracranial tumor	- cranial myeloma extending intracranially - lesions that are entirely intracranial	similar to a primary brain tumor
III	intraorbital tumor	orbit	orbital space-occupying lesion

Table 2. Involvement of Nervous System in Plasma Cell Neoplasms

Plasmacytoma involvment of petrous bone causes dysphagia secondary to lateral medullary syndrome (it is one of the brainstem vascular syndromes that occur due to the occlusion of posterior inferior cerebellar artery or one vertebral artery, which may lead to dysphagia, vertigo, vomiting, ipsilateral paralysis of soft palate, ipsilateral Horner's syndrome, ipsilateral hypotonia and ataxia, and dissociated sensory loss) and results in paralysis of the 10th and 12th cranial nerves. The body of the sphenoid and the apex of the petrous bone are the most common sites of involvement. The tumors may be either small or discrete, or they may grow to large dimensions. These lesions have a greater tendency to expand locally rather than to disseminate, a property that may be controlled by specific cytokines (Mill et al., 1980). The bone is probably the site of origin; however, they may arise from mucosa contained within the sphenoid and petrous bones, since non-osseous myelomas are common.

The cranial nerves can be affected either by local distortion or by direct destruction, such as that which occurs with invasion of the cavernous sinus or jugular foramen region. Other cause of the neuropathy with chronic and slowly progressive course may be an axonopathy with secondary demyelination. High titers of anti-MAG (myelin-associated glycoproteins) are seen in patients with neuropathy. Involvement of the 5th, 6th, and 8th cranial nerves is most common (Moossy et al., 1967).

An intracranial plasmacytoma is a rare form, which can involve the calvarium, dura or the cranial base. It could manifest with majority of neurological symptoms, such as headache, diplopia, gait disturbances, hypoesthesia and areflexia of extremities, personality disorder and many others. Intracranial plasmacytoma may be cause of acute or chronic intracerebral hemorrhage. (Goyal et al., 2006; Crowley et al., 2010)

Intraorbital localization of plasmacytoma may present with exophthalmos, increased tearing, blurred vision, also diplopia or unilateral loss of vision (Wachter et al.,2010; Brandon Hayes-Lattin et al., 2003).

2.2 Diagnosis and investigation of SBP

2.2.1 Diagnostic criteria

- single area of bone destruction due to clonal plasma cells;
- histologically normal marrow aspirate and trephine (<5% plasma cells);
- normal results on skeletal survey, including radiology of longbones;
- no anaemia, hypercalcaemia or renal impairment due to plasma cell dyscrasia;
- absent or low serum or urinary level of monoclonal immunoglobulin (level of >20 g/l suspicious of multiple myeloma);
- o additional lesions on magnetic resonance imaging (MRI) scan of the spine.

(United Kingdom Myeloma Forum. Guidelines on the diagnosis and management of solitary plasmacytoma of bone, extramedullary plasmacytoma and multiple solitary plasmacytomas: 2009 update).

2.2.2 The recommended investigations

- full blood count
- biochemical screen including electrolytes and corrected calcium
- serum immunoglobulin levels
- serum and urine protein electrophoresis and immunofixation
- serum free light chain assay
- full skeletal survey
- MRI of spine and pelvis (or skeletal survey by MR where this facility exists)
- bone marrow aspirate and trephine
- PET scanning may be useful in selected patients.

(United Kingdom Myeloma Forum. Guidelines on the diagnosis and management of solitary plasmacytoma of bone, extramedullary plasmacytoma and multiple solitary plasmacytomas: 2009 update).

2.2.3 Laboratory

SBP should be diagnosed by tissue biopsy. Fine needle aspirate is inadequate. (United Kingdom Myeloma Forum. Guidelines on the diagnosis and management of solitary plasmacytoma of bone, extramedullary plasmacytoma and multiple solitary plasmacytomas: 2009 update).

Percutaneously guided biopsy of the spine is usually possible either by fluoroscopy or CT. All diagnoses should be made or reviewed by specialist haematopathologists in accordance with NICE guidelines for improving outcomes in haematological cancers (NHS NICE Improving outcomes in haematological cancers 2003. www.nice.org.uk).

When a bone tumor is encountered which is histopathologically diagnosed as 'small round cell tumor', the differential diagnosis includes Ewing sarcoma, osteosarcoma of small cell type, malignant lymphoma, plasmacytoma, metastatic small cell lung cancer and so on.

The bone marrow of patients with SPB should have no clonal plasma cells. But some patients may demonstrate up to 10 percent clonal plasma cells, and are considered as having both SPB and monoclonal gammopathy of undetermined significance (MGUS). These patients may have a higher risk of progression to symptomatic myeloma. If patients suspected to have SPB have 10 percent or more clonal plasma cells in the bone marrow, they should be considered to have Durie-Salmon stage I myeloma rather than SPB.

Immunophenotyping. Monoclonality and /or an aberrant plasma cell phenotype should be demonstrated with useful markers being CD19, CD56, CD27, CD117 and cyclin D1 (Rawstrom A.C, 2008).The immunophenotyping of bone marrow plasma cells in SBP has not been investigated so far and since a significant number of these patients progress to multiple myeloma. It is possible that the bone marrow of patients with SBP might contain neoplastic PC at the time of diagnosis, which may correlate with risk of progression to multiple myeloma. Maayke et al. demonstrated by flow cytometry, that aberrant phenotype plasma cells present at distant bone marrow sites in 67% of patients with solitary plasmacytoma of bone (Maayke et al., 2010). In the report of Bhaskar et al., plasma cells were easily identified based on dual expression of CD38 and CD138 in the bone marrow aspirates and varied from 0.17% to 1.05%. The neoplastic as well as normal PC were seen in the bone marrow aspirates of all the cases at the time of diagnosis and ranged from 0.10% to 0.70% and 0.06% to 0.49% of all the bone marrow cells respectively (Bhaskar et al., 2009). The authors suggest, that aberrant immunophenotype rather than the light chain restriction pattern was useful in identification of low number of neoplastic plasma cells in the bone marrow as the $\kappa:\lambda$ ratio was normal in all the samples (range: 0.5% to 1.6%). However, small number of cases studied and the relatively short duration of follow-up preclude a definitive opinion on value of these findings at this time. But given the ease of flow cytometric quantitative detection and enumeration of neoplastic PC in the bone marrow, additional studies for prognostic value determination are needed.

Cytogenic. Cytogenetic studies in SBP reveal loss in chromosome 13, 1p, 14q, gain in 19p, 9q, 1q and IL-6 is considered as the principal growth factor in the pathogenesis (Christopher DM Fletcher. Diagnostic histopathology of tumors. Volume 2, 2nd edition. Churchill Livingstone).

M-protein and serum free light chain assay. The presence of monoclonal protein (M protein) in the serum or urine has been noted in 24%-72% of patients in various series (Dimopoulos MA, 2000, 2002). In experience of M.D.Anderson Cancer Center (Weber D. 2005), among 63 consecutive previously untreated patients with SBP, 62% had a serum M protein, 13% had only Bence Jones protein (BJP), and 25% had non-secretory disease. Paraprotein values were usually very low, with only 11 of 37 patients with a serum M protein > 1 g/dL (high value 2.2 g/dL) and the highest urine BJP was 0.7 g/day.

Recently, free light chain assays have provided a measurable parameter to follow in approximately 65% of patients previously diagnosed with "nonsecretory" multiple myeloma by standard electrophoretic studies (Drayson MT, 2001). In report of Frassica et al. on 46 patients with SBP, 25 (54%) had a detectable serum or urine M-protein, 4 patients had an M-protein in both serum and urine, while 1 patient had only Bence Jones proteinuria (Frassica et al., 1989). The M-protein may decrease with successful therapy of SBP, and it has been reported that complete disappearance of the M-protein 1 year after therapy is associated with prolonged disease stability (Liebross et al., 1998; Wilder et al., 2002).

Uses of the serum free light chain (SFLC) assay has the prognostic value in solitary plasmacytoma (Dispenzieri et al., 2008): an abnormal serum immunoglobulin free light chain (FLC) ratio at diagnosis may identify risk of progression to myeloma in patients with solitary bone plasmacytoma. The risk of progression at 5 years was 44% in patients with an abnormal serum FLC ratio at diagnosis compared with 26% in those with a normal FLC ratio. There is a risk stratification model using the 2 variables of FLC ratio and M-protein level (patients with a normal FLC ratio at baseline and M protein level less than 0.5 g/dL) at 1 to 2 years following diagnosis ; with either risk factor abnormal (intermediate risk); and with both an abnormal FLC ratio and M protein level of 0.5 g/dL or higher (high risk). The corresponding progression rates at 5 years were significantly different in the low, intermediate, and high groups: 13%, 26%, and 62%, respectively (Dingli et al., 1979-1983).

2.2.4 Imaging studies in diagnosis of solitary plasmocytoma

The purposes of imaging in the diagnosis and management of plasmacytoma includes:

- detection of extramedullary or/and intramedullary foci of the disease;
- exclusion of additional lesions and bone marrow involvement;
- evaluation of risk of pathological fractures;
- guiding needle biopsy;
- planning radiotherapy and surgery.

Although definitive radiotherapy usually eradicates the local disease, the majority of patients will develop multiple myeloma because of the growth of previously occult lesions which have not been detected by conventional radiography. So that, diagnosis of solitary plasmacytoma needs accurate exclusion of additional bone or soft-tissue foci and bone marrow involvement.

X-ray examination. Osteolytic lesions are generally diagnosed by radiographic analysis. Plain radiography is everywhere available and allows to visualize large areas of the skeleton. In case of solitary plasmacytoma detection, standard radiography examination, as for multiple myeloma staging, should be performed. The skeletal survey should include a posteroanterior view of the chest, antero-posterior and lateral views of the cervical spine, thoracic spine, lumbar spine, humeri and femora, antero-posterior and lateral views of the skull and antero-posterior view of the pelvis. (Grade C recommendation; level IV evidence, Guidelines for the use of imaging in the management of myeloma. British Society for Haematology, 2007).

The weakness of radiographic detection is in relatively low sensitivity: it may reveal lytic disease only when over 30% of the trabecular bone has been lost (Snapper & Khan, 1971), so, 10-20% of lesions are missed. Certain parts of the skeleton are difficult to assess accurately, such as the sternum, ribs and scapulae. In addition, this technique also provides an inadequate assessment of generalised osteopenia (Scane et al, 1994).

Due to the limitations of standard radiographic analysis, magnetic resonance imaging (MRI) and/or computed tomography (CT) have been used for early detection of myeloma-associated bone destruction.

Magnetic resonance imaging. MRI is the preferred imaging modality for the initial assessment and for the follow-up of the osseous and extraosseous extent of SPB.

MRI of the thoracic and lumbosacral spine in the diagnosis of SBP was prospectively evaluated by several studies (Moulopoulos et al, 1993, 1997, 2005). It was shown, that MRI of thoraco-lumbar spine can reveal additional abnormalities more accurate than standard X-rays. After standard local radiotherapy of SBP, patients with additional lesions by pretreatment spinal MRI show earlier progression to systemic disease than those with a negative MR imaging survey at diagnosis.

Typical focus of plasma cell infiltration have a low signal intensity on T1-weighted images and a high signal intensity on T2-weighted and STIR (short time inversion recovery) images (Libshitz et al, 1992) and generally show enhancement on gadolinium-enhanced images. Bone marrow involvement has no specificity of the findings by MRI. The next findings can exist: focal or diffuse changes, variations of the norm; also images of BM can reflect an alternative pathological or physiological process such as iron loading (Isoda et al, 2001), amyloid deposition (Baur et al, 1998) or reactive marrow hyperplasia.

Thus, most investigators agree that a negative MRI of the thoraco-lumbar spine is a prerequisite for the diagnosis of SBP. MRI should be part of the staging procedures in patients with SBP, to better assess both the extent of the local tumor and the revealing of occult lesions elsewhere.

Recommendations for MRI in diagnosis of myeloma and plasmocytoma according to quidelines for the use of imaging in the management of myeloma (British Society for Haematology, 2007)

- Urgent MR imaging is the diagnostic procedure of choice to assess suspected cord compression in myeloma patients even in the absence of vertebral collapse (Grade B recommendation; level IIB evidence).
- MR imaging of the whole spine should be performed in addition to the skeletal survey as part of staging in all patients with an apparently solitary plasmacytoma of bone irrespective of site of index lesion (Grade B recommendation; level IIB evidence).

- MR imaging should be used to clarify the significance of ambiguous CT findings, as these two imaging techniques can give complementary information (Grade C recommendation; level IV evidence).

The new diagnostic criteria recommend MRI scanning to include the pelvis. Whole body MR imaging is emerging but currently impractical because of the logistics of long imaging time. (Guidelines on the diagnosis and management of solitary plasmacytoma of bone and solitary extramedullary plasmacytoma, United Kingdom Myeloma Forum,2009)

Computed tomography. Computed tomography provides an advantage in selected situations. Owing to the high levels of radiation exposure, CT cannot be used for screening purposes. Conventional CT has higher sensitivity than plain radiographs for detecting small lytic lesions; it can provide a high predictive value in the clarification of suspicious areas on plain films, and areas, difficult for visualization, such as ribs, sternum and scapulae.

CT should be considered in patients who remain symptomatic despite having no evidence of osteolysis on the skeletal survey.

Urgent CT may be used to establish the presence of suspected cord compression in cases where MR imaging is unavailable.

CT can accuratly depict the extent of associated soft tissue masses and can direct needle biopsy for histological diagnosis (Kyle, 1985) and forms the basis for radiotherapy and surgery.

Recommendations for CT in diagnosis of myeloma and plasmocytoma according to quidelines for the use of imaging in the management of myeloma (British Society for Haematology, 2007)

- Urgent CT may be used to establish the presence of suspected cord compression in cases where MR imaging is unavailable, impossible due to patient intolerance or contraindicated e.g. intraorbital metallic foreign bodies or cardiac pacemakers (Grade B recommendation; level III evidence).
- CT of the spine may be considered to clarify the presence or absence of bone destruction in cases of clinical concern where MR is negative (Grade B recommendation; level III evidence).
- CT should be used to clarify the significance of ambiguous plain radiographic findings, such as equivocal lytic lesions, especially in parts of the skeleton that are difficult to visualise on plain radiographs, such as ribs, sternum and scapulae(Grade B recommendation; level III evidence).
- CT may identify lesions that are negative on plain radiography, and should be considered in patients who remain symptomatic despite having no evidence of osteolysis on the skeletal survey (Grade B recommendation; level III evidence).
- CT is indicated to delineate the nature and extent of soft tissue disease, and where appropriate, tissue biopsy may be guided by CT scanning (Grade B recommendation; level IIB evidence).

Positron-emission tomography. PET/CT studies are more sensitive than other imaging modalities for localizing extramedullary sites of the disease. At the present time, it is fair to conclude that clinical experience of PET imaging in patients with plasma cell dyscrasias is in evolution.

Recommendations for PET in diagnosis of myeloma and plasmocytoma according to quidelines for the use of imaging in the management of myeloma (British Society for Haematology, 2007)

- Based on currently available evidence, PET imaging cannot be recommended for routine use in the management of myeloma patients.
- Either technique may be useful in selected cases that warrant clarification of previous imaging findings, but such an approach should ideally be made within the context of a clinical trial (Grade C recommendation; level IV evidence).
- The evidence for the sensitivity of PET scanning is most convincing in the setting of extramedullary disease. It is therefore reasonable to consider PET scanning in this setting, to clarify the extent of extramedullary disease, in cases where other imaging techniques have failed to clarify the situation (Grade B recommendation; level III evidence).
- If the decision to perform PET scanning has been taken, it is advisable to avoid undertaking the procedure within 4 weeks of chemotherapy or 3 months of radiotherapy (Grade B recommendation; level III evidence).

However, PET/CT has been included as an option in the diagnosis and monitoring of myeloma patients within NCCN guidelines (NCCN, 2011)

Whole-body F-18 FDG PET has the potential to detect the early phase of bone marrow involvement in patients with EMP and unsuspected sites of bone involvement in patients with SBP (Kato et al, 2000; Schirrmeister et al, 2002), upstaging the extent of the disease and significantly affect the therapeutic decisions. According to Schirrmeister et al ., 60% of patients with known focal osteolytic lesions on plain radiography were upstaged as a result of PET imaging (Schirrmeister et al., 2002).

PET demonstrated a 93% sensitivity for focal lesions and a 84–92% sensitivity for diffuse lesions; the specificity ranged from 83–100% in patients with diffuse FDG uptake (Schirrmeister et al , 2002). False positive PET scans may arise from inflammatory changes due to chemotherapy within the previous 4 weeks or radiotherapy within the previous 2–3 months (Juweid & Cheson, 2006); also due to active infection (Mahfouz et al, 2005).

2.3 Treatment of solitary bone plasmacytoma

Radical radiotherapy remains the treatment of choice for SBP. Knobel et al confirmed excellent local disease control with radiotherapy alone in their review of 206 patients with SBP. (Knobel et al) Local relapse occurred in 21(14%) out of 148 patients who received radiotherapy alone compared with 4(80%) out of 5 patients who were treated with surgery +/- chemotherapy. Surgery (radiotherapy versus partial or complete resection and radiotherapy) did not influence the 10-year probability of local control. Median dose was 40Gy. No dose response relationship was observed for doses higher than 30Gy regardless of tumour size, however this was a retrospective analysis. Previous studies and BCSH recommend radical radiotherapy for SBP encompassing the tumor volume shown on MRI with a margin of at least 2 cm and treating to a dose of 40Gy in 20 fractions with a higher dose of 50Gy in 25 fractions being considered for SBP>5cm. Surgery is not indicated for SBP, but some patients may require decompressive laminectomy, spine fusion or intramedullary rod fixation of a long bone (United Kingdom Myeloma Forum. Guidelines on the diagnosis and management of solitary plasmacytoma of bone, extramedullary plasmacytoma and multiple solitary plasmacytomas: 2009 update).

Bisphosphonates are not recommended for the patients with SBP, except in setting of underlying osteopenia (ASCO's Guideline on Bisphosphonates for Multiple Myeloma, 2009).

2.4 Natural history and prognosis

The majority of patients with apparent SBP continue to develop myeloma and approximately 5% of all patients with multiple myeloma have an initial diagnosis of solitary plasmacytoma (Bolek et al. 1996).

The rare cancer network published data on 206 patients with SBP, the largest series to date, in 2006 (Knobel, 2006). Despite treatment, 104 of 206 (50.4%) patients developed myeloma with a median time to development of 21 months (range, 2-135 months). 5 and 10 year projected probabilities of developing myeloma were 51% (95% CI, 43-59%) and 72% (95% CI, 62-82%). Age>60 years was the only independent predictor of development of myeloma in this study. Prognostic value of the persistence of a monoclonal band after treatment could not be assessed due to lack of data. Multivariate analysis of prognostic factors in a series of 60 patients from the MD Anderson Hospital concluded that persistence of a monoclonal band for more than one year after radiotherapy was an adverse prognostic factor (Wilder R.B, 2002). Dengli et al. retrospectively analysed stored serum of 116 patients taken at time of diagnosis of SBP between 1960 and 1995. An abnormal SFLC ratio was found in 54 (47%) patients and was associated with a higher risk of progression to myeloma (p=0.039) and an adverse overall survival (p=0.033) (Dingli D.,2006). Combining the results of the SFLC ratio at diagnosis with the serum monoclonal protein levels 1-2 years after diagnosis the researchers constructed a risk stratification model (Table 3). Additionally, plasma cells with neoplastic phenotype demonstrable by flow cytometry at bone marrow sites distant to solitary plasmacytoma would also appear to predict for progression to myeloma (Hilli Q.A.,2007). Genetic factors that have prognostic significance in myeloma such as del 13q and t(4;14) have, as yet, no proven value in solitary lesions.

Variables	Risk group	5 year progression rate
Normal SFLC ratio Monoclonal protein < 5 g/l	Low	13%
Either variable abnormal	Intermediate	26%
Abnormal SFLC ratio Monoclonal protein >5 g/l	High	62%

Table 3. Risk stratification model for SBP progression to myeloma using SFLC and monoclonal protein level (Dingli D.,2006).

The prognosis after progression to multiple myeloma is also poorer for osseous plasmacytoma than for extra-medullary plasmacytoma as evidenced by multiple retrospective studies. These differences suggest a difference in the biological behavior of the two types of tumor, which is further augmented by immunohistochemical staining and flow cytometry analysis. The biological differences found in such studies include higher population of aneuploid cells, proliferating cell-nuclear antigen index, and S-phase fraction (Knowling et al.,1983; Bataille et al.,1981; Frassica et al., 1989).

3. Solitary extramedullary plasmacytoma

3.1 Epidemiology and clinically-laboratory features

Solitary extramedullary (soft tissue) plasmacytomas (EMP, SEP) are less common than SBP but carry a better prognosis as the majority can be cured by local radiotherapy (Dimopoulos et al., 1999). Although SEP can arise throughout the body almost 90% arise in the head and neck, especially in the upper respiratory tract including the nasal cavity, sinuses, oropharynx, salivary glands and larynx (Brinch et al, 1990; Wax et al,1993; Susnerwala et al, 1997; Liebross et al, 1999; Galieni et al,2000). The next most frequent site is the gastro-intestinal tract. Approximately 10% of extramedullary plasmacytomas occur in the gastrointestinal tract (Nolan et al., 2005); there are also reports about pancreatic an liver involvment (Manmeet et al.,2010).

A variety of other sites can rarely be involved, including testis, bladder, urethra, breast, ovary, lung, pleura, thyroid, orbit, brain, skin, adrenal glands, retroperitoneum, central nervous system, spleen and the lymph nodes (Cavanna et al, 1990; Rubin et al, 1990; Matsumiyama et al, 1992; Nonamura et al, 1992; Wong et al, 1994; Adkins et al, 1996; Fischer et al, 1996; Tuting & Bork, 1996; Emery et al, 1999; Muscardin et al, 2000; di Chiara et al, 2001; Ahmed M et al., 2009; Kahara et al., 2001; Pantelidou et al., 2005).

A monoclonal paraprotein is detected in the serum and/or urine in fewer than 25% of patients (Table 1). Local recurrence rates of <5% have been quoted after radiotherapy (Liebross et al, 1999). The risk of distant relapse appears to be <30%, i.e. significantly less than with SBP (Mayr et al,1990). At least two-thirds of patients survive for >10 years (Brinch et al, 1990; Galieni et al,2000).

3.1.1 Extramedullary plasmacytoma of the head and neck region

The head and neck region is the most common site for arising of EMP. About 80% of EMPs occur in the submucosa of the upper aerodigestive tract (Zheng, 2005). The most common site is the sinonasal region. Korolkowa et al. reported that 40% occur in the nasal cavity and paranasal sinus, 20% in the nasopharynx and 18% in the oropharynx (Korolkowa et al., 2004). Other sites are nasopharynx, salivary glands, thyroid glands, tonsils, cervical lynphnodes and larynx. Involvement of neighboring regions such as orbit, palate, skin or scull base can also occur.

The patients mainly manifested as local masses and relevant symptoms; by spreading of the tumor, adjacent bone erosions may occur.

The symptoms are non-specific and depends on site and spread of the tumor. The most common findings are swelling, airway obstructions; in case of sinonasal region it could be nasal obstruction (often, unilateral), nasal discharge, recurrent epistaxis and facial pain.

Also such symptoms as a sore throat and dysphonia to haemoptoea can be found (Straetmans et al., 2008), more rarely cranial nerve palsy and neck lymphadenopathy.

Clinical manifestations of plasmacytoma of the oral cavity consist of jaw pain, tooth pain, paresthesia, swelling, exophytic soft tissue growth, mobility of teeth, migration of teeth, hemorrhage, burning mouth syndrome and pathologic fracture of the involved bone (Feller et al., 2006). Solitary plasmacytoma affecting the mouth and the jaws are uncommon. The mandible is more frequently involved than the maxilla and the bony lesions of both have a predilection for the posterior areas of the jaws. (Feller et al., 2006).

3.1.2 Plasmacytoma of the gastrointestinal tract

Primary plasmacytoma of the gastrointestinal tract is a rare entity (approximately 10%).

All the segments of the gastro-intestinal tract may be involved with the small intestine being the most common followed by stomach, colon and esophagus. (Krishnamoorthy et al., 2010)

Symptoms are nonspecific, including anorexia, weight loss, epigastric discomfort or gastrointestinal bleeding (Krishnamoorthy et al., 2010); dyspepsia, vomiting and dysphagia for solids in case of esophagus affection (Chetty et al., 2003).

Symptoms of intestinal involvement may include abdominal pain, intestinal obstruction, diarrhea or perforated peritonitis. Jaundice due to extrahepatic biliary obstruction by gastroduodenal plasmacytoma is described. (Unverdi et al., 2010)

On endoscopy, gastrointestinal plasmacytoma commonly present as nodular mass; other findings are ulcerated mass or diffusely thickened mucosal fold (Krishnamoorthy et al., 2010).

Most common findings on barium enema examination include polypoid mass or constricting lesion with or without mucosal or submucosal infiltration. Other less common findings include superficial ulcers, polyps (single or multiple) or intussusception (Gupta et al., 2007).

In several cases, local amyloidosis associated with plasmacytoma of GIT is described. (Carneiro et al., 2009; Nicholl et al., 1991)

3.1.3 Cutaneous plasmacytoma

Extramedullary plasmacytomas of the skin are extremely rare and they can be divided into primary cutaneous plasmacytoma (PCP) and metastatic cutaneous plasmacytoma (MCP). While in multiple myeloma cutaneous plasmacytoma represents 5-10% of cases, PCP is extremely rare variant of plasma cell disorder (Corazza et al.,2002).

Primary cutaneous plasmacytoma is defined as monoclonal proliferation of plasma-cells that arises primarily in the skin without evidence of systemic disease. In contrast, MCP arises from lymphatic or vascular spread of tumour or, more frequently, by direct extension from underlying bone lesions. However, it can also be seen distinct from a bony focus and even as the initial manifestation of the disease with or without evidence of coexisting MM.

Any area of the skin can be involved, but it has been reported most frequently on the trunk and abdomen followed by face, scalp, neck and extremities. Unusual localizations have been described related to MCP, including scrotum, eyelid, tongue and perianal region. (Alvarez-Twose et al., 2008)

Morphologically, cutaneous plasmacytomas usually consist of erythematous nodules that may ulcerate or plaques dome-shaped and smooth-surfaced ranging from 1 to 5cm in diameter. Histopathology reveals the typical pattern represented by a dense monomorphic dermal plasmacytic infiltrate which is usually separated from the overlying epidermis by a border line. Immunohistochemical staining shows the typical monoclonality of the neoplastic cells. Plasmacytoma must also be differentiated from plasma cell infiltrates accompanying other tumors or from reactive granulomas (Corazza et al.,2002).

Cutaneous plasmacytomas should be considered a sign of poor prognosis in plasma cell disorders because they generally occur late in the course of the disease. In case of multiple myeloma, cutaneous metastasis in usually indicates aggressive behavior and short survival (Pereira et al., 2008).

3.2 Diagnosis and investigation of SEP

3.2.1 Diagnostic criteria

- Single extramedullary mass of clonal plasma cells
- Histologically normal marrow aspirate and trephine
- Normal results on skeletal survey, including radiology of long bones
- No anaemia, hypercalcaemia or renal impairment due to plasma cell dyscrasia
- Absent or low serum or urinary level of monoclonal immunoglobulin

(United Kingdom Myeloma Forum. Guidelines on the diagnosis and management of solitary plasmacytoma of bone, extramedullary plasmacytoma and multiple solitary plasmacytomas: 2009 update)

3.2.2 Laboratory

Less than one-quarter of patients have evidence of a low level of monoclonal protein in serum or urine by electrophoresis and/or immunofixation, and (similar to experience

with SBP) are require normal levels of uninvolved immunoglobulins to confirm the absence of occult disease elsewhere (Liebross et al., 1999). The free light chain assays should also prove useful in monitoring such patients, particularly those classified with non-secretory features. In addition, patients should have no sign of underlying myeloma by bone survey and chemistries should reveal no abnormalities attributable to plasma cell dyscrasia (Weber et al., 2005).

Extramedullary plasmacytoma are characterized by a 'myeloma-like' immunophenotype (Boll et al., 2010). It was demonstrated that the infiltrate consists entirely of plasma cells and that there is no B cell component. In this regard CD138, MUM1/IRF4, CD20 and PAX5 are the most useful markers although it should be recognised that CD20 and PAX5 are sometimes expressed in plasma cell malignancies. Monoclonality and /or an aberrant plasma cell phenotype should be demonstrated with useful markers being CD19, CD56, CD27, CD117 and cyclin D1 (Rawstrom A.C.,2008; Stephens E.A., 2005).

EMP may express B-cell markers, such as CD79a and CD20, and MM may express germinal centre B-cell (GCBC)-associated microRNAs, such as miR-93 and miR-181b. The presence of CD19 and lack of miR-223 suggested aberrant B-cell differentiation in CD19(+) /miR-223(-)

phenotype could be used to distinguish EMP from the CD19(-) /miR-223(+) phenotype of MM (Yu et al., 2011). Immunocytochemistry demonstrated monoclonal expression of light immunoglobulin chains in all cases which, together with demonstration of CD 38 positivity (Tani et al., 1999).

Extramedullary plasmacytoma showed absence of cyclin D1 and infrequent expression of CD56. Furthermore, extramedullary plasmacytomas were characterized by weaker staining for Bcl-2 protein and rare overexpression of p21 and p53. In comparison to extramedullary multiple myeloma, extramedullary plasmacytoma showed a more mature morphology and lower proliferation indices. There was no association between the phenotypic parameters investigated and clinical outcome in extramedullary plasmacytoma (Kremer et al., 2005).

Some non-Hodgkin lymphomas show marked plasmacytic differentiation. In such cases, it may be difficult to differentiate these lymphomas from plasmacytoma or myeloma, especially with limited diagnostic material. However, there may be immunophenotypic differences in the plasma cells in these disorders that distinguish them. The analysis of the immunophenotypes of neoplastic plasma cells in 41 cases of B-lineage non-Hodgkin lymphoma and compares them with those in plasma cell myeloma revealed that plasma cells in lymphoma were significantly more likely to express CD19, CD45, and surface immunoglobulin and less likely to express CD56 than those in myeloma (Seegmiller et al., 2007).

It was shown, that CD19 and CD56 expression can be used reliably to distinguish these entities. Some extramedullary plasmacytomas showed lymphoma-like phenotypes, suggesting that, in reality, they may represent non-Hodgkin lymphomas with extensive plasmacytic differentiation (Seegmiller et al., 2007). EMP must be distinguished from reactive plasmacytoma, plasma cell granuloma and lymphoma (MALT, marginal zone, and immunoblastic).

Boll et al. detailed clinico-pathological assessment of a cohort of 26 patients with EMP. All cases were characterized by a monomorphic plasma cell infiltrate showing strong uniform expression of both CD138 and MUM1/IRF4. There was no obvious B-cell component identified either by morphology or immunohistochemistry. Two cases did express CD20 but they both lacked PAX5 expression. With respect to the antigens aberrantly expressed in myeloma plasma cells; CD56 and CD117 expression was documented in 58% (15/26) and 29% (5/17) of cases respectively while loss of CD27 was documented in 63% (12/ 19). Aberrant expression of at least one of these antigens was demonstrable in 92% of assessable cases (22/24). Authors believe that this data along with other recently published studies strongly suggest that EMP should be considered part of the spectrum of plasma cell disorders rather than lymphoma (Boll et al., 2010).

Staining with T-cell markers is unusual but reports of plasmacytomas staining with CD43 and CD45RO do exist (Petruch et al., 1992). Rare cases are described, which were positive for myeloid markers such as CD13, CD33, CD38, and CD138 (Shin et al., 2001). Cytokeratin immunoreactivity in plasmacytomas is generally considered to be rare (Sewell et al., 1986)

Bink et al. studied 38 cases of this type of neoplasm by fluorescence in situ hybridization. Fourteen cases (37%) contained IGH breaks, including six with a t(4;14) translocation. No translocations t(11;14), t(14;16), t(8;14), nor breaks involving MALT1, BCL6 or FOXP1 were found. Loss of 13q (40%), as well as chromosomal gains (82%), were common. There was no correlation between chromosomal alterations and clinical features or local relapse. Cytogenetically, extramedullary plasmacytoma and multiple myeloma are closely related. However, the distribution of IGH translocation partners, with the notable absence of t(11;14), is different (Bink et al., 2008).

Plasma cells have low proliferative activity, making cytogenetic studies inherently difficult to perform. However, numerical and structural chromosomal aberrations have been described in 20 to 60 percent of newly diagnosed multiple myeloma patients (Durie et al., 1992). Complex karyotypes with multiple chromosomal gains and losses are the most frequent changes, but translocations, deletions, and mutations have all been reported. Monosomy or partial deletion of 13 (13q14) is the most common finding, occurring in 15 to 40 percent cases. Deletion of 17p13, associated with allelic loss of p53, is reported in 25 percent of cases, and may predict a poor outcome (Konigsberg et al., 2000).

The most common structural abnormality is a t(11;14)(q13q32) translocation, resulting in over-expression of cyclin D1, occurring in 10 to 31 percent of cases (Menke et al., 2001;).

Aalto et al. demonstrated chromosome 13 loss in 8/9 EMP cases assessed by comparative genomic hybridization (Aalto et al., 1999). Similarly Bink et al found a high incidence of 13q loss (40%) and IGH rearrangements (37%) amongst 38 cases assessed by FISH based assays (Bink et al., 2008). They also demonstrated a relatively high incidence of the t(4;14)(p16;q32) but no cases with the t(11;14)(q13;q32) and high incidence of chromosome gains (82%) but no evidence of rearrangements of MALT1, BCL6 or FOXP1 (Bink et al, 2008).

3.2.3 Imaging studies

CT or MRI scanning is required to delineate the extent of the lesion but the role of MRI scanning of other areas in the staging of SEP has not been evaluated. There are different meanings. According to guidelines on the diagnosis and management of solitary plasmacytoma of bone and solitary extramedullary plasmacytoma (United Kingdom Myeloma Forum. Guidelines on the diagnosis and management of solitary plasmacytoma of bone, extramedullary plasmacytoma and multiple solitary plasmacytomas: 2009 update), MRI of the spine is not considered to be necessary for the diagnosis of SEP. But other authors find it useful for the accurate staging of EMP, similar to SBP.

3.3 Treatment of solitary extramedullary plasmacytoma

Solitary extramedullary plasmacytoma are highly radiosensitive tumours. Local control rates of 80–100% are consistently reported with moderate doses of radiotherapy (Mayr et al, 1990; Bolek et al, 1996; Jyothirmayi et al, 1997; Liebross et al, 1998).

Solitary extramedullary plasmacytoma should be treated by radical radiotherapy encompassing the primary tumour with a margin of at least 2 cm. The cervical nodes should be included if involved. The first echelon cervical nodes should be included in SEP of Waldeyer's ring. For SEP up to 5 cm a radiotherapy dose of 40 Gy in 20 fractions is recommended. For bulky SEP of >5 cm, a higher dose of up to 50 Gy in 25 fractions is recommended.

Radiotherapy alone is the treatment of choice for head and neck SEP. Radical surgery should be avoided in head and neck SEP. For SEP at other sites complete surgical removal should be considered if feasible. Patients with involved surgical margins should receive adjuvant radiotherapy. No recommendation for adjuvant radiotherapy can be made for patients who have undergone complete surgical excision with negative margins.

Adjuvant chemotherapy should be considered in patients with tumours >5 cm and those with high grade tumours. Chemotherapy is indicated for patients with refractory and/or relapsed disease. Therapy as for MM is indicated (United Kingdom Myeloma Forum. Guidelines on the diagnosis and management of solitary plasmacytoma of bone, extramedullary plasmacytoma and multiple solitary plasmacytomas: 2009 update).

3.4 Natural history and prognosis

In most series, < 10% of patients have local recurrence of disease and the 10-year disease free and overall survival ranges from 50-80%, for the 30%-50% of patients who develop disease progression to myeloma. This occurs after a median of 1.5-2.5 years and their clinical course at progression is similar to those of patients diagnosed with de novo symptomatic myeloma (Weber D, 2005). Because of the small number of patients in most series, any statistically significant risk factors for development of myeloma are not clear and are further complicated by the inclusion of patients over many decades during which treatment and diagnostic modalities have become more refined and are likely to impact prognosis. In some series, bulky disease > 5 cm may have prognostic significance (Tsang, 2001).

4. Multiple solitary plasmacytomas

Multiple solitary plasmacytomas, which may be recurrent, occur in up to 5% of patients with an apparently solitary plasmacytoma and may involve soft tissue or bone.

4.1 Diagnostic criteria

- Absent or low serum or urinary level of monoclonal immunoglobulin
- More than one localized area of bone destruction or extramedullar tumor of clonal plasma cells which may be recurrent
- Normal bone marrow
- Normal skeletal survey and MRI of spine and pelvis
- No related organ or tissue impairment

(United Kingdom Myeloma Forum. Guidelines on the diagnosis and management of solitary plasmacytoma of bone, extramedullary plasmacytoma and multiple solitary plasmacytomas: 2009 update).

4.2 Treatment

Treatment approaches to patients with multiple solitary plasmacytomas are variable and it is likely the choice of therapy will be influenced by factors such as patient age, sites of recurrence, numbers of lesions and disease free interval. Recurrent solitary plasmacytoma out with the original site of radiotherapy, in the continuing absence of systemic disease, may be treated with additional radiotherapy. Patients with more extensive disease or early relapse may benefit from systemic therapy +/- autologous stem cell transplantation, as indicated for myeloma, with small cases series suggesting long term disease control (Dimopouloos, 2003). Newer agents including thalidomide and bortezomib have also been used successfully, prior to transplantation, in small numbers of patients with relapsed plasmacytoma (Chim, 2005; Katodritou, 2007; Pantelidou, 2006).

5. References

Christopher DM Fletcher. *Diagnostic histopathology of tumors*. Volume 2, 2nd edition. Churchill Livingstone

Jaffe E.S., Harris N.L., Stein H., Vardiman J.W. (Eds.). (2001). World Health Organization Classification of Tumours, Pathology and Genetics, Tumours of Haematopoietic and Lymphoid Tissues. Lyon: IARC press

Snapper, I. & Khan, A. (1971) Myelomatosis: fundamentals and clinical features. University Park Press, Baltimore.

Aalto, Y., Nordling, S., Kivioja, A.H., Karaharju, E., Elomaa, I. &Knuutila, S. (1999) Among numerous DNA copy number changes, losses of chromosome 13 are highly recurrent in plasmacytoma. *Genes, Chromosomes and Cancer*, 25, 104–107

Ahmed M, Al-Ghamdi A, Al-Omari M, Aljurf M, Al-Kadhi Y. (2009) Autologous bone marrow transplanation for extramedullary plasmacytoma presenting as adrenal incidentaloma. *Ann Saudi Med* 29:219-22;

Adkins, J.W., Shields, J.A., Shields, C.L., Eagle, Jr, R.D., Flanagan, J.V. & Campanella, P.C. (1996) Plasmacytoma of the eye and orbit. *International Ophthalmology*, 20, 339–343.

Alvarez-Twose I.et al. Metastatic cutaneous plasmacytoma presenting as a perianal giant mass (2008) *Dermatology Online Journal* 14 (9)

Bataille R, Sany J. (1981) Solitary myeloma: clinical and prognostic features of a review of 114 cases. *Cancer.*;48:845-851

Baur, A., Stabler, A., Lamerz, R., Bartl, R. & Reiser, M. (1998) Light chain deposition disease in multiple myeloma: MR imaging features correlated with histopathological findings. *Skeletal Radiology*, 27, 173–176.

Bhaskar A, Gupta R, Sharma A., Kumar L, Jain P. (2009) Analysis of bone marrow plasma cells in patients with solitary bone plasmacytoma. *Cancer Therapy* Vol 7, 49-52.

Bink K, Haralambieva E, Kremer M, Ott G, Beham-Schmid C, de Leval L, Peh SC, Laeng HR, Jütting U, Hutzler P, Quintanilla-Martinez L, and Fend F.(2008) Primary extramedullary plasmacytoma: similarities with and differences from multiple myeloma revealed by interphase cytogenetics. *Haematologica* 93(4):623-626

Bolek, T.W., Marcus, R.B. & Mendenhall, N.P. (1996) Solitary plasmacytoma of bone and soft tissue. *International Journal of Radiation Oncology, Biology, Physics*, 36, 329–333.

Boll M et al (2010) - Extramedullary plasmacytoma are characterized by a 'myeloma-like' immunophenotype and genotype and occult bone marrow involvement. *British Journal of Haematology*, 2010, 151: 525–531

Brinch, L., Hannisdal, E., Foss Abrahamsen, A., Kvaloy, S. & Langholm, R. (1990) Extramedullary plasmacytomas and solitary plasma cell tumours of bone. *European Journal of Haematology*, 44, 131–134.

Brinch, L., Hannisdal, E., Foss Abrahamsen, A., Kvaloy, S. & Langholm, R. (1990) Extramedullary plasmacytomas and solitary plasma cell tumours of bone. *European Journal of Haematology*, 44, 131–134.

Cavanna, L., Fornari, F., Civardi, G., Di Stasi, M., Sbolli, G., Foroni, R., Voltolini, F. & Buscarini, L. (1990) Extramedullary plasmacytoma of the testicle. Sonographic appearance and ultrasonically guided biopsy. Blut, 60, 328–330.

Carneiro F.P. (1991) Extramedullary plasmocytoma associated with a massive deposit of amyloid in the duodenum. Postgrad Med J 67, 1075 - 1077

Chang, M.Y., Shih, L.Y., Dunn, P., Leung, W.M. & Chen, W.J. (1994) Solitary plasmacytomas of bone. *Journal of the Formosa Medical Association*, 93, 397–402.

Chetty R, Bramdev A, Reddy AD.(2003). Primary extramedullary plasmacytoma of the esophagus. *Ann Diagn Pathol.* Jun;7(3):174-9.

Chim C.S., Ooi G.C., Loong F., Au A.W.M., Lie A.K.W. (2005) Bortezomib in primary refractory plasmacytoma. *Journal of Clinical Oncology*;23:2426-2428

Corazza M et al. (2002) Primary cutaneous plasmacytoma on chronic lymphoedema. *European Journal of Dermatology.* Volume 12, Number 2, 191-3.

D Dingli, R A. Kyle, S. V Rajkumar, G S. Nowakowski, D R. Larson, J P. Bida, M A. Gertz, T M. Therneau, L. J Melton, III, A Dispenzieri, and J A. Katzmann.(2006) Immunoglobulin free light chains and solitary plasmacytoma of bone. *Blood.* 108(6): 1979–1983

di Chiara, A., Losito, S., Terracciano, L., di Giacomo, R., Iaccarino, G.& Rubolotta, M.R. (2001) Primary plasmacytoma of the breast. *Archives of Pathology and Laboratory Medicine*, 125, 1078–1080.

Dimopouloos M.A.,Papadimitriou C., Anagnostopoulos A., Mitsibounas D., Fermand J.P. (2003). High dose therapy with autologous stem cell transplantation for solitary plasmacytoma complicated by local relapse or isolated distant recurrenceю *Leukaemia and Lymphoma*;44:153-155

Dimopoulos, M.A., Moulopoulos, L.A., Maniatis, A. & Alexanian, R.(2000) Solitary plasmacytoma of bone and asymptomatic multiple myeloma. *Blood*, 96, 2037–2044.

Dingli D., Kyle R.A., Rajkumar V., Nowakowski G.S., Larson D.R., Bida J.P., Gertz M.A., Therneau T.M., Melton L.J., Dispenzieri A., Katzmann J.A. (2006) Immunoglobulin free light chains and solitary plasmacytoma of bone. *Blood*;108:1979-1983

Dispenzieri A, Kyle R, Merlini G, Miguel JS, Ludwig H, Hajek R, Palumbo A, Jagannath S, Blade J, Lonial S, Dimopoulos M, Comenzo R, Einsele H, Barlogie B, Anderson K, Gertz M, Harousseau JL, Attal M, Tosi P, Sonneveld P, Boccadoro M, Morgan G, Richardson P, Sezer O, Mateos MV, Cavo M, Joshua D, Turesson I, Chen W, Shimizu K, Powles R, Rajkumar SV, Durie BG; International Myeloma Working Group. (2009) International Myeloma Working Group guidelines for serum-free light chain analysis in multiple myeloma and related disorders. Leukemia. 23(2):215-24.

Durie, BG (1992) Cellular and molecular genetic features of myeloma and related disorders. Hematol *Oncol Clin North Am*; 6:463-477

E Tani, G C Santos , E Svedmyr , L Skoog.(1999) Fine-needle aspiration cytology and immunocytochemistry of soft-tissue extramedullary plasma-cell neoplasms . - *Diagnostic Cytopathology*,- Vol 20, Issue 3, pp 120–124

Feller L et al. (2006) Extramedullary myeloma in an HIV-seropositive subject. Literature review and report of an unusual case. *Int J Radiat Oncol Biol Phys* 64:210-7.

Fischer, C., Terpe, H.J., Weidner, W. & Schulz, A. (1996) Primary plasmacytoma of the testis. Case report and review of the literature. *Urologia Internationalis*, 56, 263–265.

Frassica DA, Frassica FJ, Schray MF, Sim FH, Kyle RA. (1989) Solitary plasmacytoma of bone: Mayo Clinic experience. *Int J Radiat Oncol Biol Phys.*;16: 43-48

Frassica DA, Frassica FS, Schray MF, et al. (1989) Solitary plasmacytoma of bone: Mayo Clinic experience. *Int J Radiat Oncol Biol Phys.*16:43-48

Galieni, P., Cavo, M., Pulsoni, A., Avvisati, G., Bigazzi, C., Neri, S.,Caliceti, U., Benni, M., Ronconi, S. & Lauria, F. (2000) Clinical outcome of extramedullary plasmacytoma. *Haematologica*, 85,47–51.

Galieni, P., Cavo, M., Pulsoni, A., Avvisati, G., Bigazzi, C., Neri, S.,Caliceti, U., Benni, M., Ronconi, S. & Lauria, F. (2000) Clinical outcome of extramedullary plasmacytoma. Haematologica, 85, 47–51. in multiple myeloma and related disorders eukemia 1-10

Gupta V. et al (2007) Primary isolated extramedullary plasmacytoma of colon. *World Journal of Surgical Oncology* 5:47

Isoda, H., Kojima, H., Shimizu, K., Kurokawa, H., Ikeda, K., Sawada,S., Sakaida, N. & Okamura, A. (2001) Multiple myeloma: short T2 on MR imaging. *Clinical Imaging*, 25, 141–143.

Jyothirmayi, R., Gangadharan, V.P., Nair, M.K. & Rajan, B. (1997) Radiotherapy in the treatment of solitary plasmacytoma. *British Journal of Radiology*, 70, 511–516.

Kahara T, Nagai Y, Yamashita H, Nohara E, Kobayashi K, Takamura T. (2001) Extramedullary plasmacytoma in the adrenal incidentalom. *Clin Endocrinol* 55:267-270;

Kato, T., Tsukamoto, E., Nishioka, T., Yamazaki, A., Shirato, H.,Kobayashi, S., Asaka, M., Imamura, M. & Tamaki, N. (2000) Early detection of bone marrow involvement in extramedullary plasmacytoma by whole-body F-18 FDG positron emission tomography. *Clinical Nuclear Medicine*, 25, 870–873.

Katodritou E., Speletas M., Pouli A., Tsitouridis J., Zervas K., Terpos E. (2007) Successful treatment of extramedullary plasmacytoma of the cavernous sinus using a combination of intermediate dose of thalidomide and dexamethasone. *Acta Haematologica*; 117:20-23

Krishnamoorthy N, Bal MM, Ramadwar M, Deodhar K, Mohandas KM. (2010) A rare case of primary gastric plasmacytoma: an unforeseen surprise. J Cancer Res Ther. 6(4):549-51.

Kyle, R.A. (1985) Multiple myeloma: current therapy and a glimpse of the future. *Scandinavian Journal of Haematology*, 35, 38–47.

Knobel D., Zouhair A. et al. (2006) Prognostic factors in solitary plasmacytoma of bone: a multicenter rare cancer network study. *BMC Cancer*;6:118

Knowling MA, Harwood AR, Bergsagel DE.(1983) Comparison of extramedullary plasmacytomas with solitary and multiple plasma cell tumors of bone. *J Clin Oncol.* 1:255-262;

Konigsberg, R, Zojer, N, Ackerman, J, et al.(2000) Predictive role of interphase cytogenetics for survival of patients with multiple myeloma. *J Clin Oncol*; 18:804-812

Korolkowa O, Osuch-Wójcikiewicz E, Deptała A, Suleiman W. (2004) Extramedullary plasmacytoma of the head and neck, *Otolaryngol Pol.* 58(5):1009-12. [Article in Polish]

Kremer M, Ott G, Nathrath M, Specht K, Stecker K, Alexiou C, Quintanilla-Martinez L, Fend F J. (2005) Primary extramedullary plasmacytoma and multiple myeloma: phenotypic differences revealed by immunohistochemical analysis. *Pathol.*2005(1):92-101

Libshitz, H.I., Malthouse, S.R., Cunningham, D., MacVicar, A.D. & Husband, J.E. (1992) Multiple myeloma: appearance at MR imaging. Radiology, 182, 833–837.

Liebross RH, Ha CS, Cox JD, Weber D, Delasalle K, Alexanian R. (1998) Solitary bone plasmacytoma: outcome and prognostic factors following radiotherapy. *Intl J Radiat Oncol Biol Phys.*;41: 1063-1067;

Liebross RH, Ita CS, Cox JD, et al. (1999) Clinical Course of extramedullary plasmacytoma. *Radiother Oncol.*;52:245-249

Liebross, R.H., Ha, C.S., Cox, J.D., Weber, D., Delasalle, K. & Alexanian, R. (1999) Clinical course of solitary extramedullary plasmacytoma. *Radiotherapy Oncology*, 52, 245–249.

Maayke Boll, Elizabeth Parkins, Sheila J. M. O'Connor,Andy C. Rawstron, Roger G. Owen, (2010) - Extramedullary plasmacytoma are characterized by a 'myeloma-like' immunophenotype and genotype and occult bone marrow involvement. *British Journal of Haematology*, 151, 525–531.

Manmeet S. Padda,a Tiffani Milless,b Adebowale J. Adeniran,c Sepi Mahooti,c and Harry R. Aslaniana. (2010) Pancreatic and Gastric Plasmacytoma Presenting with Obstructive Jaundice, Diagnosed with Endoscopic Ultrasound-Guided Fine Needle Aspiratio. *Case Rep Gastroenterol.* Sep-Dec; 4(3): 410–415

Matsumiyama, K., Kanayama, Y., Yamaguchi, S., Ueyama, W., Iwasaki, M. & Osafune, K. (1992) Extramedullary plasmacytoma (EMP) of urinary bladder. *Urology*, 40, 67–70.

Mayr, N.A., Wen, B.-C., Hussey, D.H., Burns, C.P., Staples, J.J., Doornbos, J.F. & Vigliotti, A.P. (1990) The role of radiation therapy in the treatment of solitary plasmacytomas. *Radiotherapy and Oncology*, 17, 293–303.

McLain, R.F. & Weinstein, J.N. (1989) Solitary plasmacytomas of the spine: a review of 84 cases. *Journal of Spinal Disorders*, 2, 69–74.

Menke, DM, Horny, HP, Griesser, H, et al. (2001)Primary lymph node plasmacytomas (plasmacytic lymphomas). *Am J Clin Pathol*; 115:119

Mill WB, Griffith R. (1980) The role of radiation therapy in the management of plasma cell tumors. *Cancer.* 45:647-652

Moulopoulos, L.A. & Dimopoulos, M.A. (1997) Magnetic resonance imaging of the bone marrow in hematologic malignancies. *Blood*, 90,2127-2147.

Moulopoulos, L.A., Dimopoulos, M.A., Weber, D., Fuller, L., Libshitz,H.I. & Alexanian, R. (1993) Magnetic resonance imaging in the staging of solitary plasmacytoma of bone. *Journal of Clinical Oncology*, 11, 1311-1315.

Moulopoulos, L.A., Gika, D., Anagnostopoulos, A., Delasalle, K., Weber, D., Alexanian, R. & Dimopoulos, M.A. (2005) Prognostic significance of magnetic resonance imaging of bone marrow in previously untreated patients with multiple myeloma. *Annals of Oncology*, 16, 1824-1828.

Muscardin, L.M., Pulsoni, A. & Cerroni, L. (2000) Primary cutaneous plasmacytoma: report of case with review of the literature. *Journal of the American Academy of Dermatology*, 43, 962-965.

Nolan KD, Mone MC, Nelson EW. (2005) Plasma cell neoplasms. Review of disease progression and report of a new variant. *Surg Oncol.* 14:85-90

Nonamura, A., Mizukami, Y., Shimizu, J., Oda, M., Watanabe, Y., Kamimura, R., Takashima, T. & Kitagawa, M. (1992) Primary extramedullary plasmacytoma of the lung. *Internal Medicine*, 31, 1396-1400.

Pantelidou D, C.Tsatalasa, D.Margaritis, A.J.Karayiannakis, V.Kaloutsi, E.Spanoudakis, I.Katsilieris, E.Chatzipaschalis, E.Sivridis, G.Bourikas (2005). Extramedullary plasmacytoma: report of two cases with uncommon presentation. Ann Hematol;84:188-191

Pantelidou D., Tsatalas C., Margaritis D., Anastasiadis A.G., Kaloutsi V., Argyropoulou P., Prassopoulos P., Bourikas G. (2006) Successful treatment of lymph node extramedullary plasmacytoma with bortezomib. *Annals of Hematology*;85:188-190

Pereira M.A. et al. (2008).Cutaneous metastatic plasmacytomas with tropism for a previously injured limb. *Dermatology Online Journal* 14 (9)

Petruch UR, Horny HP, Kaiserling E. (1992) Frequent expression of haemopoietic and non-haemopoietic antigens by neoplastic plasma cells: an immunohistochemical study using formalin-fixed, paraffin-embedded tissue. *Histopathology* .20:35-40

Rubin, J., Johnson, J.T., Killeen, R. & Barnes, L. (1990) Extramedullary plasmacytoma of the thyroid associated with a serum monoclonal gammopathy. *Archives of Otolaryngology - Head and Neck Surgery*,116, 855-859.

Seegmiller A.C, Xu Y, McKenna R.W. and Karandikar N.J.(2007) Immunophenotypic Differentiation Between Neoplastic Plasma Cells in Mature B-Cell Lymphoma vs Plasma Cell Myeloma .*J Clin Pathol* 127:176-181.

Sewell HF, Thompson WD, King DJ. (1986) IgD myeloma/immunoblastic lymphoma cells expressing cytokeratin. *Br J Cancer* 53:695-696

Shin J.S, G A. Stopyra, M. J. Warhol, H. A.B. Multhaupt (2001). Plasmacytoma with Aberrant Expression of Myeloid Markers, T-cell Markers, and Cytokeratin. *J Histochem Cytochem* vol. 49 no. 6: 791-792

Scane, A.C., Masud, T., Johnson, F.J. & Francis, R.M. (1994) The reliability of diagnosing osteoporosis from spinal radiographs. Age Ageing, 23, 283-286.

Schirrmeister, H., Bommer, M., Buck, A.K., Muller, S., Messer, P.,Bunjes, D., Dohner, H., Bergmann, L. & Reske, S.N. (2002) Initial results in the assessment of multiple myeloma using 18F-FDG PET. *European Journal of Nuclear Medicine and Molecular Imaging*, 29, 361-366.

Schirrmeister, H., Buck, A.K., Bergmann, L., Reske, S.N. & Bommer, M. (2003) Positron emission tomography (PET) for staging of solitary plasmacytoma. *Cancer Biotherapy & Radiopharmaceuticals*, 18, 841–845.

Straetmans J, Stokroos R.(2008) Extramedullary plasmacytomas in the head and neck region. *Eur Arch Otorhinolaryngol.*Nov;265(11):1417-23.

Susnerwala, S.S., Shanks, J.H., Banerjee, S.S., Scarffe, J.H., Farrington, W.T. & Slevin, N.J. (1997) Extramedullary plasmacytoma of the head and neck region: clinicopathological correlation in 25 cases. *British Journal of Cancer*, 75, 921-927.

The International Myeloma Working Group. Criteria for the classification of monoclonal gammopathies, multiple myeloma and related disorders: a report of the International Myeloma Working Group. (2003) *British Journal of Haematology*; 121:749-757

Tsang, R.W., Gospodarowicz, M.K., Pintilie, M., Bezjak, A., Wells, W.,Hodgson, D.C. & Stewart, A.K.I. (2001) Solitary plasmacytoma treated with radiotherapy: impact of tumour size on outcome. *International Journal of Radiation Oncology, Biology, Physics*, 50, 113–120.

Tuting, A.U. & Bork, K. (1996) Primary plasmacytoma of the skin. *Journal of the American Academy of Dermatology*, 34, 386–390.

United Kingdom Myeloma Forum. Guidelines on the diagnosis and management of solitary plasmacytoma of bone and solitary extramedullary plasmacytoma (2004). *British Journal of Haematology*, 124, 717–726

Unverdi S, Köklü S, Tuncer F, Duranay M. (2010) Gastroduodenal plasmacytoma presenting with jaundice. *South Med J.* Feb;103(2):159-61.

Vaicys, C., Schulder, M., Wolansky, L.J. & Fromowitz, F.B. (1999) Falco-tentorial plasmacytoma. Case report. *Journal of Neurosurgery*, 91, 132–135.

Wax, M.K., Yun, K.N. & Omar, R.A. (1993) Extramedullary plasmacytomas of the head and neck. *Otolaryngology – Head and Neck Surgery*, 109, 877–885.

Weber D.M. (2005) Solitary Bone and Extramedullary Plasmacytoma. *Hematology.* : 373-376

Wilder RB, Ha CS, Cox JD, Weber D, Delasalle K, Alexanian R. (2002). Persistence of myeloma protein for more than one year after radiotherapy is an adverse prognostic factor in solitary plasmacytoma of bone. *Cancer*;94: 1532-1537

Wong, K.F., Chan, J.K., Li, L.P., Yau, T.K. & Lee, A.W. (1994) Primary cutaneous plasmacytoma - report of two cases and review of the literature. *American Journal of Dermatopathology*, 16, 391–397.

Yu SC, Chen SU, Lu W, Liu TY, Lin CW. Expression of CD19 and lack of miR-223 distinguish extramedullary plasmacytoma from multiple myeloma. *Histopathology.* 2011 Mar 14. doi: 10.1111/j.1365-2559.2011.03793.x. [Epub ahead of print]

NHS NICE Improving outcomes in haematological cancers 2003. Available from http://www.nice.org.uk

United Kingdom Myeloma Forum. Guidelines on the diagnosis and management of solitary plasmacytoma of bone, extramedullary plasmacytoma and multiple solitary plasmacytomas: 2009 update (2009) Available from http://www.bloodmed.com/contentimage/guidelines/3454.pdf

11

Multiple Myeloma and Dentistry

Ajaz Shah, Suhail Latoo and Irshad Ahmad
Govt. Dental College Srinagar, University of Kashmir, India

1. Introduction

Multiple myeloma (MM) is a malignant neoplasm of plasma cells that is characterized by the production of pathologic M proteins, bone lesions, kidney disease, hyperviscosity, and hypercalcemia. MM occurs more frequently in patients between 50 and 80 years of age, with a mean age of 60 years and man are more affected than women (1). Systemic symptoms are due to bone pain pathologic fractures, renal failure, hypercalcemia, weight loss, fatigue, weakness, fever, thrombocytopenia, neutropenia, diarrhea, orthostatic hypotension and infections (2, 3). Initial findings are bone pain in 68% of patients, anemia in 62%, renal insufficiency in 55%, hypercalcemia in 30%, hepatomegaly in 21%, and splenomegaly in 5%. (4)

2. Oral and maxillofacial manifestations

Oral and maxillofacial lesions in patients with multiple myeloma are not uncommon, but multiple myeloma is often overlooked. Because the symptoms are many, the disease proves difficult to diagnose. Approximately 5 to 30% of myeloma patients have lesions in the jaw. Incidental discovery of lesions in the jaw may be the first evidence of this disease. Although uncommon, an initial presentation of multiple myeloma may reveal oral or maxillofacial symptoms. The oral manifestations of MM are the first sign of the disease in about 14% of the patients. (5)

The patient may experience pain, swelling, numbness of the jaws, epulis formation, or unexplained mobility of the teeth. (6 -11)

More than 30% of patients with MM develop osteolytic lesions in the jaw (9). Osteolytic lesions are more frequent in the mandible than in the maxilla, especially in the posterior teeth region, ramus and condylar process, presumably because of greater hematopoietic activity in these areas. (6,7) The radiographic appearance of the lesions is generally punched out osteolytic lesions (60%). In most instances, the lesions appear unassociated with the apices of the teeth.(6,12) (Figure 1) From the radiological point of view, MM can exhibit three distinct radiographic aspects in the skeletal system, including, in the maxillaries (9):

1. Bone with no apparent alteration
2. Multiple radiolucent areas
3. Generalized bone rarefaction
4. Osteoporotic alterations

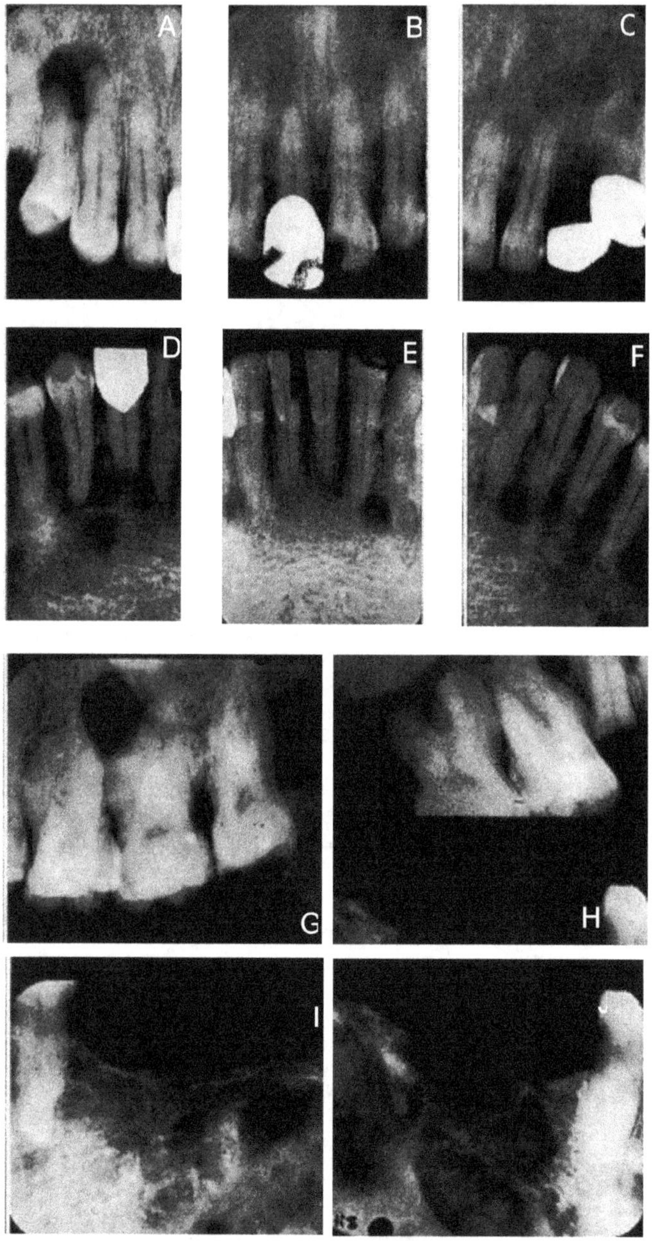

Fig. 1. Radiographs showing osteolytic lesions caused by MM in different regions of maxilla and mandible.

Skull lesions are more common than jaw lesions. Multiple radiolucent lesions of varying size, with ill-defined margins and a lack of circumferential osteosclerotic activity, should suggest this diagnosis (Figure 2). (6)

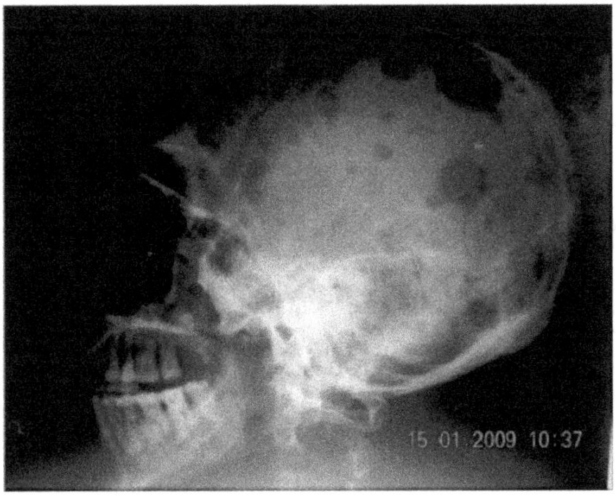

Fig. 2. Lateral Skull view showing multiple punched out radiolucent lesion

Extraosseous lesions also occur in a significant number of patients (Figure 3) although a majority of the lesions are asymptomatic.

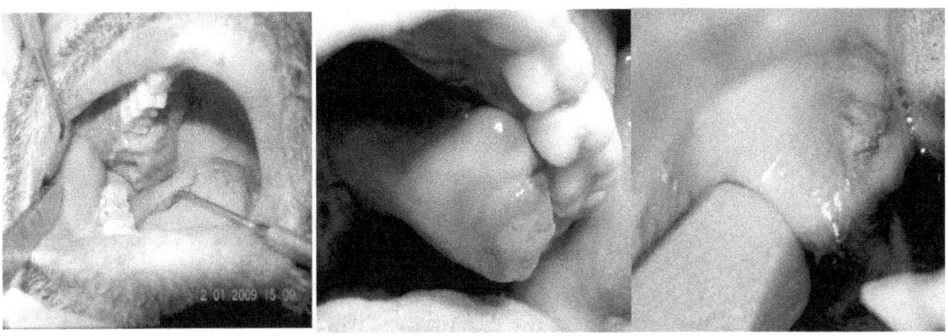

Fig. 3. Extraosseous presentations of MM

Amyloidosis as an additional complication has been reported in 6% to 15% of patients with multiple myeloma. Oral manifestations occur in nearly 39% of primary amyloidosis patients in which multiple myeloma associated lesions consist a small portion (13-15). Rarely oral amyloidosis may be the first symptom of multiple myeloma (16-18). The amyloid deposits in oral mucosa of primary amyloidosis patients presents as papules, nodules and plaques(13-15,19). These lesions may interfere with speech, chewing, swallowing and ability to close mouth. Amyloid involvement of oral tissue is rather rare, and the tongue is the most encountered subsite (20). Macroglossia, usually seen in primary amyloidosis, occurs in approximately 20% of patients (21,22). It seems that almost all secondary amyloidosis originates from reactive systematic conditions (23). Even though macroglossia is known to be the most common manifestation, mucosal nodules are considered to be more specific signs indicative of amyloidosis of the tongue since tongue enlargement can also occur in the absence of amyloidosis (19). Amyloid deposition in the salivary glands may cause xerostomia. In late stages, lesions may even lead to oropharyngeal blokage (24). Presence of amyloidosis in multiple myeloma patients is usually associated with poor survival. The median survival time in these patients is assumed to be about 4 months and death usually occurs as a complication of amyloidosis effecting major organ systems (25). Tongue biopsy is an excellent method of diagnosis. When a dentist/dental specialist is requested to take a biopsy specimen to detect amyloidosis, the specimen must include muscle tissue from the mucobuccal fold or tongue.

3. Dental management

Patients in long-term remission can undergo dental treatment, while patients with advanced or relapsed disease with reserved prognosis should receive palliative or urgent treatment only. Dental treatment should be performed always after consultation with the specialist, as it can be modified by certain aspects of the therapy and of the disease prognosis (26).

It is very important to carry out a detailed history. This should include the diagnosis and status of the neoplasia, the nature and duration of previous and ongoing treatment, prognosis, comorbid medical conditions, current medications, past dental history, and prior history of oral and non-oral infections (27).

All patients with MM should undergo comprehensive oral and dental evaluation in which is important to (26):

1. Evaluate for presence of petechiae, ecchymosis, gingival hemorrhage, tooth mobility, tooth migration, facial pain, and/or paresthesia, indicative of local manifestations of MM.
2. Evaluate for presence of dental/periodontal disease as a risk factor for development of osteonecrosis of the jaw (ONJ) and/or bacteraemia.
3. Evaluate radiographs (panoramic and periapicals, as indicated) for evidence of osteolytic lesions (if detected, refer for further radiographic evaluation) and to determine potential risk for developing osteonecrosis of the jaw (ONJ).

Dental treatment of these patients should be performed before starting the chemo/radiotherapy, treating any teeth with pulpal and periapical pathology, periodontal abscess, pericoronaritis, gross clinical caries and periodondontal disease. In the case of patients scheduled for autologous hematopoietic cell transplant, dental treatment should be avoided during the 3 days when stem cells are mobilized and harvested to minimize contamination secondary to iatrogenic transient bacteremia (27).

The main problems in dental treatment of patients with MM are:

1. **Tendency to bleed**

Hemorrhages are the dentist's major concerns when treating a patient with MM. Bleeding may result from several causes, including thrombocytopenia, abnormal platelet function, abnormal coagulation, or hyperviscosity. Intraoral bleeding manifests as petechiae and ecchymoses, and occasionally hematoma formation. These lesions do not require treatment, and large hematomas should not be excised due to risk of hemorrhage.

For routine operative care where bleeding is not anticipated, treatment can generally be provided in even severely thrombocytopenic patients ($\leq$ 10,000/ mm^3)without the need for transfusions.

If surgery is necessary, recent results of platelet count, bleeding time, prothrombin time, and partial thromboplastin time should be obtained. Depending on the extent of surgery, coordination of platelet transfusion the day of the procedure may be indicated, although single tooth extractions can generally be managed by an experienced clinician with localized measures even with levels as low as 15,000 cells/mL (27).

2. **Increased risk of infection**

Patients with compromised lymphocyte function or low neutrophil count due to their malignancy or secondary to myelosuppressive chemotherapy are prone to newly acquired infections and/or exacerbation or reactivation of latent infections (27-29). In many cases the clinical presentation of oral infections may be atypical compared to what would normally be expected in a healthy patient population. Use of diagnostic tools, including cultures, cytological smears, and tissue biopsies, is critical in identifying pathogens and guiding appropriate therapies (27).

a. Dental infections:

Oral prophylaxis, oral hygiene instruction and elimination of oral sources of infection before beginning cancer treatment, can significantly reduce the risk of infectious complications (27,29). Odontogenic infections of pulpal and periodontal origin are frequently encountered and should be suspected in the presence of orofacial pain, large restorations, gross clinical caries, and periapical radiolucency. Dental radiographs must be obtained for any suspected odontogenic infection. Endodontically treated teeth with a radiographically adequate seal can become symptomatic during severe neutropenia, and while these may be initially managed with antibiotics, in most cases extraction is indicated. Similarly, chronic periodontal disease can become acutely exacerbated with or without the traditional clinical signs of inflammation and swelling. Treatment includes broad-spectrum antibiotics, chlorhexidine rinses, scaling and curettage, and extraction of hopeless teeth. Extractions should be performed as early as possible prior to beginning therapy to allow maximum healing. Prior to extractions or any other invasive procedures the platelet and absolute neutrophils counts must be reviewed and appropriate measures taken to minimize risk of complications (27).

b. Opportunistic infections:
   i. **Viral infections:** Primary infection or reactivation of herpes family viruses is common in these patients, especially during intensive chemotherapy and in the context of advanced disease. Herpex simplex virus is the most common viral infection in these patients and typically presents as single or multiple painful ulcerative lesions that may involve any oral mucosal surface. Varicella-zoster virus (VZV) reactivation is less common. Treatments for both infections include acyclovir, valacyclovir or famciclovir, the latter appearing to have an advantage in preventing post-herpetic neuralgia following VZV infections (27,29).
   ii. **Fungal infections:** Oropharingeal candidiasis is the most common fungal infection in cancer patients. Candidiasis can present as pseudomembranous (the most common), erythematous, hyperplastic, or angular cheilitis. Symptoms include generalized discomfort, dysgeusia, xerostomia, and burning. Initial episodes can be treated with topical azoles or nystatin for 7 to 14 days; in severe cases, systemic therapy should be considered with 100 to 200 mg/day of fluconazole or itraconazole for 7 to 14 days or long-term for prophylaxis, especially in recurrent cases. In patients with nonhealing solitary ulcerations, deep fungal infections (aspergillus, zygomyces, and histoplasma)

should be considered, the management of which requires aggressive therapy with intravenous azoles, amphotericin B, and the echinocandins (27,29).

3. **Risk of developing osteonecrosis of jaws (ONJ)**

In MM patients treated with radiotherapy or intravenous bisphosphonates there is a risk of developing osteonecrosis of jaws. The unique environment of the oral cavity could explain why the maxilla and mandible are solely involved. It can be hypothesized that patients who have received long-term bisphosphonate therapy may have a compromised blood supply to their maxilla and mandible. When dental extractions are performed on this group of patients, the open bony wound with a compromised healing ability cannot cope with the presence of oral microflora.The extraction wound then becomes infected and progresses into osteomyelitis due to the poor healing ability of the tissues. It then develops into osteonecrosis. It should be noted that all other bones in the skeleton are well enclosed in the soft tissue and thus protected from a resident microflora. (30)

Preventive recommendations

A comprehensive recent medical history is essential before commencing any dental treatment. Identifying the risk factors in the medical history is mandatory and will help the patient's overall well-being and safety. Patients taking radiotherapy or potent bisphosphonates for more than one year, particularly for bone conditions other than osteoporosis, and those on concomitant steroids appear to be at highest risk of developing ONJ. Other factors that appear to further increase the risks include: residual multiple myeloma or another malignancy; hypoproteinemia; renal impairment from disease or drugs; and/or chemotherapy.

The treatment plan for a patient who has been on radiotherapy or bisphosphonate therapy should involve restorative dentistry, limited non-surgical periodontics and endodontics to control dental decay, periodontal disease and periapical inflammation. Patients who have dentures should have well maintained soft liners to minimize trauma to the oral mucosa or leave their dentures out. Failing soft liners would be more irritating than a hard but smooth denture.

Extraction and all types of surgery should be avoided. If an extraction is mandatory, for example an infected vertically split tooth, then the tooth should be extracted with minimal bony damage or exposure. Although there is no research to validate it, prophylactic antibiotics and suturing the socket to close the wound are advised. As a novel approach the authors have been using orthodontic elastic bands to exfoliate teeth. This results in a slow extraction over a few weeks which allows the oral mucosa to migrate down the tooth as it exfoliates so there is no open wound.(31,32)

There are conflicting reports regarding dental implants. Experimental studies show a positive effect of bisphosphonates on the bone around implants in experimental animals and humans (33, 34 35) . Failure of osteintegration in a patient who had successfully integrated implants but then commenced on bisphosphonate therapy has been reported.(36) Current advice is that placement of implants is best avoided if the patient has serious bone disease and are on potent doses. Osteoporotic patients on lower doses need a full informed consent before proceeding. Patients on bisphosphonate therapy with existing implants ↓should be regularly clinically and radiographically monitored. Increased bone density around the implant, similar to that shown around the socket in may occur. If bone pain or loss of integrity occurs the superstructure should be removed and the implant left submerged.(36)

Bone surgery must be avoided as the bone is exceedingly dense and avascular necrosis may occur.

Full dental assessment and treatment planning should occur prior to the patient commencing radiotherapy or bisphosphonate therapy (Table 1). (37)

Prior to radiotherapy/ bisphosphonate therapy

↓

Referral for dental assessment
Establish dental fitness
– Eliminate caries (extractions, restorations)
– Establish healthy periodontium (scaling, extractions)

↓

Commence radiotherapy/bisphosphonate therapy

↓

Regular monitoring of oral health
Clinical examination
Radiology
Dental – maintain oral health
– avoid extractions, avoid dentures

Table 1. Preventive strategy for OJN

Therapeutic recommendations

The first step is to establish the diagnosis if a patient on radiotherapy/bisphosphonate therapy presents with a non-healing oral wound. This requires an accurate medical and dental history. Patients with diabetes and immunocompromised patients can have delayed wound healing. Once the diagnosis of ONJ is made the treating medical practitioner, oral and maxillofacial surgeon and dentist need to confer to establish a management plan. At present there is no simple single effective treatment for ONJ. (38-42)

The first approach should be non-surgical with the use of antiseptic mouth rinses and antibiotics to prevent or treat secondary infection. Removable appliances lined with a periodontal pack that passively cover the bony defect can be inserted to protect the site from further trauma and may aid mucosal covering of the exposed bone.(37,42)

If the exposed bone is painful or there is significant secondary infection, localized surgical debridement without primary reconstruction can be considered. Minimal mucoperiosteal flap reflection to preserve the blood supply to underlying bone should be used. The problem is that the whole skeleton is involved. Resection to a normal bleeding bone margin cannot be undertaken as for osteoradionecrosis. Bone grafting, either as a free graft or by microvascular transfer, involves affected bone. There is a risk that there could be two problem areas, the donor graft site as well as the recipient jaw site. Major re-section surgery should be avoided if at all possible. (38-42)

In summary, for established cases it is recommended that treatments begin with the recognition that palliation and control of secondary infection are the primary goals. Control of progression has been obtained in most cases with long-term or intermittent courses of a penicillin or second generation cephalosporin, chlorhexidine mouthwash and periodic minor debridement of soft-textured sequestrating bone and wound irrigation (Table 2).

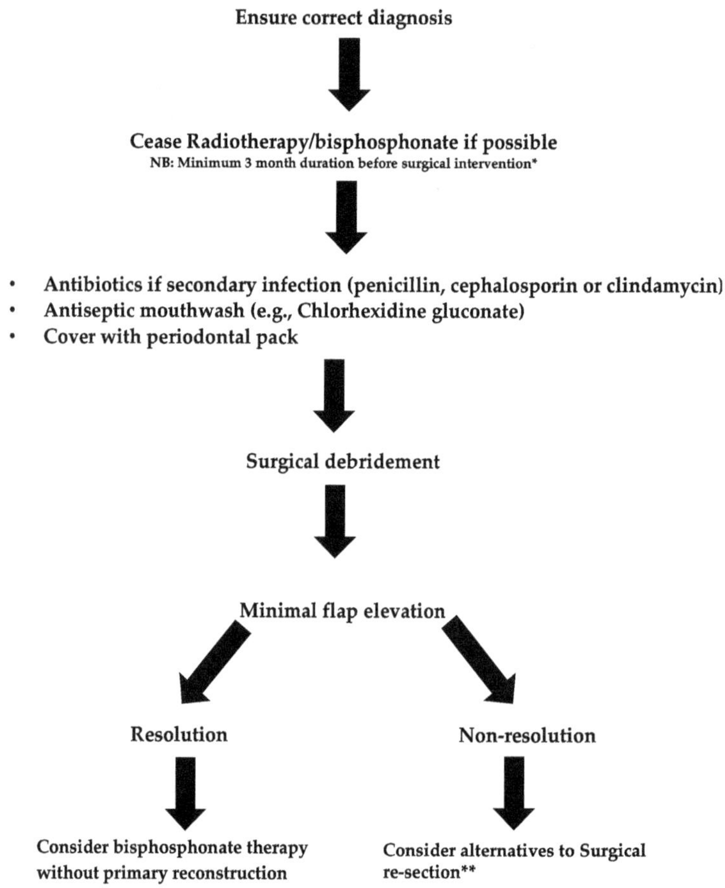

*It is probable that this time span is too short.
**Extreme caution is recommended at this point

Table 2. Therapeutic management of ONJ

4. Anemia

Patients with severe anemia often complain of that they fatigue easily and may not be able to tolerate time-consuming dental treatment.

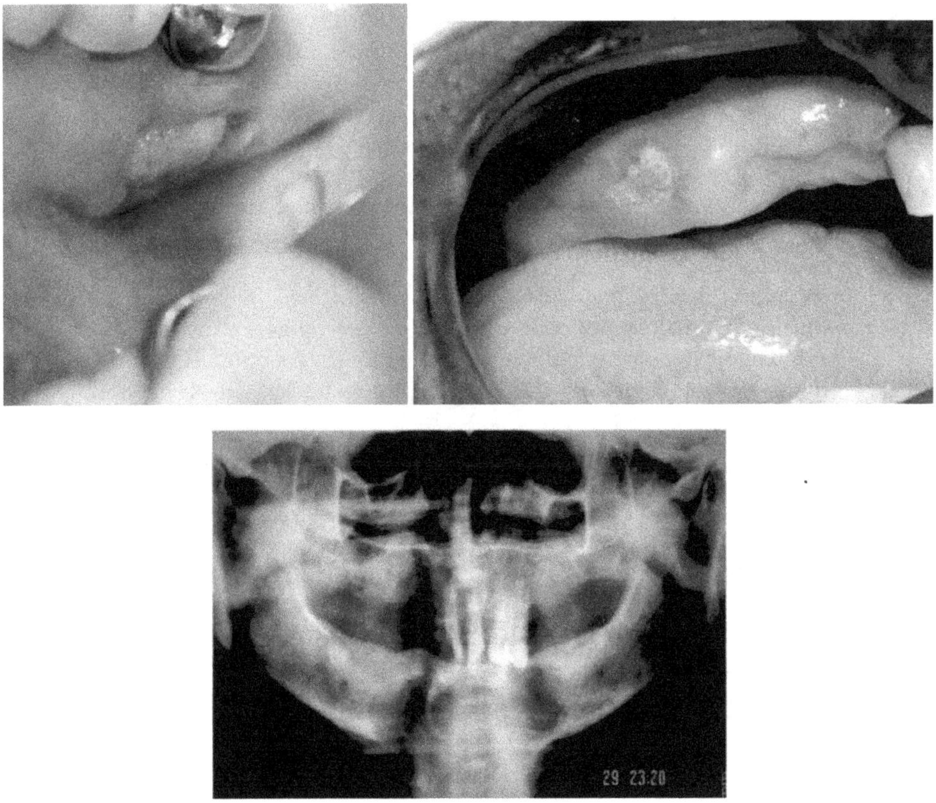

Fig. 4. Clinical and radiographic presentations of ONJ

The need for blood products and the appropriate venue for dental treatment should be discussed with the patient's oncologist, as these patients may require continuous monitoring of vital signs and blood counts perioperatively (26).

5. Corticosteroids treatment

Patients receiving high-dose systemic corticosteroids may display evidence of secondary adrenal insufficiency. Adrenal crises secondary to insufficiency are rare in the dental setting, and steroid supplementation before nonsurgical dental procedures is not recommended. Steroid supplementation before oral surgery is usually recommended. The amount, duration, and venue for supplementation should be determined by both the dental specialist performing the procedure and the patient's oncologist (26).

6. Secondary malignancy

Patients treated for MM are at high risk for relapse of primary disease as well as developing secondary malignancies. Considering the increased risk of second primary cancer of the head and neck in the survivors of MM, and the fact that squamous cell carcinoma is the most common second primary solid malignancy after allogeneic hematopoietic cell transplant, oral health care professionals play a critical role in the long-term surveillance of this patient population (27).

7. **Specific considerations**
   - Patients with renal dysfunction may require modified dosing intervals of medications (26).
   - In patients with multiple myeloma, it is important to evaluate for presence of hard/soft tissue masses that could indicate deposition of plasma cells and/or light chain associated amyloid, and biopsy if necessary (26).
   - Patients with multiple myeloma and significant bone pain, especially in the back, may need frequent breaks and may require frequent repositioning during dental procedures (26).
   - In patients undergoing orthodontic treatment, the removal of orthodontic appliances and delivery of retainers is recommended, as well as the postponement of orthodontic treatment until the patient has finished immunosuppressive therapy and the risk of hematologic relapse requiring further intervention is reduced (43,44).

Considerations in dental treatment of patients with MM are summarized in table 3.

Prior to dental treatment	During dental treatment
1. Patients in long-term remission can undergo dental treatment, while patients with advanced or relapsed disease with reserved prognosis should receive palliative or urgent treatment only. 2. Dental treatment should be performed always after consultation with the specialist 3. It is important to carry out a detailed history, a comprehensive oral and dental evaluation and a complete radiographic exam. 4. Dental treatment should be performed before starting the chemo/radiotherapy.	1. Bleeding tendency 2. Increased risk of infection 3. Risk of developing osteonecrosis of the jaw. 4. Anemia 5. Corticosteroids treatment 6. Secondary malignancies 7. Specific considerations

Table 3. Considerations in dental treatment of patients with MM

3. References

[1] Kyle RA, Gertz MA, Witzig TE, Lust JA, Lacy MQ, Dispenzieri A etal. Review of 1027 patients with newly diagnosed multiple myeloma. Mayo Clin Proc 2003; 78:21-33.

[2] Currie WJ, Hill RR, Keshani DK. An unusual cause of maxillary tuberosity enlargement. Br Dent J 1994;177:60-2.

[3] Zachriades N, Papanicolaou S, Papavassiliou D, Vairaktaris E, Triantafyllou D, Mezitis M. Plasma cell myeloma of the jaws. Int J Oral Maxillofac Surg 1987;16:510-5.

[4] Kyle RA. Multiple myeloma: review of 869 cases. Mayo Clin Proc 1975;50:29-40.

[5] Epstein JB, Voss NJ, Stevenson-Moore P. Maxillofacial manifestations of multiple myeloma. An unusual case and review of the literature. Oral Surg Oral Med Oral Pathol 1984;57:267-71.

[6] Lee SH, Huang JJ, Pau WL, Chan CP. Gingival mass as the primary manifestation of multiple myeloma. Oral Surg Oral Med Oral Pathol 1996;82:75- 79.

[7] Lambertenghi-Deliliers G, Bruno E, Cortellezzi A, Fumagalli L, Morosini A. Incidence of jaw lesions in 193 patients with multiple myeloma. Oral Surg Oral Med Oral Pathol 1988;65:533–537.

[8] Seoane J, Aguirre-Urizar JM, Esparza-Gómez G, Suárez-Cunqueiro M, Campos-Trapero J, Pomareda M. The spectrum of plasma cell neoplasia in oral pathology. Med Oral. 2003 Aug-Oct;8(4):269-80.

[9] Epstein JB, Voss NJ, Stevenson-Moore P. Maxillofacial manifestations of multiple myeloma. An unusual case and review of the literature. Oral Surg Oral Med Oral Pathol. 1984 Mar;57(3):267-71.

[10] Mozaffari E, Mupparapu M, Otis L. Undiagnosed multiple myeloma causing extensive dental bleeding: report of a case and review. Oral Surg Oral Med Oral Pathol Oral Radiol Endod. 2002 Oct;94(4):448-53.

[11] Reboiras López MD, García García A, Antúnez López J, Blanco Carrión A, Gándara Vila P, Gándara Rey JM. Anaesthesia of the right lower hemilip as a first manifestation of multiple myeloma. Presentation of a clinical case. Med Oral. 2001 May-Jul;6(3):168-72.

[12] Pinto L SS, Campagnoli EB, Leon JE, etal. Maxillary lesion presenting as a first sign of multiple myeloma. Case report.Med Oral Patol Oral Cir Bucal 2007; 12: E344-7.

[13] Reinish EI, Raviv M, Srolovitz H, Gornitsky M. Tongue, primary amiloidosis and multiple myeloma. Oral Surg Oral Med Oral Pathol 1994; 77: 121-125.

[14] Jacobs P, Sellars S, King HS. Massive macroglossia, amyloidosis and myloma. Postgrad Med J 1988; 64: 696-8.

[15] Van Der Wal, Logmans SH, Van Der Kwast WAM, Van Der Vaal I. Amyloidosis of the tongue: A clinical and postmortem study. J Oral Pathol 1984; 13: 632-639.

[16] Kielts TR. Amyloidosis of the buccal mucosa as diagnostic precursor in multiple myeloma: Report of a case. J Am Dent Assoc. 1964; 69: 701.

[17] Flick WG, Lawrence FR. Oral amyloidosis as initial symptom of multiple myeloma. Oral Surg 1980; 49: 18-20.

[18] Babajews A. Occult multiple myeloma associated with amyloid of the tongue. Br J Oral Maxillofac Surg. 1985; 23: 298-303.

[19] Raubenheimer EJ, Dauth J, Pretorius FJ. Multiple myeloma and amyloidosis of the tongue. J Oral Pathol 1988; 17: 554-9.

[20] Rutger I, Martijn R, Peter C, Theo M. Amyloidosis of the tongue as a paraneoplastic marker of plasma cell dyscrasia. Oral Surg Oral Med Oral Pathol 2002;94:444-447.

[21] Smith A, Speculand B. Amyloidosis with oral involvement. Br J Oral Maxillofac Surg 1985;23:435–444.

[22] Yusa H, Yoshida H, Kikuchi H, Onizawa K. Dialysis-related amyloidosis of the tongue. J Oral Maxillofac Surg 2001;59:947–950.

[23] Mardinger O, Rotenberg L, Chaushu G, Taicher S. Surgical management of macroglossia due to primary amyloidosis. Int J Oral Maxillofac Surg 1999; 28:129-131.

[24] Daoud MS, Lust JA, Kyle Ra, Pittelkow MR. Monoclonal gammopathies and associated skin disorders. J Am Acad Dermatol 1999; 40: 507-515.

[25] Salisbury PL, Jacoway RJ. Oral amyloidosis: a late complication of multiple myeloma. Oral Surg Oral Med Oral Pathol 1983; 56: 48.

[26] Stoopler ET, Vogl DT, Stadtmauer EA. Medical management update: multiple myeloma. Oral Surg Oral Med Oral Pathol Oral Radiol Endod. 2007;103:599-609.

[27] Mawardi H, Cutler C, Treister N. Medical management update: Non-Hodgkin lymphoma. Oral Surg Oral Med Oral Pathol Oral Radiol Endod. 2009;107:e19-33.

[28] Raut A, Huryn JM, Hwang FR, Zlotolow IM. Sequelae and complications related to dental extractions in patients with hematologic malignancies and the impact on medical outcome. Oral Surg Oral Med Oral Pathol Oral Radiol Endod. 2001;92:49-55.

[29] Heimdahl A. Prevention and management of oral infections in cancer patients. Support Care Cancer. 1999;7:224-8.

[30] Melo MD, Obeid G. Osteonecrosis of the maxilla in a patient with a history of bisphosphonate therapy. J Can Dent Assoc 2005;71:111-113.

[31] Lawler B, Sambrook PJ, Goss AN. Antibiotic prophylaxis for dentoalveolar surgery: is it indicated? Aust Dent J 2005;50 Suppl 2:S54-S59.

[32] Arvier J, Tideman H, Vickers P. Foreign bodies and gingival lesions. Aust Dent J 1987;32:285-287.

[33] Yoshinari M, Oda Y, Inoue T, Matsuzaka K, Shimono M. Bone response to calcium phosphate-coated and bisphosphonateimmobilized titanium implants. Biomaterials 2002;23:2879- 2885.

[34] Duarte PM, deVasconcelor Gurgel BC, Sallum AW, Filho GR, Sallum EA, Nociti FH. Alendronate therapy may be effective in the prevention of bone loss around titanium implants inserted in estrogen deficient rats. J Periodontal 2005;76:107-114.

[35] Degidi M, Piatelli A. Immediately loaded bar-connected implants with an anodized surface inserted in the anterior mandible in a patient treated with disphosphonates for osteoporosis: a case report with a 12 month follow up. Clin Implant Dent Relat Res 2003;5:269-272.

[36] Starck WJ, Epker BN. Failure of osseointegrated dental implants after disphosphonate therapy for osteoporosis: a case report. Int J Oral Maxillofac Implants 1995;10:74-78.

[37] Expert Panel Recommendations for the prevention, diagnosis and treatment of osteonecrosis of the jaws. June 2004. (Submitted for publication). Available www.novartis.com.au

[38] Ruggiero SL, Mehrotra B, Rosenberg TJ, Engroff SL. Osteonecrosis of the jaws associated with the use of bisphosphonates: a review of 63 cases. J Oral Maxillofac Surg 2004;62:527-534.

[39] Tarassoff P, Csermak K. Avascular necrosis of the jaws: risk factors in metastatic cancer patients. J Oral Maxillofac Surg 2003;61:1238-1239.

[40] Marx RE. Pamidronate (Aredia) and zoledronate (Zometa) induced avascular necrosis of the jaws: a growing epidemic. J Oral Maxillofac Surg 2003;61:1115-1117.

[41] Migliorati CA. Bisphosphonates and oral cavity avascular bone necrosis. J Clin Oncol 2003;21:4253-4254.

[42] Carter GD, Goss AN, Doecke C. Bisphosphonates and avascular necrosis of the jaw: a possible association. Med J Aust 2005;182:413-415.

[43] Sheller B, Williams B. Orthodontic management of patients with hematologic malignancies. Am J Orthod Dentofacial Orthop. 1996;109:575-80.

[44] Isaac AM, Tholouli E. Orthodontic treatment for a patient who developed acute myeloid leukemia. Am J Orthod Dentofacial Orthop. 2008;134:684-8.

12

Renal Disease in Multiple Myeloma

Guray Saydam, Fahri Sahin and Hatice Demet Kiper
Ege University Hospital,
Dept. of Internal Medicine
Turkey

1. Introduction

Renal involvement is a common feature of Multiple Myeloma (MM) that is associated with significant morbidity and shortened survival. At the time of diagnosis, some degree of renal impairment is present in about half of the cases. In some of patients dialysis is required eventually (Hutchison, 2007). A review from the US Renal Data System (USRDS) reports that the number of patients with myeloma associated end-stage renal disease (ESRD) in 2004 in the United States was 5,390, with a prevalence of 1.1%. The presence of renal involvement is commonly associated with a higher tumor burden and worse prognosis, as the severity of renal failure is highly correlated with patient survival. Based on large series in which renal function was evaluated by serum creatinine levels; 43% of 998 patients had a renal insufficiency with the serum creatinine concentrations above 1,5 mg/dl (133 μmol/L) and one-year survival was found 80% in this group, while it was 50% in the patient group who had creatinine levels more than 2,3 mg/dl (200 μmol/L) (Winearls CG,1995). In another report, 22% of 423 patients had a severe renal insufficiency with the values of creatinine concentration greater than 2 mg/dl (177 μmol/L) (Bladé J,et al.,1998). As the serum creatinine level is affected due to the attenuated muscle mass of elderly MM patient population, International Myeloma Working Group has recommended use of glomerular filtration rate calculated by Modification of Diet in Renal Diseaese (MDRD) formula for the assessment of renal functions. For the assessment of the severity of acute renal injury, RIFLE (Risk, Injury, Failure, Loss and End-stage) and AKIN (Acute Kidney Injury Network) criteria may also be used.

Renal failure is reversible in the majority of the patients and reversibility is an important prognostic factor which is associated with a long-term survival. With appropriate therapy, more than 50% patients with moderate renal insufficiency had improvement in renal functions during the first three months and it was found to be associated with better prognosis. (Knudsen et al.,2000) Successful managment of reversible precipitating factors such as dehydration, hypercalcemia, hyperuricemia, infections and use of nephrotoxic agents like contrast materials, non steroidal anti-inflammatory drugs (NSAID) and angiotensin-converting enzyme inhibitors can successfully contribute to reversal of renal failure. Initiation of early aggressive anti-myeloma therapy results in rapid decline of light chain production which can contribute significantly to renal function recovery.

Pathogenesis of renal disease in Multiple Myeloma is multifactorial . It is associated with excess production of monoclonal light chains by the neoplastic B-cell clone. Renal lesions occur primarily in tubules; however glomeruli, interstitium and blood vessels may also be involved. Myeloma cast nephropathy (Light Chain Cast Nephropathy -LCCN, Myeloma kidney) is the most prominent type of MM renal involvement and is primarily tubular. Isolated distal or proximal tubular dysfunction and acquired Fanconi Syndrome also may be seen. Glomerular lesions are usually related to AL-amyloidosis and light/heavy deposition disease. Interstitial nephritis and plasma cell infiltration demonstrate the involvement of renal interstitium. Types of pathologic lesions are basically determined by the mutated amino acid sequence of the monoclonal light chain. This was confirmed with LC injected mice that developed the same pattern of renal disease as was seen in the donor MM patient. (Solomon A, Weiss DT, Kattine AA,1991) Autopsy series of patients with myeloma found that the most frequent pathology is LCCN accounts for 40% to 60%, whereas light chain deposition disease and amyloidosis were seen in 5% and7% cases respectively. (Ivanyi B.,1989) In native renal biopsy studies of patients with myeloma and renal disease,40 to 63% had cast nephropathy, 19 to 26% had light-chain deposition disease, 7 to 30% had amyloidosis, and <1% had cryoglobulinemic renal > disease." (Ganewal D.,et al,1992 ve Montseny JJ. et al,1998) Renal biopsy is not indicated many patients for differential diagnosis to concern therapeutic options and estimation of prognosis in patients with the diagnosis of myeloma. (Kidney biopsy is generally not indicated for many of patients)

We have tried to summarize the all pathophysiological mechanisms and clinical presentations of renal involvement in MM patients in this chapter.

2. Light Chain Cast Nephropathy (myeloma kidney)

LCCN is the most common cause of renal failure associated with myeloma, which accounts for approximately 90% of the cases. (Lin J,et al,2001) Renal failure may present both acutely or chronically but it is often acute in nature and can be severe with serum creatinine levels above 7 mg/dl (Montseny J,et al,1998). Characteristic lesion is a tubulointerstitial nephritis associated with monoclonal free light chains (FLCs) leading to intra-tubular cast formation/obstruction and direct tubular toxicity. Overproduction of FLCs by the neoplastic B-cell clone plays a crucial role in causing typical renal damage characterized by tubular atrophy and tubulointerstitial fibrosis. The degree of renal impairment correlates with tubular injury but not with the extent of cast formation. (Silva FG, et al,1983)The normal amount of light chain excretion is less than 30 mg/day, however it is generally more than 1 gr/day in a myeloma patient with LCCN and can be massive (>20 gr/day) leading to nephrotic syndrome in less than 10% of the cases. The rate of FLC excretion corelates with renal insufficiency. In a demographic study of 1353 patients, 16% of the cases with < 1 gr/d FLC proteinuria had renal failure versus 47% and 63% in those with 1-10 gr/d and > 10 gr/d, respectively (p=0,001) (Knudsen LM,et al,1994) Patients with LCCN are at higher risk of developing advanced myeloma with severe anemia and hypercalcemia (Durie-Salmon stage 3).

2.1 Pathogenesis of LCCN

The main pathology is cast nephropathy ie : the presence of excess FLCs in the plasma and urine which are produced by a neoplastic clone of plasma cells. Catabolism of circulating

FLCs intrinsically occurs in the kidney. In normal individuals, serum FLCs are relatively freely filtered through the glomerulus because of their low molecular weights (22,5 kd for monomeric kappa and 45 kd for dimeric lambda) and cationic net charge. After glomerular filtration; the FLCs in the tubular fluid bind to the tandem scavenger receptor system megalin/cubilin and are endocytosed via the clathrin dependent endosomal/lysosomal pathway (Batuman V et al., 1998). Megalin and cubilin are the two major, multiligand, endocytic receptors which are highly expressed in the apical endocytic apparatus of the renal proximal tubule and they are responsible for the tubular reabsorbtion of most proteins filtered in the glomeruli. Receptor Associated Protein (RAP) is also known as a high-affinated ligand for megalin, thus, it plays a significant role in endocytic function of the proximal tubule (Verroust PJ et al.,2002). Endocytic uptake of FLCs is followed by the hydrolisation and degradation in the lysosomes, and after acidifying in vesicles, the released aminoacids pass through basement membrane and re-circulate back to the system (Leheste et al., 1999)

In Multiple Myeloma, over-production of FLCs exceeds the reabsorbation capacity of the proximal tubules and results in the presence of FLCs in the distal nephron and overflow light chain proteinuria (Bence Jones proteinuria). Tamm-Horsfall Mucoprotein (THMP, also known as Uromodulin) is a renal epithelial glycoprotein which is secreted by the cells of the thick ascending limb of the loop of Henle and it forms the gel-like matrix of urinary casts. Over-concentrated FLCs bind to a specific peptide domain on THMP and constitutes the waxy cast formation that aggregates in distal tubules leading to tubular obstruction. Some factors may promote cast formation, such as dehydration (by stasis in tubules), hypercalcemia, acidosis, radiocontrast medications (by interacting with light chains) and furosemide (by increasing luminal sodium chloride). Increasing intra-luminal pressure reduces the glomerular filtration rate, therefore by the loss of metabolism related to GFR, circulating concentration FLCs increases also in the tubules. This circumstance triggers a vicious cycle in the pathogenesis of myeloma kidney. Intra-tubular cast formation usually results in tubular rupture and necrosis that precipitates interstitial inflammatory nephritis (Hill GS et al.,1983) Interstitial fibrosis and tubular atrophy follow : this fact can be accepted as the main pathology underlying the renal impairment related to cast nephropathy. Direct tubular toxicity is one of the another basic mechanisms leads to LCCN and dose-dependent toxicity can be occur in the proximal tubuler epithelial cells (PTEC) by light chains, resulting in tubular necrosis. Type of light chain is also important to determine the degree and the localization of renal injury for the reason that nephrotoxicity may differ based on the characteristics of the light chains. THMP interacts with the hyper-variable regions of the light chains and shows variable affinity to different types (Sanders et al., 1990). This phenomenon can explain why some patients have a severe renal disease with smaller amount of light chains and some have minimal renal dysfunction with larger rates. It is also well known that kappa and lambda light chains are both toxic to the tubule ephitelium but lambda is more associated with amyloidosis whereas kappa is frequently involves in Light Chain Deposition Disease (LCDD) and acquired adult's Fanconi's syndrome.

Recent studies in last decade put emphasis on the role of proximal tubule cells in the pathogenesis of cast nephropathy. These studies have demonstrated that proximal tubular endocytosis of light chains induces pro-inflammatory and inflammatory cytokine releasing such as IL-6, IL-8, TNF alfa and monocyte chemotactic protein-1 (MCP-1). It has also been suggested that these cytokines and chemokines are mediated by activated transcription factors like NF-kappa β which are signalled through the MAPKs ERK 1/2, JNK and p38. (Sengul S et al., 2002,2003). This inflammatory process results in interstitial fibrosis and tubular damage which is associated most probably with the additon of incremental Transforming Growth Factor β (TGF-β) production (Keeling J, Herrera GA, 2007). There are still ongoing studies to clarify the molecular mechanisms involved in cast nephropathy and further studies are needed to have a clear understanding.

2.2 Diagnosis of LCCN

According to a renal biopsy study of 259 elderly patients who had unexplained renal failure, LCCN was found in 40% of patients with previously undiagnosed myeloma (Haas M,et al,2000). On this basis, LCCN should be considered in any patient over age 40 who presents with unexplained renal failure. Urine dipstick test is usually inadequate to detect FLCs, because it is primarily sensitive for albumin but insensitive for Bence Jones protein. Therefore, sulfosalicylic acid (SSA) which detects all proteins should be chosen to detect FLCs by the assessment of turbidity. A remarkably positive SSA test when dipstick is relatively negative supports the presence of non-albumin proteins like Bence Jones protein in the urine.Serum protein electrophoresis (SPEP) and urine protein electrophoresis (UPEP) should be performed initially in every patient with suspected myeloma. To confirm the diagnosis by measuring the amount and type of the monoclonal protein, immunofixation of serum and 24 h urine collection are also recommended especially in patients with normal protein electrophoretic pattern in cases with strong suspicion for myeloma. FLC assays which reveal the quantification of serum FLC levels, κ/λ ratio and urinary FLC excretion should be obtained on every patient and these assays are particularly important in non-secretory myeloma patients whom serum and urine immunofixation analysis is negative.

For a definitive diagnosis, renal biopsy is generally needed. Pathologic findings of LCCN basically include the demonstration of prominent tubular casts in distal nephron. With light microscopy, in hematoxylin and eosin-stained sections, the casts are brightly eosinophilic and usually seem large and "brittle" because they are typically lamellated/fractured and also surrounded by macrophages and multinucleated giant cells of foreign-body type diagnostically. The other staining properties of the casts are classified as Periodic acid-Schiff (PAS) negative, fuchsinophilic with Masson's trichrome and less frequently Congo red positive. Immunofluorescence microscopy can differentiate the light chain with THMP from the other serum proteins.

2.3 Prognosis and treatment of LCCN

Multiple Myeloma is a progressive and incurable disease and median survival is about 6 months or less if it is not treated. In the past decade, by the advances in the myeloma treatment, median survival has increased from an average of 3 years to >5 years. Renal function is an important prognostic factor for MM and renal failure is associated with a worse prognosis as the others like lower serum albumin and higher β-2 microglobulin levels. Severity and reversibility of renal impairment is also important in prognosis. In patients who present with a plasma creatinine concentration of <1,5 mg/dl (130 μmol/L), the one-year survival was 80%, compared with 50% for patients with a creatinine level of

>2.3 mg/dl (200 µmol/L) (Winearls CG, 1995). In cast nephropathy, renal failure is often reversible by appropriate management of the precipitating factors and early aggressive treatment to reduce FLC production. Many studies suggest that renal recovery is closely related with a better prognosis and similar outcomes who have a normal renal function at diagnosis (Bladé J.et al, 1998), however, on the contrary some claims it is not associated with a favorable outcome (Kastritis et al,2007). Renal dysfunction due to LCNN is usually presents in acute nature and some factors may contribute to reduce GFR by inducing cast precipitation or may be the main cause of acute renal failure (ARF). First of all, an appropriate supportive care should be administered to correct the precipitating factors lead to ARF and it should be followed by a specific anti-myeloma therapy.

Autologous Stem Cell Transplantation in LCCN

The use of autologous stem cell transplantation (ASCT) for patients with myeloma and renal insufficiency has been studied in last decade. Many of these patients are considered ineligible for ASCT because of a high risk of treatment-related toxicity.

In a retrospective study of 81 patients with multiple myeloma and renal failure (plasma creatinine >2mg/dl), 60 patients underwent transplantation with melphalan 200 mg/m^2, and the remaining 21 had a reduction of the melphalan dose to 140 mg/m^2 because of excessive toxicity. The treatment-related mortality rate after the first ASCT was 6% and the 3-year event-free and overall survival rates were 48 and 55%, respectively. The degree of toxicity was acceptable and stem cell collection or engraftment were not negatively affected by renal failure (Badros A,et al,2001). In another large study from Mayo Clinic, it has revealed that creatinine level did not affect complete response rate and time to progression (17 months), but patients with creatinine levels above 2 mg/ml had a higher day-100 mortality rate (13% vs.3%) and a shorter overall survival rate (31 vs 47 months) than those with normal renal function. Platelet engraftment was also significantly delayed for patients with renal insufficiency. In conclusion; ASCT may reverse renal failure in patients with multiple myeloma but it must be used with caution in selected patients with an appropriate dose adjustment of melphalan.

3. Other causes of ARF and prevention and supportive care

3.1 Volume depletion

Hypovolemia facilitates cast precipitation by increasing FLC concentration in tubule lumen and lower urine flow contributes to intratubular obstruction. Some of myeloma patients present with acute oliguric renal failure and vigorous fluid therapy should be immediately initiated to replace volume depletion. The goals of fluid therapy are to increase the urine formation and tubule flow rate to prevent intratubular cast precipitation and obstruction. Isotonic or one-half isotonic saline is generally used to administer the hydration regimen with an initial infusion rate of 150 ml/h to achieve a high urine output at least 3 lt/day. Close monitoring should be carried out therefore some patients who have renal or heart failure may develop volume overload. In such cases, hydration regimen should be modified and if it is essential, a loop diuretic may be used to forced diuresis. Adequate hydration usually reverses the pre-renal component of ARF and oliguric status generally responses to therapy preferably in the first 24 hours.

3.2 Hypercalcemia

Hypercalcemia occurs in more than 25 %of myeloma patients in the course of the disease and 15 %of patients have mild hypercalcemia with serum calcium level 11.0-13.0 mg/dl at diagnosis. Moderate or severe hypercalcemia may also be seen and may contribute to ARF. Hypercalcemia is the second most common cause of renal failure in MM (Blade J, Rosinol L.,2005). As the other malignancy-related hypercalcemias, some osteoclast activating factors and bone resorbing cytokines like lymphotoxin, interleukin-6, interleukin 1-β and a parathyroid related protein are produced by neoplastic cells and results in increased bone resorption (Kitazawa R,et al,2002). Elevated calcium concentration in renal tubules cause intratubular calcium deposition and vasoconstriction in renal vasculature. Decreased glomerular filtration rate induces cast precipitation and probably augments the toxicity of FLCs (Smolens P,et al,1987). Hypercalcemia may also causes nephrogenic diabetes insipidus which is characterized by ADH resistance and with the impairment of renal concentrating ability, polyuria and polydipsia may develop. Increased diuresis results in hypovolemia and aggravates the pre-renal component of renal failure. Renal dysfunction due to hypercalcemia is usually reversible and management strategy should be based on to correct serum calcium concentration. In mild asymptomatic hypercalcemia which can be described as <14 mg/dl (4 mmol/L), initially intravenous hydration should be preferred. Loop diuretics should not be used in myeloma-related hypercalcemia because of their facilitating effect on cast nephrotoxicity by increasing luminal sodium chloride. If there is no response to the fluid therapy within 12 hours, a bisphosphonate should be administered while considering renal functions. Although bisphosphonates are very useful and effective in the management of malignancy-related hypercalcemia, they must be used with caution in myeloma patients because of their nephrotoxicity and the risk of subsequent hypocalcaemia. In addition, beside their hypocalcemic effect, it has been shown that bisphosphonates reduce the incidence of skeletal events and improve life quality (Berenson JR,et al, 1998). Pamidronate (a dose of 60 to 90 mg as a 2 hours infusion) and Zoledronic acid (a dose of 4 mg, as a 15 minutes infusion) are the most common bisphosphonates in clinical use and regimen may be repeated at intervals of 2 or 4 weeks if necessary. Serum calcium and creatinine levels should be monitorized regularly and appropriate dose adjustment should be done in patients with severe renal impairment and vitamin D deficiency. For moderate or severe hypercalcemia, anti-myeloma therapy which includes steroids should be promptly initiated. Calcitonin may also help to reduce serum calcium concentrations without the risk of severe hypocalcemia and nephrotoxicity.

3.3 Nephrotoxic drugs

Some drugs and radiocontrast materials should not be used in myeloma patients because of their nephrotoxic potential, especially in the state of volume depletion.

3.3.1 Intravenous radiocontrast solutuions

Contrast induced nephropathy (CIN) is defined as an acute reduction in renal function due to iodinated contrast media administration and it is one of the most common cause of hospital-acquired acute renal failure. Patients with myeloma are at high risk group to develop renal impairment secondary to radiocontrast using and especially in the setting of hypovolemia, contrasts may precipitate acute renal failure in the rate of approximately 1.5 percent (McCarthy CS, Becker JA, 1992). These agents induce light chain precipitation in the tubules and furthermore they may also interact with light chains and contribute to intra-tubular obstruction. However, recent studies suggest that myeloma patients with normal creatinine and low β2-microglobulin levels (< 2.8 mg/L) are at low risk for developing CIN and radiocontrast administration is safe in this group (Pahade JK,et al,2011). Nevertheless, the removal or avoidance of iodinated contrast agents should be preferred primarily but if it is not possible, adequate hydration should be performed during and after the procedure as well as using of low-osmolar or iso-osmolar radiocontrast media.

3.3.2 Non-steroid anti-inflammatory drugs and others

NSAIDs basicly block the production of prostaglandins (PGs) via inhibition of cyclooxygenase enzyme activitiy (COX-1 and COX-2). By the suppression of vasodilatatory PGs, renal vasoconstriction occurs and it leads to a reduction in the renal blood flow and glomerular filtration rate which may contribute to ARF. PGs blockage also leads to salt and water retention by the inhibition of chloride reabsorbtion and antidiuretic hormone (ADH). NSAIDs also can develop papillary necrosis and chronic interstitial nephritis. Patients with hypercalcemia or lower renal blood flow due to congestive heart failure, chronic renal failure or any other cause of hypovolemia and sodium depletion, have higher risk for worsening renal functions after using NSAIDs (Murray MD,et al,1995). Thus, NSAID therapy in patients with myeloma should be administered carefully and avoided if possible to prevent further renal damage.

ACE inhibitors, angiotensine receptor blockers (ARBs), diuretics and aminoglycosides are the other nephrotoxic agents that affect renal functions adversely in myeloma patients and should be stopped or avoided if possible.

3.4 Hyperuricemia

Hyperuricemia due to increased nucleic acid turnover, is present in upto 50% myeloma patients at diagnosis. It may also be seen as a result of chemotherapy even though tumor lysis syndrome and acute uric acid nephropathy are rare in multiple myeloma. Adequate hydration, alkalinization of the urine and prophylactic use of allopurinol can overcome this complication significantly.

3.5 Hyperviscosity syndrome

Hyperviscosity syndrome is a group of symptoms results from increased blood viscosity due to the excessive amounts of circulating proteins and commonly occurs in association with paraprotein disorders, such as Waldenström macroglobulinemia (IgM) and rarely multiple myeloma (IgA,IgG3,kappa). It is classically manifested by spontaneous bleeding from mucous membranes due to impaired platelet function, neurologic and pulmonary symptoms as a result of ischemia in brain and lung tissue and visual defects related to rehinopathy. Although this syndrome rarely affects the kidneys permanently, it may also lead to acute renal failure occasionally. Plasmapheresis may be used to decrease viscosity significantly and also exchange transfusions and hydration may be administered in the treatment strategy.

4. Therapy modalities for myeloma kidney

4.1 Plasmapheresis

Extracorporeal removal of nephrotoxic light chains from the blood seems to be a reasonable approach in cast nephropathy and plasma exchange has been widely used in clinical practice to decrease serum FLC concentrations. However, there is no convincing evidence about the benefit of plasmapheresis in acute renal failure in multiple myeloma and conflicting outcomes have been reported by many studies ((Zuchelli P,et al,1988, Clark WF,et al,2005, Leung N,et al,2008) .

Currently, plasmapheresis is indicated for patients with acute renal failure due to myeloma cast nephropathy to assist in the rapid removal of circulating excess FLCs and must be done together with dexamethasone-based regimens to limit production of new light chains. Renal biopsy is primarily needed to confirm tissue diagnosis but in emergency conditions presence of very high levels of FLCs in the serum or urine may prompt initiation of plasmapheresis. Standart regimen includes five to seven exchanges within seven or ten days and may be repeated if necessary.

4.2 Dialysis

Dialysis is an alternative approach to remove FLCs from circulation but it is generally insufficient for large amounts of light chains. Both hemodialysis and peritoneal dialysis may be administered in patients with acute or chronic renal failure, however, plasmapheresis is relatively more effective in the way of light chain reduction acutely.

Recently, newer protein permeable and larger pored hemodialysis membranes that remove the FLCs more efficiently has been developed and studies focused on these high- cut off (HCO) dialysers. It has been demonstrated that daily, extended hemodialysis using the Gambro HCO 1100 dialyzer which has an effective cut-off for <50 kd proteins, could remove continuously large quantities of FLC (Hutchinson CA,et al,2007). A following pilot study handled by same team in 2009 concluded that in dialysis-dependent acute renal failure secondary to cast nephropathy, patients who received uninterrupted chemotherapy and extended HCO-HD had sustained reductions in serum FLC levels and independent renal function recovered in 74 percent of patients. An interruption in chemotherapy was found to be associated with unfavorable outcomes and therefore it was hard to distinguish the benefits of chemotherapy and HCO dialysis separately.

The **EU**ropean trial of free **LI**ght chain removal by ex**TE**nded haemodialysis in cast nephropathy (EuLITE) is a very recent prospective, randomised controlled, multicenter clinical trial of HCO dialysis versus conventional dialysis in patients with with cast nephropathy, dialysis dependent acute renal failure and de novo multiple myeloma who all receive bortezomib, doxorubicin and dexamethasone as chemotherapy (Hutchinson CA,et al,2008). This study is ongoing and if it suggests that if efficacious, this therapy will offer clinicians new options in the management of these patients.

4.3 Anti-myeloma treatment

4.3.1 Conventional chemotherapy

Renal dysfunction in myeloma patients usually indicates high tumor burden and aggressive disease and it is important to initiate an early, effective therapy to provide a remission and renal reversal immediately. Alkylator-based conventional chemotherapy with Melphalan-Prednisone (MP) was usually reserved for patients who are ineligible for ASCT because of advanced age >70 and/or severe comorbidities (Rajkumar SV,Kyle RA,2005). MP regimen is also insufficient in renal function recovery and dose adjustment problems due to the renal elimination of melphalan limit the efficacy of therapy. In a study of Nordic Myeloma Study Group ,by the treatment with alkylating agents and standard dose steroids, reversal of renal failure was found in 58% of patients, whereas 40% of patients with a creatinine 2.3mg/dl achieved a normal renal function (Knudsen LM,et al,2000).

Combination chemotherapies like Vincristin+ Doxorubicin+ Dexamethasone (VAD),or Cyclophosphamide + Dexamethasone, or Dexamethasone alone are more preferable regimens by clinicians to achieve a rapid control of the disease. Dose modification is not needed in renal failure because of low renal excretion of mentioned agents. From a single instution study in 94 patients who had renal failure with myeloma, renal function recovery was observed in 26% of cases by conventional combination chemotherapy. Median survival for these patients was 28.3 months, compared with 3.8 months for those with irreversible renal failure ($P<0.001$). Furthermore, survival was not significantly different in patients with renal recovery vs those with normal renal function ($P=0.97$). Response rate to chemotherapy was found to be considerably lower in patients with renal failure than those with normal renal function (39% versus 56%; $P<0.001$). However, if patients dying within the first 2 months of treatment were excluded, there was no significant differences in the response rate between patients with renal failure and those with normal renal function. This result can be explained by high rate of early mortality in patients with renal failure accounting for 30% within first two months. Combination chemotherapy was also found to be more effective than MP or CP regimens with the response rates relatively 50% versus 24% ($P=0.03$) even though survivals were similar (Blade J,et al,1998).

4.3.2 High-dose dexamethasone-based regimens

High-dose dexamethasone-based regimens are alternatively safe and effective for newly diagnosed myeloma patients with renal impairment. In the first study of pulse dexamethasone therapy in previously untreated patients, the overall response rate was 43% similar to VAD and serious complications were considerably fewer, 4% versus 27% (Alexanian R,et al,1992). In a series of 41 myeloma patients with renal impairment treated with high-dose dexamethasone, rate of renal function recovery was found 73% which was higher than the reversal rate of standart dose steroid included alkylator-based regimens. This study concluded that high-dose dexamethasone was effective even in one-half of patients with negative prognostic factors in terms of reversal such as massive proteinuria, cast nephropathy and severe renal insufficiency. It is also suggested that combination with novel biologic agents, such as thalidomide and/or bortezomib also can provide a more rapid improvement in renal function (Kastritis E,et al,2007).

4.3.3 Novel agents

Overall survival in multiple myeloma has improved remarkably in the last decade with the introduction of three novel agents used in both denovo and relapsed MM; Thalidomide, Bortezomib and Lenalidomide (Kumar SK,et al,2008). Combination of bortezomib and high-dose dexamethasone is considered as the primary treatment option for myeloma patients with renal impairment and improves renal function rapidly in most patients. Incorporation of mechanical removal of serum FLCs may also provide an additive benefit to this combination for patients with acute renal failure due to myeloma cast nephropathy. Thalidomide is also therapeutic choice for the patients with severe renal impairment; however there is limited experience and data about it. Lenalidomide can reverse renal dysfunction in a subgroup of myeloma patients with mild or moderate renal impairment, thus it is effective and safe if administered at reduced doses according to renal function.

4.3.3.1 Thalidomide

Since the relationship between bone marrow angiogenesis and disease progression in myeloma has been well established, anti-angiogenic drug thalidomide has been demonstrated to be useful in the treatment of myeloma. Thalidomide is the first immunomodulatory drug (Imid) with proven anti-myeloma activity. No dose adjustment is required for the patients with renal impairment owing to the fact that it is not excreted in kidneys.

In a study of 20 patients with stage III relapsed or refractory myeloma and chronic renal failure, treatment with thalidomide alone or in combination with dexamethasone resulted in 12 of 15 responsive patients who recovered to normal renal function. Furthermore two patients who were dialysis-dependant showed a reduction in serum creatinine. Toxicity profile of thalidomide with or without dexamethasone was not significantly different among the patients with renal failure and normal renal function. Thus, it has concluded that thalidomide can be safely administered in patients with advanced myeloma and renal failure (Tosi P,et al,2004). In another study reversal of renal failure observed in 80% of previously untreated patients who received thalidomide in combination with high-dose dexamethasone with or without bortezomib (Kastritis E,et al,2007). Although many studies indicate similar toxicity in any level of renal dysfunction, some reports have suggested that toxic effects of thalidomide as severe neuropathy, constipation, lethargy and bradycardia are more frequent in patients with a serum creatinine level over 3mg/dl (Pineda-Roman M, Tricot G,2007). Treatment with thalidomide has been also reported in association with severe hyperkalemia in small part of patients with renal impairment (Harris E,et al,2003). More recently in a study of highcut off haemodialysis with thalidomide therapy, 14 of 19 patients recovered renal function and became independent of dialysis (Hutchison CA,et al,2009).

4.3.3.2 Lenalidomide

Lenalidomide is a small molecule analogue of thalidomide and a second generation immunomodulatory drug which is highly effective in patients with relapsed or refractory myeloma, especially in combination with dexamethasone or alkylator agents. It is mainly excreted in kidneys by both glomerular filtration and active tubular reabsorption and dose adjustment is required for the patients with renal impairment. Therefore, data on the efficacy of lenalidomide in myeloma patients with severe renal failure is limited, because most of studies excluded patients with serum creatinine >2 mg/dl.

MM-009 and MM-010 phase 3 studies that compared Lenalidomid plus dexamethasone versus dexamethasone alone in patients with relaps or refractory myeloma demonstrated that there was no difference in disease response rates between patients with any degree of renal impairment and with normal renal function. In moderate or severe renal impairment, 72% of the patients had an improvement in their renal function with Len+Dex, although there was an increased incidence of thrombocytopenia in patients with creatinine clearance <50 ml/min (Dimopoulos MA,et al,2010). In the following study of same researchers, patients treated by Len+Dex at a dose adjusted according to renal function, 3 of 12 patients with renal impairment (25%) achieved complete renal response and 2 (16%) achieved minor renal response, moreover there were no differences in the incidence of adverse events among patients with and without renal dysfunction. A Spanish retrospective analysis reported that with the combination of Len+Dex, response rate was 57% in 15 dialysis-dependent myeloma patients ;one patient became independent of dialysis (Roig M,2009). In a phase II study which included treatment-naive patients who received Len+Dex showed that patients with a baseline Cr Cl< 40 ml/ min were 8.4 times more likely to require lenalidomide dose reduction due to grade 3 or higher myelosupression (Niesvizky R,et al,2007). Eventually available data suggest that lenalidomide may be safely administered to patients with renal impairment at the recommended reduced dose based on renal function with similar anti-myeloma activity and without significant additional toxicity. Recommended administration of lenalidomide is described as no dose reduction for CrCl<50 ml/min, reduce the dose to 10 mg/d in patients with CrCl 30-50 ml/min; to 15 mg every other day in patients with CrCl<30 ml/min not on dialysis and to 5 mg once daily in patients requiring dialysis.

4.3.3.3 Bortezomib

Bortezomib is the first proteasome inhibitor with proven activity in both newly diagnosed and relapsed or refractory myeloma. It may be used alone or in combination with steroids and other chemotherapeutic agents safely in patients with renal failure because its pharmacokinetics are independent of renal clearance and no dose adjustment is required.

In the SUMMIT (Study of Uncontrolled Multiple Myeloma Managed with Proteasome Inhibition Therapy) and CREST (Clinical Response and Efficacy Study of Bortezomib in the Treatment of Relapsing Multiple Myeloma) phase 2 trials; overall response rates were found 45% in patients with CrCl>80 ml/min and 25% in those with CrCl<50 ml/min. Toxicity and discontinuation rates were similar between the patients with renal impairment and normal renal function (Jagannath S, et al, 2005). In APEX (Assessment of Proteasome Inhibition for Extending Remissions), a phase III study, bortezomib versus high-dose dexamethasone was assessed in terms of efficacy and safety in patients with relapsed myeloma with varying degrees of renal impairment. Time to progression (TTP) and overall survival (OS) were similar between the subgroups with CrCl>50 ml/min and <50 ml/min, although there was insignificant trend toward shorter TTP and OS in patients with CrCl 50 ml/min or below. OS was significantly shorter in dexamethasone-treated patients with any degree of renal dysfunction (P=0.003), indicating that bortezomib is more effective than dexamethasone in overcoming the poor prognostic effect of renal failure. Toxicity of bortezomib was similar between subgroups (San Miguel JF,et al,2008).

In a retrospective analysis of 24 relapsed or refractory myeloma patients who were all dialysis-dependent, overall response rate was reported 75% with complete or near complete renal response (CR or nCR) rate of 30%. Three patients became dialysis-independent after bortezomib therapy and safety profile of bortezomib was found similar in any stage of renal impairment (Chanan-Khan AA,et al,2007). In a phase II study that assessed the efficacy of BDD (bortezomib + doxorubicin + dexamethasone) therapy in patients with multiple myeloma with light chain-induced acute renal failure, myeloma response and renal response were obtained in 72% and 62% of patients respectively. Survivals were not different between patients with and without renal response but was lower in previously treated patients (P <0 .001) (Ludwig H,et al,2009).

VISTA (Velcade as Initial Standard Therapy in multiple myeloma: Assessment with melphalan and prednisone) is the largest analysis of a phase III trial comparing VMP (bortezomib+melphalan+prednisone) and MP (melphalan+prednisone) combinations in myeloma patients with renal impairment. Response rates were higher and TTP and OS longer with VMP versus MP across renal cohorts. Response rates in VMP arm and TTP in both arms did not appear significantly different between patients with CrCl ≤ 50 or >50 ml/min; OS appeared slightly longer in patients with normal renal function in both arms. Renal impairment reversal was seen in 49 of 111 (44%) patients receiving VMP versus 40 of 116 (34%) patients receiving MP. In both arms, rates of grade 3 and 4 adverse events appeared higher in patients with renal impairment; with VMP, rates of discontinuations or bortezomib dose reductions due to adverse effects did not appear affected (Dimopoulos MA,et al,2009).

According to the consensus statement on behalf of the International Myeloma Working Group, high dose dexamethasone and bortezomib are the recommended treatment for MM in patients with any degree of renal impairment especially for those with light chain cast nephropathy.

5. Light chain amyloidosis (Primary, AL amyloidosis)

Light-chain amyloidosis (AL) is the most common form of systemic amyloidosis in western countries, with an estimated incidence of 0.8 per 100,000 person years. This entity is characterized by tissue deposits of insoluble immunoglobulin light chain fragments which polymerize into extracellular amyloid fibrils with a typical β-pleated sheet secondary structure. Amyloid deposits derived from light chains accumulate in normal tissues like most commonly in the kidney, heart, liver and peripheral nervous system, resulting in structural organ dysfunction. It may be associated with an underlying plasma cell disorder like multiple myeloma, Waldenström Macroglobulinemia or MGUS (monoclonal gammopathy of undetermined significance). It is more commonly derived from the variable region of lambda light chain than kappa (75% vs. 25%) and rarely seen in association with heavy chains (AH-amyloidosis). Renal involvement is the most common manifestation in about 60–74% of cases and usually presents as nephrotic syndrome with progressive worsening of renal function (Kyle RA, Gertz MA,1995, Obici L,et al,2005). All compartments of the kidney may be involved though predominant localisation is glomerulus. Renal failure at presentation is seen in 20% of patients generally observed with massive proteinuria and progresses to end-stage renal disease (ESRD) in ~40% of patients over a median time of 35 months (Bergesio F,et al,2008). In approximately 10% of patients, amyloid deposition occurs in the renal vasculature or tubulointerstitium rather than glomeruli, resulting in renal dysfunction without significant proteinuria.

5.1 Pathogenesis of AL amyloidosis

AL amyloid fibrils are derived from the N-terminal region of monoclonal immunoglobulin light chain which contains a variable (VL) domain. It is postulated that certain amino acid sequences for λ light chains change the thermodynamic stability and hydrophoby of the protein, leading to increased potential of fibril forming. It has been shown that λ VI light chains are more specifically associated with AL-amyloidosis (Solomon A,et al,1982). Furhermore posttranslational modifications of the light chains, such as glycosylation, may promote the amyloidogenic potential by protecting the fibril from degradation. β-pleated sheets are mainly responsible for the aggregation of light chains to form oligomers which do not dissolve in normal proteolysis and these aggregates are stabilized with other proteins, including glycosaminoglycans, proteoglycans, serum amyloid P (SAP), fibronectin and apolipoprotein E.

Mesangium is the initial site of the glomerular injury and amyloid fibrils replace the normal mesangial matrix by endocytosis of mesangial cells and transporting into lysosomes. Extracellular amyloid fibrils also stimulate the activation of matrix metalloproteinases (MMPs) and inhibit TGF- β as a regulator of matrix production, result in decreased synthesis of mesangial matrix. Tissue architecture is destroyed by amyloid deposits with its secondary effects on matrix and also direct toxicity, thus glomerular damage occurs which leads to renal failure.

5.2 Diagnosis of AL amyloidosis

AL amyloidosis is a rare disorder and it is difficult to diagnose because of nonspecific early clinic manifestations before specific organ failure occurs. Its diagnosis should be suspected in any patient with non-diabetic nephrotic syndrome, peripheral neuropathy, hypertrophic cardiomyopathy, hepatomegaly and macroglossia, especially when they are associated in a patient with typical age of >60 and male sex.

All amyloidosis-suspected patients need the diagnosis which is confirmed histologically. Abdominal subcutaneous fat aspiration is recommended as the initial minimal invasive diagnostic procedure and when it is combined with bone marrow biopsy, amyloid deposits may be identified in 90% of patients. If both examinations are negative, then a renal biopsy may be indicated and diagnostic in >95% of patients with manifest renal disease. Histopathological assessment characteristically contains congo red-positive staining leads to the apple-green birefringence under the polarized light microscopy. Amyloid deposits are always seen as diffuse amorphous hyaline material in glomeruli especially in mesangium and also in the wall of blood vessels. Electrophoresis with serum (71% sensitivity) and urine (84% sensitivity) immunofixation needs to be performed in all patients . after confirming the histopathologic diagnosis, to differentiate the type of amyloidosis Quantitative Ig measurement, Ig-free light chain λ and κ testing, 24-hour urine total protein measurement (more than 0.5 g per day; mainly albumin), complete blood count, creatinine level, alkaline phosphatase level, measurement of troponin, brain natriuretic peptide, or N-terminal pro-brain natriuretic peptide levels, and echocardiography should be the following examinations for a complete diagnosis of AL amyloidosis.

5.3 Prognosis and treatment of AL amyloidosis

The survival of patients with amyloidosis is considerably variable, depending on some prognostic factors like the presence of coexisting myeloma, the number of organs involved especially the presence and severity of cardiac involvement, and response to therapy. Although the median survival is ranging from 12 to 18 months in different series, by the developments in treatment approaches, quality of life and survival have been considerably improved. In a retrospective analysis of 147 patients with AL amyloidosis, 20 patients had concurrent multiple myeloma and patients with both AL and myeloma had a significantly worse prognosis than those with AL alone with OS as 14 versus 32 months (Pardanani A,et al,2003). In a prospective study of 220 patients with primary systemic amyloidosis, the most important prognostic factor was reported as cardiac involvement and it was associated with the poorest prognosis with median survival less than 6 months. Nephrotic syndrome and renal failure were also poor prognostic factors with median survival rates of 15 and 16 months respectively, compared with 26 months in patients with normal renal function (P=0.007) (Kyle RA,et al,1997)

Standart cytotoxic chemotherapies have been widely used in last decades to inhibit the production of amyloidogenic light chains which usually include melphalan and prednisone or high dose dexamethasone. In a few small studies; combination of melphalan+prednisone achieved a reduction or complete resolution of proteinuria and improvement in renal function (Cohen J,et al,1975, Benson MD,1986). In a phase 2 study of 45 patients who were ineligible for ASCT, the combination of high-dose dexamethasone with melphalan was found more effective with a hematological response of 67% and functional organ improvement as 48% (Palladini G,et al,2004).

Although thalidomide is poorly tolerated by amyloidosis patients and treatment-related toxicity is frequent, with dose escalation, thalidomide+dexamethasone can be considered an option, alone or in combination with cyclophosphamide for the treatment of patients who relapse after melphalan-dexamethasone or ASCT. In a trial of 75 patients which compared the safety and efficacy of CTD in standart and attenuated doses, organ responses were found in 31% of the 48 hematologic responders, but no patient with ESRD became dialysis independent and no objective cardiac responses were observed. (Wechalekar AD,et al,2007) Lenalidomide also has been combined with dexamethasone in the treatment of AL amyloidosis and a phase 2 trial demonstrated that haematologic response rate was 67% and 41% of the patients with renal involvement experienced more than 50% reduction in urinary protein excretion without worsening of renal function (Sanchorawala V,et al,2007). Recent studies have suggested that bortezomib with or without dexamethasone is significantly active in AL amyloidosis and induces rapid responses and high rates of hematologic and organ responses. In a retrospective report which includes the AL patients who were treated or untreated previously, overall response rates were found 81% and 76% respectively, with bortezomib+dexamethasone combination (Kastritis E,et al,2010). In a case report of an AL patient who have stage V renal disease with hemodialysis support and age above 65 years, relatvelygood response with acceptable tolerance has been shown with bortezomib+high-dose dexamethasone regimen (Mello RA,et al,2011).

In a selected patient group who are eligible for ASCT, by using a risk-adapted approach such as dose escalation of melphalan in patients with renal dysfunction, use of myeloablative chemotherapy followed by ASCT may be the most successful approach. In a study of 123 AL patients treated with high-dose melphalan followed by ASCT, renal response was noted in 43.4% of the patients with a better survival. It was also found that the severity of proteinuria was an independent predictor of renal response after ASCT and the recovery of renal function and prevention of ESRD after ASCT depended on the the degree of preexisting damage to the kidney (Leung N,et al,2007).

6. Monoclonal Immunoglobulin Deposition Disease (MIDD)

Nonamyloidotic monoclonal Ig deposition disease (MIDD) is characterized by deposition of monoclonal Ig subunits in kidney with an excess accumulation of extracellular matrix, leading to nodular sclerosing glomerulopathy, interstitial fibrosis, proteinuria, and renal insufficiency. According to the Ig deposition type, three subtypes of MIDD have been described, including light chain DD (LCDD), light-and heavy-chain (LHCDD) and heavy chain DD (HCDD). LCDD is the most prevalent subtype and found in 5% of patients with myeloma at autopsy series (Ivanyi B,1990). The most common cause is myeloma with the ratio of 65%, however 32% of cases are not associated with a manifested haematologic disorder. Although they are similar entities, in comparison to AL amyloidosis, the deposited light chains are kappa chains in 85% of LCDD cases, do not have a fibrillar organization and do not bind congo red. The majority of patients have a severe renal insufficiency with a median serum creatinine level of 3.8 mg/dl and usually tend to present with a higher serum creatinine concentration and lower rate of protein excretion than patients with AL amyloidosis (Harris AA,et al,1997). Cardiac, hepatic or small intestinal involvement also may be seen in MIDD.

6.1 Pathogenesis of MIDD

Initial process in MIDD usually includes the interaction between abnormal kappa chain (κ-I or κ-IV) and the mesangial cells of the glomerulus. Light chains were shown to stimulate the mesangial proliferation and secretion of transforming growth factor-beta (TGF-β) (Zhu L,et al,1995). TGF-β increases the production of collagen IV, laminin, and fibronectin which are deposited in the extracellular matrix (ECM) of the kidneys and also decrease the levels of collagenase, metalloproteinases, serin protease and other enzymes that degrades matrix proteins. Progressive light chain deposition and accumulation of ECM components inevitably lead to organ fibrosis and dysfunction. In MIDD, deposits predominantly localized in the tubular basement membranes and Bowman's capsule rather than in the glomeruli, though nodular glomerulosclerosis is present 60% of cases associated with a nephrotic range proteinuria. Tubular lesions are characterized by the deposition of a granular, punctuate, eosinophilic, periodic acid-Schiff (PAS)-positive, ribbon-like material along the interstitial side of the tubular basement membrane in electron microscopy. Glomerular lesions are usually associated with diffuse mesangial expansion by PAS positive and Congo red negative nonfibrillar matrix that focally forms nodules. Deposits may also be seen in renal vasculature with same staining properties.

6.2 Diagnosis of MIDD

LCDD should be considered in the differential diagnosis of any patients with nephrotic syndrome and renal insufficiency of unknown origin. Standart testing procedure should be administered initially as in other plasma cell dyscrasias, and in most of the patients, elevated ratio of κ/λ free light chains in the serum and urine and a predominance of κ light chain-positive plasma cells on bone marrow biopsy help to confirm LCDD diagnosis. However, approximately 25% of patients have no demonstrable light chain in serum or urine by immunoelectrophoresis or immunofixation. A definitive diagnosis of LCDD is based on renal biopsy with elaborate histological examination and electron microscopy. Characteristic light microscopic, immunofluorescence, and electron microscopic findings which are mentioned before are the important keys for the diagnosis.

6.3 Prognosis and treatment of MIDD

The median survival of a patient with MIDD is 4 years, with survival at 1 yr and 8 yr of 66% and 31%, respectively. In largest studies, the variables that were independently associated with a worse patient survival were shown as age, initial creatinine, underlying multiple myeloma, and extrarenal LC deposition. Median time to progression to ESRD was reported to be 2.7 years and the 5-year uremia free survival was 37%. The only variables that were independently associated with renal survival were age and degree of renal insufficiency at presentation (Pozzi C,et al,2003). Renal and patient survivals were significantly worse in patients with LCDD who had coexisting cast nephropathy (Lin J,et al,2001).

Therapy of MIDD is similar to that for multiple myeloma and the main goal is to reduce Ig production in order to preserve renal function and improve survival. Combination of melphalan and prednisone has been used, but the response rates have been low with an 5 yr patient and renal survival of 70% and 37%, respectively. In patients with a serum creatinine < 4 mg/dl at presentation, stabilization or improvement in renal function after chemotherapy was found 60%, whereas 82% of patients with a serum creatinine >4 mg/dl progressed to ESRD despite therapy (Heilman RL,et al,1992). A combination of high-dose melphalan and autologous stem cell transplantation was reported to improve renal function without excessive morbidity or mortality. The largest study of ASCT in MIDD revealed that, serum creatinine improved by 50% or more in 4 of 11 patients and the nephrotic syndrome resolved in all, after ASCT (Royer B,et al,2004). In another study, patients who survived ASCT, high-dose chemotherapy and ASCT led to a median reduction in proteinuria of 92% and median improvement in GFR as 95% (Lorenz EC,et al,2008). Renal transplantation is associated with recurrence of LCDD in the transplanted kidney and effective chemotherapy or ASCT should be administered concurrently to control the underlying plasma cell dyscrasia. It is well established that bortezomib decreases TGF-β expression through inhibiting the NFκB pathway, thus recent researches focus on bortezomib-based chemotherapy in the treatment of MIDD and it appears to be safe and effective for the patients with renal dysfunction (Gharwan H, Truica CI,2011).

7. Renal tubular dysfunction

Multiple myeloma is the most common cause of proximal renal tubular acidosis in the adult. The toxic effect of light chains may be limited to tubular dysfunction and presented without renal insufficiency. This entity commonly occurs with kappa light chains. Some biochemical characteristics in the variable domain of the light chain has the capacity for resistance to protease degradation and a tendency to accumulate in tubule epithelial cells and form intracellular crystal formation. By the released intracellular lysosomal enzymes and the direct toxic effects of light chains, tubular damage occurs and clinic presentation includes the symptoms of Fanconi syndrome. Proximal renal tubular acidosis with loosing the potassium, phosphate, uric acid and bicarbonate resuting in aminoaciduria, renal glycosuria, hypophosphatemia, hyperchloremic metabolic acidosis, hypokalemia, proteinuria of tubular origin, and hypouricemia. Osteomalacia, chronic renal failure and chronic acidosis are the most common manifestations of Fanconi syndrome related to light chains. Episodes of dehydration may be seen due to polyuria and polydipsia. Furthermore, myeloma kidney may be aggravated with proximal dysfunction because of reduced light chain reabsorption and elevated precipitation in the distal nephron. With appropriate therapeutic management of underlying myeloma and vitamin D, calcium, and phosphorus supplementation for osteomalasic patients, considerable improvement can be obtained.

8. Conclusion

As we have tried to summarize above, kidney should be accepted one of the main targets in the course of myeloma especially in the diagnosis and treatment. Early diagnosis and prevention could result in preventing many renal complications and potential hazards during treatment period and if planned, stem cell transplantation.

9. References

Alexanian R, Dimopoulos MA, Delasalle K, Barlogie B. Primary dexamethasone treatment of multiple myeloma. Blood. 1992 Aug 15;80(4):887-90.

Badros A, Barlogie B, Siegel E, Roberts J, Langmaid C, Zangari M, Desikan R, Shaver MJ, Fassas A, McConnell S, Muwalla F, Barri Y, Anaissie E, Munshi N, Tricot G. Results of autologous stem cell transplant in multiple myeloma patients with renal failure. Br J Haematol. 2001 Sep;114(4):822-9.

Batuman V, Verroust PJ, Navar GL, et al. Myeloma light chains are ligands for cubilin (gp280). Am J Physiol. 1998;275:F246-F254.

Benson MD. Treatment of AL amyloidosis with melphalan, prednisone, and colchicine. Arthritis Rheum. 1986 May;29(5):683-7.

Berenson JR, Lichtenstein A, Porter L, Dimopoulos MA, Bordoni R, George S, Lipton A, Keller A, Ballester O, Kovacs M, Blacklock H, Bell R, Simeone JF, Reitsma DJ, Heffernan M, Seaman J, Knight RD. Long-term pamidronate treatment of advanced multiple myeloma patients reduces skeletal events. Myeloma Aredia Study Group. J Clin Oncol. 1998 Feb;16(2):593-602.

Bergesio F, Ciciani AM, Manganaro M, Palladini G, Santostefano M, Brugnano R, Di Palma AM, Gallo M, Rosati A, Tosi PL, Salvadori M; Immunopathology Group of the Italian Society of Nephrology. Renal involvement in systemic amyloidosis: an

Italian collaborative study on survival and renal outcome. Nephrol Dial Transplant. 2008 Mar;23(3):941-51. Epub 2007 Oct 19.

Bladé J, Fernández-Llama P, Bosch F, Montolíu J, Lens XM, Montoto S, Cases A, Darnell A, Rozman C, Montserrat E. Renal failure in multiple myeloma: presenting features and predictors of outcome in 94 patients from a single institution. Arch Intern Med. 1998 Sep 28;158(17):1889-93

Bladé J, Rosiñol L. Renal, hematologic and infectious complications in multiple myeloma. Best Pract Res Clin Haematol. 2005;18(4):635-52. Review

Chanan-Khan AA, Kaufman JL, Mehta J, Richardson PG, Miller KC, Lonial S, Munshi NC, Schlossman R, Tariman J, Singhal S. Activity and safety of bortezomib in multiple myeloma patients with advanced renal failure: a multicenter retrospective study. Blood. 2007 Mar 15;109(6):2604-6. Epub 2006 Nov 30.

Clark WF, Stewart AK, Rock GA, Sternbach M, Sutton DM, Barrett BJ, Heidenheim AP, Garg AX, Churchill DN; Canadian Apheresis Group. Plasma exchange when myeloma presents as acute renal failure: a randomized, controlled trial. Ann Intern Med. 2005 Dec 6;143(11):777-84. Erratum in: Ann Intern Med. 2007 Mar 20;146(6):471.

Cohen HJ, Lessin LS, Hallal J, Burkholder P. Resolution of primary amyloidosis during chemotherapy. Studies in a patient with nephrotic syndrome. Ann Intern Med. 1975 Apr;82(4):466-73.

Dagher F, Sammett D, Abbi R, Tomasula JR, Delaney V, Butt KM. Renal transplantation in multiple myeloma. Case report and review of the literature. Transplantation. 1996 Dec 15;62(11):1577-80.

Dimopoulos MA, Richardson PG, Schlag R, Khuageva NK, Shpilberg O, Kastritis E, Kropff M, Petrucci MT, Delforge M, Alexeeva J, Schots R, Masszi T, Mateos MV, Deraedt W, Liu K, Cakana A, van de Velde H, San Miguel JF. VMP (Bortezomib, Melphalan, and Prednisone) is active and well tolerated in newly diagnosed patients with multiple myeloma with moderately impaired renal function, and results in reversal of renal impairment: cohort analysis of the phase III VISTA study. J Clin Oncol. 2009 Dec 20;27(36):6086-93. Epub 2009 Oct 26.

Dimopoulos MA, Terpos E. Lenalidomide: an update on evidence from clinical trials. Blood Rev. 2010 Nov;24 Suppl 1:S21-6.

Gertz MA, Lacy MQ, Dispenzieri A, Hayman SR, Kumar S, Leung N, Gastineau DA. Impact of age and serum creatinine value on outcome after autologous blood stem cell transplantation for patients with multiple myeloma. Bone Marrow Transplant. 2007 May;39(10):605-11. Epub 2007 Mar 19.

Gharwan H, Truica CI. Bortezomib-based chemotherapy for light chain deposition disease presenting as acute renal failure. Med Oncol. 2011 Apr 9. [Epub ahead of print]

Haas M, Spargo BH, Wit EJ, Meehan SM: Etiologies and outcome of acute renal insufficiency in older adults: A renal biopsy study of 259 cases. *Am J Kidney Dis* 35 : 433–447, 2000

Harris AA, Wilkman AS, Hogan SL, et al. Amyloidosis and light chain deposition disease in renal biopsy specimens: Pathology, laboratory data, demographics and frequency (abstract). J Am Soc Nephrol 1997; 8:537A.

Harris E, Behrens J, Samson D, Rahemtulla A, Russell NH, Byrne JL. Use of thalidomide in patients with myeloma and renal failure may be associated with unexplained hyperkalaemia. Br J Haematol. 2003 Jul;122(1):160-1.

Heilman RL, Velosa JA, Holley KE, Offord KP, Kyle RA. Long-term follow-up and response to chemotherapy in patients with light-chain deposition disease. Am J Kidney Dis. 1992 Jul;20(1):34-41.

Hill GS, Morel-Maroger L, Mery JP, Brouet JC, Mignon F: Renal lesions in multiple myeloma: Their relationship to associated protein abnormalities. *Am J Kidney Dis* 2 : 423–438, 1983

Hutchison CA, Bradwell AR, Cook M, Basnayake K, Basu S, Harding S, Hattersley J, Evans ND, Chappel MJ, Sampson P, Foggensteiner L, Adu D, Cockwell P. Treatment of acute renal failure secondary to multiple myeloma with chemotherapy and extended high cut-off hemodialysis. Clin J Am Soc Nephrol. 2009 Apr;4(4):745-54. Epub 2009 Apr 1.

Hutchison CA, Cockwell P, Reid S, Chandler K, Mead GP, Harrison J, Hattersley J, Evans ND, Chappell MJ, Cook M, Goehl H, Storr M, Bradwell AR. Efficient removal of immunoglobulin free light chains by hemodialysis for multiple myeloma: in vitro and in vivo studies. J Am Soc Nephrol. 2007 Mar;18(3):886-95. Epub 2007 Jan 17.

Hutchison CA, Harding S, Mead G, Goehl H, Storr M, Bradwell A, Cockwell P. Serum free-light chain removal by high cutoff hemodialysis: optimizing removal and supportive care. Artif Organs. 2008 Dec;32(12):910-7.

Iványi B. Frequency of light chain deposition nephropathy relative to renal amyloidosis and Bence Jones cast nephropathy in a necropsy study of patients with myeloma. Arch Pathol Lab Med. 1990 Sep;114(9):986-7.

Iványi B. Renal complications in multiple myeloma. Acta Morphol Hung. 1989;37(3-4):235-43.

Jagannath S, Barlogie B, Berenson JR, Singhal S, Alexanian R, Srkalovic G, Orlowski RZ, Richardson PG, Anderson J, Nix D, Esseltine DL, Anderson KC; SUMMIT/CREST Investigators. Bortezomib in recurrent and/or refractory multiple myeloma. Initial clinical experience in patients with impared renal function. Cancer. 2005 Mar 15;103(6):1195-200.

Kastritis E, Anagnostopoulos A, Roussou M, Gika D, Matsouka C, Barmparousi D, Grapsa I, Psimenou E, Bamias A, Dimopoulos MA. Reversibility of renal failure in newly diagnosed multiple myeloma patients treated with high dose dexamethasone-containing regimens and the impact of novel agents. Haematologica. 2007 Apr;92(4):546-9.

Kastritis E, Wechalekar AD, Dimopoulos MA, Merlini G, Hawkins PN, Perfetti V, Gillmore JD, Palladini G. Bortezomib with or without dexamethasone in primary systemic (light chain) amyloidosis. J Clin Oncol. 2010 Feb 20;28(6):1031-7. Epub 2010 Jan 19.

Keeling J, Herrera GA. The mesangium as a target for glomerulopathic light and heavy chains: pathogenic considerations in light and heavy chain-mediated glomerular damage. Contrib Nephrol. 2007;153:116-34.

Kitazawa R, Kitazawa S, Kajimoto K, Sowa H, Sugimoto T, Matsui T, Chihara K, Maeda S. Expression of parathyroid hormone-related protein (PTHrP) in multiple myeloma. Pathol Int. 2002 Jan;52(1):63-8. Review.

Knudsen LM, Hippe E, Hjorth M, Holmberg E, Westin J: Renal function in newly diagnosed multiple myeloma: A demographic study of 1353 patients. The Nordic Myeloma Study Group. *Eur J Haematol* 53 : 207–212, 1994

Knudsen LM, Hjorth M, Hippe E: Renal failure in multiple myeloma: Reversibility and impact on the prognosis. Nordic Myeloma Study Group. *Eur J Haematol* 65 : 175-181, 2000

Kumar SK, Dingli D, Lacy MQ, Dispenzieri A, Hayman SR, Buadi FK, Rajkumar SV, Litzow MR, Gertz MA. Autologous stem cell transplantation in patients of 70 years and older with multiple myeloma: Results from a matched pair analysis. Am J Hematol. 2008 Aug;83(8):614-7.

Kyle RA, Gertz MA, Greipp PR, Witzig TE, Lust JA, Lacy MQ, Therneau TM.A trial of three regimens for primary amyloidosis: colchicine alone, melphalan and prednisone, and melphalan, prednisone, and colchicine. N Engl J Med. 1997 Apr 24;336(17):1202-7.

Kyle RA, Gertz MA. Primary systemic amyloidosis: clinical and laboratory features in 474 cases. Semin Hematol. 1995 Jan;32(1):45-59.

Leheste JR, Rolinski B, Vorum H, Hilpert J, Nykjaer A, Jacobsen C, Aucouturier P, Moskaug JO, Otto A, Christensen EI, Willnow TE. Megalin knockout mice as an animal model of low molecular weight proteinuria. Am J Pathol. 1999 Oct;155(4):1361-70.

Leung N, Dispenzieri A, Lacy MQ, Kumar SK, Hayman SR, Fervenza FC, Cha SS, Gertz MA. Severity of baseline proteinuria predicts renal response in immunoglobulin light chain-associated amyloidosis after autologous stem cell transplantation. Clin J Am Soc Nephrol. 2007 May;2(3):440-4. Epub 2007 Apr 4.

Leung N, Gertz MA, Zeldenrust SR, Rajkumar SV, Dispenzieri A, Fervenza FC, Kumar S, Lacy MQ, Lust JA, Greipp PR, Witzig TE, Hayman SR, Russell SJ, Kyle RA, Winters JL. Improvement of cast nephropathy with plasma exchange depends on the diagnosis and on reduction of serum free light chains. Kidney Int. 2008 Jun;73(11):1282-8. Epub 2008 Apr 2

Lin J, Markowitz GS, Valeri AM, Kambham N, Sherman WH, Appel GB, D'Agati VD. Renal monoclonal immunoglobulin deposition disease: the disease spectrum. J Am Soc Nephrol. 2001 Jul;12(7):1482-92

Lorenz EC, Gertz MA, Fervenza FC, Dispenzieri A, Lacy MQ, Hayman SR, Gastineau DA, Leung N. Long-term outcome of autologous stem cell transplantation in light chain deposition disease. Nephrol Dial Transplant. 2008 Jun;23(6):2052-7. Epub 2008 Jan 4.

Ludwig, H. *et al.* Bortezomib-doxorubicin-dexamethasone (BDD) in patients with acute light chain induced renal failure (ARF) in multiple myeloma (MM). Final results of a phase II study [abstract 3862]. *Blood* 114, 1486a (2009).

McCarthy CS, Becker JA. Multiple myeloma and contrast media. Radiology. 1992 May;183(2):519-21.

Mello RA, Santos DS, Freitas-Silva MP, Andrade JA. Renal failure due to primary amyloidosis: a case report and literature review. Sao Paulo Med J. 2011 May;129(3):176-80.

Montseny JJ, Kleinknecht D, Meyrier A, Vanhille P, Simon P, Pruna A, Eladari D. Long-term outcome according to renal histological lesions in 118 patients with monoclonal gammopathies. Nephrol Dial Transplant. 1998 Jun;13(6):1438-45.

Murray MD, Black PK, Kuzmik DD, Haag KM, Manatunga AK, Mullin MA, Hall SD, Brater DC. Acute and chronic effects of nonsteroidal antiinflammatory drugs on glomerular filtration rate in elderly patients. Am J Med Sci. 1995 Nov;310(5):188-97

Niesvizky R, Naib T, Christos PJ, Jayabalan D, Furst JR, Jalbrzikowski J, Zafar F, Mark T, Lent R, Pearse RN, Ely S, Leonard JP, Mazumdar M, Chen-Kiang S, Coleman M. Lenalidomide-induced myelosuppression is associated with renal dysfunction: adverse events evaluation of treatment-naïve patients undergoing front-line lenalidomide and dexamethasone therapy. Br J Haematol. 2007 Sep;138(5):640-3

Obici L, Perfetti V, Palladini G, Moratti R, Merlini G. Clinical aspects of systemic amyloid diseases. Biochim Biophys Acta. 2005 Nov 10;1753(1):11-22. Epub 2005 Sep 2. Review.

Pahade JK, LeBedis CA, Raptopoulos VD, Avigan DE, Yam CS, Kruskal JB, Pedrosa I. Incidence of contrast-induced nephropathy in patients with multiple myeloma undergoing contrast-enhanced CT. AJR Am J Roentgenol. 2011 May;196(5):1094-101.

Palladini G, Perfetti V, Obici L, Caccialanza R, Semino A, Adami F, Cavallero G, Rustichelli R, Virga G, Merlini G. Association of melphalan and high-dose dexamethasone is effective and well tolerated in patients with AL (primary) amyloidosis who are ineligible for stem cell transplantation. Blood. 2004 Apr 15;103(8):2936-8. Epub 2003 Dec 18.

Pardanani A, Witzig TE, Schroeder G, McElroy EA, Fonseca R, Dispenzieri A, Lacy MQ, Lust JA, Kyle RA, Greipp PR, Gertz MA, Rajkumar SV. Circulating peripheral blood plasma cells as a prognostic indicator in patients with primary systemic amyloidosis. Blood. 2003 Feb 1;101(3):827-30. Epub 2002 Sep 5.

Pineda-Roman M, Tricot G. High-dose therapy in patients with plasma cell dyscrasias and renal dysfunction. Contrib Nephrol. 2007;153:182-94. Review.

Pozzi C, D'Amico M, Fogazzi GB, Curioni S, Ferrario F, Pasquali S, Quattrocchio G, Rollino C, Segagni S, Locatelli F. Light chain deposition disease with renal involvement: clinical characteristics and prognostic factors. Am J Kidney Dis. 2003 Dec;42(6):1154-63. Review.

Rajkumar SV, Kyle RA. Conventional therapy and approach to management.Best Pract Res Clin Haematol. 2005;18(4):585-601. Review.

Rajkumar SV, Kyle RA. Multiple myeloma: diagnosis and treatment. Mayo Clin Proc. 2005 Oct;80(10):1371-82. Review

Roig M, Ibanez A, Garcia I, *et al.* Activity and safety of lenalidomide and dexamethasone in multiple myeloma patients with advanced renal failure: a Spanish multicenter retrospective study. Lancet Oncol 2010; 11:29–37.

Royer B, Arnulf B, Martinez F, Roy L, Flageul B, Etienne I, Ronco P, Brouet JC, Fermand JP. High dose chemotherapy in light chain or light and heavy chain deposition disease. Kidney Int. 2004 Feb;65(2):642-8.

San Miguel JF, Schlag R, Khuageva NK, Dimopoulos MA, Shpilberg O, Kropff M, Spicka I, Petrucci MT, Palumbo A, Samoilova OS, Dmoszynska A, Abdulkadyrov KM, Schots R, Jiang B, Mateos MV, Anderson KC, Esseltine DL, Liu K, Cakana A, van de Velde H, Richardson PG; VISTA Trial Investigators. Bortezomib plus melphalan and prednisone for initial treatment of multiple myeloma. N Engl J Med. 2008 Aug 28;359(9):906-17.

Sanchorawala V, Wright DG, Rosenzweig M, Finn KT, Fennessey S, Zeldis JB, Skinner M, Seldin DC. Lenalidomide and dexamethasone in the treatment of AL amyloidosis: results of a phase 2 trial. Blood. 2007 Jan 15;109(2):492-6. Epub 2006 Sep 7.

Sanders PW, Booker BB, Bishop JB, Cheung HC. Mechanisms of intranephronal proteinaceous cast formation by low molecular weight proteins. J Clin Invest. 1990 Feb;85(2):570-6.

Sengul S, Zwizinski C, Batuman V. Role of MAPK pathways in light chain-induced cytokine production in human proximal tubule cells. Am J Physiol Renal Physiol. 2003;284:F1245-F1254.

Sengul S, Zwizinski C, Simon EE, Kapasi A, Singhal PC, Batuman V. Endocytosis of light chains induces cytokines through activation of NF-kappaB in human proximal tubule cells. Kidney Int. 2002;62:1977-1988.

Silva FG, Pirani CL, Mesa-Tejada R, Williams GS: The kidney in plasma cell dyscrasias: A review and a clinicopathologic study of 50 patients. In: *Progress in Surgical Pathology,* edited by Fenoglio C, Wolff M, New York, Masson, 1983 , pp 131–176

Smolens P, Barnes JL, Kreisberg R. Hypercalcemia can potentiate the nephrotoxicity of Bence Jones proteins. J Lab Clin Med. 1987 Oct;110(4):460-5.

Solomon A, Frangione B, Franklin EC. Bence Jones proteins and light chains of immunoglobulins. Preferential association of the V lambda VI subgroup of human light chains with amyloidosis AL (lambda). J Clin Invest. 1982 Aug;70(2):453-60.

Solomon A, Weiss DT, Kattine AA. Nephrotoxic potential of Bence Jones proteins. N Engl J Med. 1991 Jun 27;324(26):1845-51.

Tosi P, Zamagni E, Cellini C, Cangini D, Tacchetti P, Tura S, Baccarani M, Cavo M. Thalidomide alone or in combination with dexamethasone in patients with advanced, relapsed or refractory multiple myeloma and renal failure. Eur J Haematol. 2004 Aug;73(2):98-103.

Verroust PJ, Birn H, Nielsen R, Kozyraki R, Christensen EI. The tandem endocytic receptors megalin and cubilin are important proteins in renal pathology. Kidney Int. 2002;62:745-756.

Wechalekar AD, Goodman HJ, Lachmann HJ, Offer M, Hawkins PN, Gillmore JD. Safety and efficacy of risk-adapted cyclophosphamide, thalidomide, and dexamethasone in systemic AL amyloidosis. Blood. 2007 Jan 15;109(2):457-64. Epub 2006 Sep 21.

Winearls CG. Acute myeloma kidney. Kidney Int. 1995 Oct;48(4):1347-61

Zhu L, Herrera GA, Murphy-Ullrich JE, Huang ZQ, Sanders PW. Pathogenesis of glomerulosclerosis in light chain deposition disease. Role for transforming growth factor-beta. Am J Pathol. 1995 Aug;147(2):375-85.

Zucchelli P, Pasquali S, Cagnoli L, Ferrari G. Controlled plasma exchange trial in acute renal failure due to multiple myeloma. Kidney Int. 1988 Jun;33(6):1175-80.

13

Stem Cell Mobılızatıon in Multıple Myeloma

Şule Mine Bakanay and Taner Demirer
Ankara University Medical School,
Department of Hematology & Stem Cell Transplantation Unit, Ankara,
Turkey

1. Introduction

High dose melphalan supported by autologous hematopoietic cell transplantation (AHCT) has been shown to prolong survival and decrease relapse rates compared to conventional chemotherapies in elligible patients with plasma cell myeloma (PCM) (Attal et al., 1996; Child et al., 2003; Fermand et al., 2005; Koreth et al., 2007; Palumbo et al., 2004). Patients who are considered candidates for high dose therapy receive 2-4 cycles of non-melphalan containing induction therapies followed by peripheral blood progenitor cell(PBPC) mobilization and collection. Pateints proceed to high dose melphalan (200 mg/m^2) supported with AHCT. High dose melphalan and AHCT has been the gold standard treatment approach in patients with PCM younger than 65 but can be extended to mid-70's in patients otherwise in good performance status. Second AHCT has been shown to increase survival, especially those who could not achieve very good partial response (VGPR) after the first AHCT (Attal et al., 2003, Barlogie et al., 2006). Additionally, patients who had a long progression free survival after the first transplantation may benefit from salvage transplantation at relapse (Ljungman et al., 2010). These advances have mandated the mobilization and collection of PBPCs adequate for double transplants. Although not prospectively studied, the traditional minimum and optimum CD34+ cell dose limits have been $2 \times 10^6/kg$ and $\geq 4 \times 10^6/kg$ for single ; $4 \times 10^6/kg$ and $\geq$ 8-10 $x10^6/kg$ for double AHCT, respectively (Bensinger et al., 1995, Giralt et al., 2009). Therefore, successfull stem cell mobilization and collection are crucial for treatment of PCM. Risk factors such as age >60 years, the extend of prior chemotherapy or radiotherapy and prolonged disease duration are recognized predictors for poor mobilization. The induction treatment given before the process of PBPC mobilization and collection should not be toxic to the bone marrow. It has been clearly revealed over the past decades that the traditional induction regimens; vincristine, adriamycin, dexamathasone (VAD) or single agent dexamathasone have no impact on PBPC mobilization. However, today, they have been completely replaced with novel agents which are associated with better response rates. During the recent years, the impact of these novel induction agents (thalidomide, lenalidomide and bortezomib) on PBPC mobilization have been of major concern. Although the classical PBPC mobilization methods (G-CSF alone or G-CSF after chemotherapy) have been generally successful in PCM, there is still a considerable amount of mobilization failures. Studies have been focused on the investigational agents alone or in conjunction with G-CSF to imrove PBPC mobilization efficiency, prevent mobilization failures and the need for second or subsequent mobilization attempts which often delay the timely performance of the transplantation and increase the morbidity and the cost. In this chapter, we will focus on the current stem cell mobilization strategies as well as the novel mobilizing agents in PCM and the impact of novel anti-myeloma drugs on PBPC mobilization.

2. Mobilization approaches in PCM

2.1 G-CSF alone

The optimal PBPC mobilization strategy in PCM is unclear. Both growth factor alone or chemotherapy followed by growth factor (chemomobilization) have been the most frequently used approaches. In growth factor-only mobilization, recombinant human granulocyte-colony stimulating factor (G-CSF) is commonly administered at 10 µg/kg/day s.c. for 4 days , PBPCs are collected from day 5 onwards and G-CSF continued until the last day of apheresis. PBPCs are collected by continuous flow apheresis procedure often processing 2-2.5 times the patient's blood volume. CD34+ cell enumeration is performed by flow cytometry according to the ISHAGE guidelines(Sutherland et al., 1996). The stem cell product is then cryopreseved until use for AHCT. Recombinant human G-CSF is reliable, with predictable mobilization efficiency. The most common toxicities observed during G-CSF administration such as bone pain, low grade fever, headache, are generally managable. However, G-CSF may be associated with rare serious adverse events such as spontaneous splenic rupture, thrombosis, flare of autoimmune disease and precipitation of sickle crisis (Cashen et al., 2007).

2.2 G-CSF analogs

2.2.1 Filgrastim and lenograstim

Filgrastim (Neupogen, F Hoffmann-La Roche, Basel, Switzerland) and lenograstim (Granocyte, Chugai-Aventis Pharmaceuticals, France) are nonglycosylated and glycosylated analogs of recombinant human G-CSF approved for PBPC mobilization. Studies investigating the patients with hematological malignancies who underwent PBSC mobilization for AHCT could not demonstrate any difference between glycosylated and non-glycosylated G-CSF in terms of both efficacy and toxicity (Kopf et al., 2006; Lefrere et al., 1999). The glycosylation of G-CSF contributes to a greater chemical-physical stability of lenograstim: the glycosylated G-CSF is more stable and resistant to degradation. The recommended dosage of lenograstim when used alone for PBPC mobilization is 5 µ/kg/day (s.c./i.v.). On the other hand, equal doses of 10 µ/kg/day of filgrastim and lenograstim have been recommended for mobilization of CD34+ cells without associated chemotherapy. However, a recent study has suggested that lower dose (7.5 µ/kg/day) of glycosylated G-CSF may be as effective as the standard dose of non-glycosylated G-CSF for PBPC mobilization in patients undergoing AHCT (Ataergin et al., 2008).

2.2.2 Pegfilgrastim

Pegylated G-CSF (pegfilgrastim, Neulasta, Amgen Inc.,CA, USA) is currently approved by the US FDA for prevention of prolonged neutropenia after chemotherapy for nonmyeloid malignancies (Neulasta; package insert). Its potential in PBPC mobilization is currently being explored. Due to its long plasma half-life compared to unconjugated G-CSF (33 vs 4-6 hours), it has the advantage of maintaining clinically effective serum levels over about two weeks after a single 6mg s.c. administration and achieving patient compliance. Its effect is self-limited and is terminated with cellular uptake by the recovering neutrophils (Hunter et al., 2003; Molineux et al., 1999). Clinical studies have demonstrated that pegfilgrastim is at least as efficient as filgrastim in mobilizing PBPCs after chemotherapy and this effect was not dose dependent. Pegfilgrastim was associated with a more rapid leukocyte recovery and an earlier performance of the first apheresis procedure in comparison to unconjugated G-CSF in PCM patients (Bruns et al., 2006; Fruehauf et al., 2007; Stiedl et al., 2005). Additionally, in a tandem transplant study, PBPC mobilization with chemotherapy plus pegfilgrastim in 237 PCM patients, a second booster injection of 6mg pegfilgrastim on day 13 after an initial administration on day 6, improved the serum G-CSF concentrations and the mobilization results (Tricot et al., 2008). In contrast to mobilization after chemotherapy, growth factor-only mobilization requires higher doses of pegfilgrastim to provide effective serum G-CSF levels (Hosing et al., 2006; Willis et al., 2009). However, this approach is not cost-effective when compared with unconjugated G-CSF. Pegfilgrastim is well tolerated with an advese event profile similar to that of unconjugated G-CSF. Bone pain is the most common complaint and a case of splenic rupture that may not have been related to pegfilgrastim was reported in one trial (Fenk et al., 2006).

2.3 Chemomobilization

The standard chemomobilization in myeloma consists of cyclophosphamide(CY) plus growth factor (Goldschmidt et al., 1996). High dose CY has been prefered in patients who fail initial mobilization attempt with growth factor only or for patients who could not achieve at least partial remission after induction regimens with the hope to control the high tumor burden before transplantation. However, it has been demonstrated that high dose CY does not increase overall complete remission rates or improve the time to progression for patients with myeloma undergoing AHCT (Dingli et al., 2006). At our center, CY 4 gr/m^2 with the same dose MESNA to prevent hemorrhagic cystitis is administered on day 1 and recombinant human G-CSF (10 µg/kg/day, in two divided doses) is started either on day 4 or day 7. The optimal timing for G-CSF initiation has not been determined conclusively. We have demonstrated that late (day 7) administration of G-CSF was as efficient and more cost-effective than early administration (Ozcelik et al., 2009). Flow cytometric quantification of peripheral blood(PB) CD34+ cells is performed when the WBC count reaches >1000/µl from the chemotherapy induced nadir. The apheresis is started when PB CD34+ cell count exceeds 10 cells/µl and continued until adequate number of CD34+ cells are collected usually for 1-3 apheresis procedures. Transfusion support should be given to keep the pre-apheresis Hb and platelet counts at ≥ 10gr/dl and ≥ 20 000-30 000/µl, respectively.

The dose of CY reported for mobilization has ranged from 1.5 to 7 gr/m^2. Retrospective studies comparing CY doses of 4 gr/m^2 versus 7 gr/m^2 and 1.2-2 gr/m^2 versus 4 gr/m^2 have favored lower doses because of similar stem cell mobilization efficiency but with considerably lower toxicity (Fitoussi et al., 2001; Jantunen et al., 2003). In a randomized study in myeloma patients comparing single dose 7 g/m^2 with 2.4 g/m^2 , higher number CD34+ cells were collected on the first apheresis day and there was a lower consumption of

G-CSF with the lower-dose CY regimen, which also permitted collection to occur as an outpatient procedure and was more cost-effective (Petrucci et al., 2003). Hiwase et al in their retrospective analysis have demonstrated that compared with low dose (1-2 gr/m^2) CY, patients receiving intermediate dose (3-4 gr/m^2) CY were more likely to collect the CD34+ cell number (≥4 x10^6/kg) adequate for tandem transplant. Febrile neutropenia was more frequent in intermediate dose CY group (38% vs 13%) but the increased toxicity was managable and acceptable (Hiwase et al., 2007). In the light of these studies, most centers prefer 3-4 gr/m^2 CY in their chemomobilization protocol (Gertz et al., 2010a).

High dose CY plus G-CSF is very efficient for PBPC mobilization in PCM patients but when compared with growth factor-only mobilization, chemotherapy plus growth factor mobilizes higher number of PBPCs in lower number of apheresis procedures but with the cost of increased toxicity; nausea- emesis, neutropenic fever, non-staphylococal bacteremia, sepsis, hemorrhagic cystitis, cardiac toxicity, hospitalization, requirement for transfusion support and with mortality rate of 1-2%. Moreover, there is increased possibility of delayed engraftment after AHCT if transplanted early after (e.g. <30 days) stem cell procurement (Gertz et al., 2009; To et al., 1990).

With the purpose of decreasing toxicity and at least preserving the efficiency, various alternative chemomobilization protocols with or without CY have also been investigated. Addition of etoposide (2 gr/m^2) to CY (4.5 gr/m^2) mobilization in a non-randomized study, resulted in increased toxicity without significant improvement in CD34+ cell yield (Gojo et al., 2004). In CAD protocol, CY (1gr/m^2, day 1) was combined with doxorubicin (15 mg/m2, day 1-4) and dexamethasone (40 mg, day 1-4) followed by a single dose 12 mg pegfilgrastim on day 5. Eighty-eight percent of patients achieved their CD34+ cell harvest target of 7.5 x 10^6 CD34/kg following a median of two apheresis. Mobilization efficiency and engraftment following transplantation using pegfilgrastim was comparable to filgrastim and patients mobilized with CAD plus pegfilgrastim had decreased time to first apheresis (13 vs 15 days)(Fruehauf et al., 2007). The former common induction protocol VAD followed by daily G-CSF 10 µg/kg from day 10 to day 15 was found to be as effective and less toxic than high-dose CY followed by daily G-CSF 5 µg/kg from day 8 in newly diagnosed myeloma patients (Lefrère et al., 2006). Blood stem cell collection results after mobilization with combination chemotherapy containing ifosfamide, epirubicin, and etoposide (IEV) followed by G-CSF in myeloma were favorable and allowed to support a tandem transplantation procedure in younger and elder patients in 97 and 95%, respectively. Grade ¾ hematological toxicity was observed in majority of patients and extramedullary toxicity including nephrotoxicity and neurotoxicity in 5–10% (Straka et al., 2003). IEV mobilized peripheral blood stem cells more efficiently than cyclophosphamide and etoposide, achieving a threshold of 6 x 10^6 CD34/kg in 97 vs. 71% with comparable major toxicities and similar tumor response rates, although there was one treatment-related death due to septic shock in the IEV chemotherapy group (Hart et al., 2007). DCEP protocol includes dexamethasone (40 mg/d, day 1-4) , CY 400 mg/m^2, etoposide 40 mg/m^2 and cisplatin 10 mg/m^2, daily continuous infusion for 4 days and has proved to be an effective salvage therapy for relapsed/refractory myeloma patients. G-CSF 5 µg/kg/day starting 48 h after the end of DCEP has been an effective mobilization protocol with 87 and 75% of patients achieving ≥ 2 x 10^6 and >4 x 10^6 /kg CD34+ cells, respectively (Lazzarino et al., 2001). The same group of investigators compared DCEP with CY (4 g/m^2) followed by G-CSF and concluded that DCEP is better tolerated and more effective than CY for PBPC mobilization. Moreover, high-dose CY has limited anti-myeloma activity compared to DCEP. One study demonstrated the comparable efficiency and lower toxicity of shorter-infusional schedule of DCEP with respect to full-infusional schedule (Corso et al., 2002, 2005). Another study combined DCEP-short with a single dose 6mg s.c. pegfilgrastim and reported promising results (Zappasodi et al., 2008). In a pilot study, vinorelbin combined with CY 1.5 g/m^2 had similar efficiency compared to CY 4 g/m^2 in PBPC mobilization and less toxicity and no requirement for hospitalization (Annunziata et al., 2006). Melphalan i.v. 60mg/m^2 plus G-CSF 10 µg/kg/day was successful in mobilizing PBPC from myeloma patients. However, toxicity was notable and duration of mobilization was longer compared with CY 3 g/m^2 (16.5 days vs 10 days)(Gupta et al., 2005). Melphalan is a highly effective anti-myeloma drug but due to its stem cell toxicity, it is neither used for PBSC mobilization, nor recommended as an initial therapy for patients elligible for AHCT. In a retrospective analysis, single agent etoposide (1.5 g/m^2) plus G-CSF was most potent at mobilizing PBPCs compared to CY (2-4 g/m^2) plus G-CSF or G-CSF alone. Although the success rate for collecting the minimum CD34+ dose was similar in all groups, higher proportion of patients mobilized with etoposide could achieve the optimum dose required for tandem transplant. There was no difference in the progression free survival among the groups (Nakasone et al., 2009). Recently, in a retrospective single center review, intermediate dose etoposide (375 mg/m^2, day 1 and 2) followed by G-CSF was found to be highly effective in myeloma patients including the high risk patients for mobilization failure (Wood et al., 2011). However, myelosuppressive mobilization regimens neither seem to have any anti-myeloma effects nor appear to improve outcome (Attal et al., 2003). And most centers no longer routinely use CY for patients in first plateau.

3. High risk patients for mobilization failure

Although there may be variations in each center's definition of mobilization failure, generally it can be defined as lack of achievement of $\geq 2 \times 10^6$/kg CD34+ yield after 3 consecutive apheresis procedure or inability to start apheresis because of not reaching to >10 CD34+ cells/µl of PB . Extensive BM involvement with malignancy, prior radiotherapy especially to marrow-rich sites, prior treatment with alkylating agents, prior multiple chemotherapy regimens and older age have been associated with increased risk of mobilization failure (Bensinger et al., 2009; Demirer et al., 1996; Leung et al., 2010). Although the number of CD34+ cells collected decreases with increasing age, the experience has revealed that sufficient stem cell yield for ≥ 1 AHCT can be safely obtained in elderly patients up to 69-72 years (Roncon et al., 2011; Tempescul et al., 2010). On the other hand, in one retrospective study including myeloma and lymphoma patients, the total number of cycles of previous chemotherapy and previous treatment with melphalan were more significant predictors of poor mobilization than sex, age or body weight (Wuchter et al., 2010). Recently, prior prolonged exposure to novel agent lenalidomide has also been considered as a risk factor, which will be discussed later. With the current mobilization strategies about 5-10% of patients with PCM still end up with mobilization failure (Bensinger et al., 2009; Pusic et al., 2008). The classical strategy when patients fail G-CSF only mobilizations has been CY followed by G-CSF. However, this results in unnecessary exposure of the patients to chemotherapy toxicity for sole mobilization purposes, which means that novel PBPC mobilization approaches are required.

4. Novel agents for PBPC mobilization

Historically, attempts to increase the mobilization efficiency concentrated on using high doses of G-CSF or combining G-CSF with other cytokines and growth factors some of which are currently used in other indications. However, either due to inefficiency or AEs, most of these agents could not become a part of the standart mobilization. In recent years, several cytokines and chemokines have been investigated that may prove useful for amplifying yields of CD34+ cells without introducing additional toxicity. There are also investigational agents which are yet in preclinical and phase I clinical trials (Table 1) (Bakanay & Demirer, 2011).

Agents
Growth Factors Granulocyte-Macrophage Colony Stimulating Factor Recombinant human erythropoietin Recombinant human stem cell factor Recombinant human thrombopoietin Parathyroid hormone Recombinant human growth hormone
Chemokine axis mobilizers AMD3100 GRO-β analogs (SB-251353)
Other small molecules and peptides Very Late Antigen-1 antibodies Retinoic acid receptor alpha agonists Thrombopoietin receptor agonists

Table 1. Agents investigated as adjunct to G-CSF for PBPC mobilization

4.1 Plerixafor

Plerixafor (AMD3100, Mozobil, Genzyme Corporation, Cambridge, MA, USA) is a bicyclam molecule which selectively and reversibly antagonizes CXCR4 and disrupts its interaction with stromal cell derived factor-1 (SDF-1), thereby releasing hematopoietic stem cells into the circulation (Gerlach et al., 2001; Hendrix et al., 2000). Plerixafor has received approval by the US FDA and the European Medicines Evaluation Agency for use in combination with G-CSF to mobilize PBPCs for collection and subsequent AHCT in patients with NHL and PCM who previously failed mobilization with G-CSF alone (DiPersio et al. 2009a,2009b; Mozobil package insert). Plerixafor results in rapid mobilization of PBPC, which peaks at approximately 10 hours. Plerixafor has been shown to synergize with G-CSF for mobilizing stem cells in patients with PCM in various clinical conditions (Calandra et al., 2008; DiPersio et al., 2009a; Flomenberg et al., 2005; Stiff et al., 2009; Tricot et al., 2010). The results from phase II studies indicated that plerixafor added to G-CSF for PBPC mobilization from myeloma patients mobilized more CD34+ cells per day of apheresis than G-CSF alone (4.4 vs 3-3.5 fold) with 95 to 100% of the patients achieving the minimum number (≥ 2 x10^6/kg) of target CD34+ cells in a median of 1-2 apheresis days. Even the heavily pretreated patients had the median 2.5 fold increase in the PB CD34+ cells and could proceed with high dose therapy and AHCT (Stewart et al., 2009; Stiff et al., 2009). In a randomized, placebo-controlled phase III study the proportion of patients from whom ≥ 6 x10^6 CD34+ cells/kg were collected in ≤2 days of apheresis served as the primary end point. The protocol for plerixafor plus G-CSF mobilization has been summarized(Table 2). The results demonstrated that the addition of plerixafor to G-CSF resulted in a significantly higher probability of achieving the optimal CD34+ cell target for tandem transplantation in fewer days of apheresis in PCM patients without any additional toxicity(Table 3). Peripheral blood stem cells mobilized by plerixafor and G-CSF resulted in prompt and durable engraftment after AHCT(DiPersio et al., 2009a).

GCSF 10 µg/kg/day s.c. on days 1-4
Plerixafor 240 µg/kg/day s.c. started on the evening of day 4
Apheresis initiated 10 h after the first dose of plerixafor on the morning of day 5
Daily GCSF before apheresis in the morning and plerixafor in the evening
Continued until the target CD34+ cells ≥ 6 x 10^6/kg was collected or a predetermined maximum number of apheresis (4-5) was reached

Table 2. Mobilization protocol of Plerixafor plus GCSF

	Plerixafor + G-CSF N=148	Placebo + G-CSF N=154
Achieved primary end point (%)	71.6	34.4
Achieved min. collection (%)	95.9	92.9
Fold increase PB CD34/µl	4.8	1.7
Median number of apheresis days to collect the target	1	4
Median(range) collected CD34 cells x10^6/kg	10.96 (0.66-104.57)	6.18 (0.11-42.66)
Failed mobilization (%)	0	4.6

Table 3. Phase III Clinical trial of PBPC mobilization with Plerixafor plus G-CSF in PCM

There is lack of sufficient information on direct comparison of mobilization with G-CSF and plerixafor to mobilization with chemotherapy and G-CSF. In a retrospective comparison, both G-CSF plus plerixafor and CY plus G-CSF resulted in similar numbers of cells collected as well as costs of mobilization and clinical outcomes (Shaughnessy et al., 2011). For the patients from whom sufficient number of CD34+ cells could not be collected after the first mobilization attempt with G-CSF alone, a second(rescue) mobilization has been traditionally attempted with chemotherapy plus G-CSF. However, instead of chemomobilization, a rescue stem cell mobilization with G-CSF and plerixafor can be offered in patients who only require PBPC mobilization and collection without any need for further tumor reduction. In compassionate use programs, plerixafor has been used successfully in myeloma patients who were either proven or predicted to be poor mobilizers. About 75% of the patients could be rescued after failure from chemotherapy (Basak et al., 2011a; Calandra et al., 2008; Duarte et al., 2011). Plerixafor plus G-CSF can also be an option for myeloma patients who had received a previous AHCT and who require a repeated mobilization for a second transplantation. In a recent study, successful mobilization of PBPCs was performed in a similar proportion of the previously transplanted patients and other patients who had not undergone ASCT (70% vs 82.6%) (Basak et al., 2011b).

Plerixafor combined with chemotherapy and G-CSF in a recent open-label, multicenter trial on 40 patients with PCM and NHL, also proved to be a feasible method of stem cell mobilization. However, further studies are warranted to evaluate the exact timing of incorporating plerixafor into chemomobilization (Dugan et al., 2010). Table 4 gives a single center approach to mobilization in the era of novel mobilizing agent, plerixafor (Gertz, 2010b). In one single center experience, preemptive use of plerixafor was successful in patients who had either PB CD34+ counts <10/µl at the time of marrow recovery or poor yield of first apheresis CD34+ <1x 10^6 /kg (Jantunen et al., 2011). Similarly, a promising approach with growth factor and patient-adapted use of plerixafor has been recently suggested to be superior to chemotherapy and growth factor for autologous PBPC mobilization. The preemptive use of plerixafor using the PB CD34+ cell count on day 4 of G-CSF administration and the collection target to decide between continuing G-CSF only or adding plerixafor to the mobilization regimen may potentially reduce the percentage of failure in first-line mobilizations (Costa et al., 2011a, 2011b). A recent study demonstrated that the quantity of CD34+ cells collected on day 1, rather than the PB CD34+ cell count, might identify patients unlikely to achieve adequate stem cell collection for AHCT and suggested that patients who collect <0.70 x10^6 CD34+ cells/kg on day 1 could be considered for treatment modifications such as adding plerixafor (Duong et al., 2011).

G-CSF 10 µg/kg single dose x 4 days If collecting for 1 transplant: if CD34+ < 10 x 10^6/L, add plerixafor If collecting for >1 transplant: if CD34+ < 20 x10^6/L, add plerixafor
If relapsed or primary refractory myeloma or circulating plasma cells: CY 1.5 g/m^2 x 2 days, begin G-CSF 5 µg/kg on day 3 Check CD34+ when WBC >1000 x 10^6/L. If CD34+ < 10 x 10^6/L continue to check for three consecutive days. If CD34 remains < 10 x10^6/L, begin plerixafor

Table 4. The Mayo Clinic Rochester approach to PBPC mobilization in myeloma

Plerixafor is well tolerated and adverse events are usually mild and transient. The most common adverse events are diarrhea, nausea, vomiting, flatulance and injection-site reactions, fatigue, arthralgia, headache, dizziness and insomnia. Severe adverse events such as hypotension and dizziness after drug administration and thrombocytopenia after apheresis are very rare (DiPersio et al., 2009, Mozobil package insert). No case of splenic rupture due to plerixafor has been reported to date. No evidence of tumor cell mobilization could be demonstrated after plerixafor in PCM and NHL patients(Fruehauf et al., 2010). A plerixafor dose reduction to 160 μg/kg in patients with a creatinine clearance value ≤ 50 mL/min is recommended (Douglas et al., 2011; MacFarland et al., 2010; Pinto et al., 2010). Plerixafor addition to G-CSF has undoubtedly increased the number of patients who could proceed with high dose therapy and AHCT. Plerixafor incorporation in the first line mobilization protocols in patients who are predicted poor mobilizers will eliminate the need for further mobilization attempts and the cost-effectiveness of such approaches should be clarified. Recently, the International Myeloma Working Group(IMWG) have proposed some strategies to overcome the risk factors for poor PBPC mobilization in PCM (Giralt et al., 2009) (Table 5).

Risk Factor	Proposed strategy
Age>60	Consider plerixafor
History of melphalan exposure	Consider upfront chemomobilization or plerixafor
Extensive prior therapy and prolonged disease duration	Harvest early between cycles 2-4 Consider upfront plerixafor or chemomobilization Assess marrow for secondary dysplastic changes before collection
Extensive radiotherapy to marrow bearing tissue	Consider collection before radiotherapy Consider upfront chemomobilization or plerixafor Assess marrow for secondary dysplastic changes before collection

Table 5. Strategies proposed by IMWG to overcome the risk factors for poor PBPC mobilization in PCM

5. The effect of novel induction protocols on PBPC mobilization in PCM

Until the last decade, the standard first line therapy for PCM has been either VAD or single agent dexamethasone. These therapies clearly do not have any adverse effects on PBPC mobilization from the bone marrow. However, they have been replaced by more efficient novel agents such as IMIDs (thalidomide and lenalidomide) and proteosome inhibitor bortezomib. Novel induction agents in myeloma are effective as first line therapy enhancing the quality of responses prior to AHCT and by controlling the tumor load at diagnosis they decrease the early mortality and prolong the overall survival. With the novel induction agents, the time from diagnosis to planned AHCT is shorter and most patients can achieve ≥ VGPR after the transplantation which eliminates the need for tandem AHCT for most patients. In fact it also neccesitates re-exploration of the role of first line AHCT in selected patients, moving AHCT to a second line position. The novel agents are also used as adjuncts to transplant conditioning regimen or as maintenance therapy after transplant (Dimopoulos et al., 2007; Harousseau et al., 2010; Kumar et al., 2009; Rajkumar et al., 2006).

5.1 Thalidomide

The IMIDs have antiangiogenesis, immunomodulatory activity and direct cyctotoxic affects on myeloma cells. Pretransplant treatment with IMIDs appear to have no impact on engraftment kinetics suggesting that both thalidomide and lenolidomide do not have qualitative effects on stem cells. Thalidomide was the first IMID to be used in PCM and initial therapy with thalidomide-dexamethasone (thal/dex) was superior to dexamethasone alone (Rajkumar et al., 2006). Although there has been controversial reports, most studies have shown no impact of thalidomide on stem cell mobilization and >80% of patients who received thal/dex were able to collect adequate stem cells for tandem transplant (Cavo et al., 2005). In a phase III randomized study, patients treated with induction regimen TAD (Thalidomide, doxorubicine, dexamethasone) had fewer CD34+ cell collection following CAD plus G-CSF mobilization than patients who received VAD as induction. However, the number of CD34+ cells were sufficient to support double AHCT in 82% of TAD treated patients (Breitkreutz et al., 2007). However, in a recent study thalidomide in combination with CY and dexamethasone (CTD) as induction regimen had significantly (49%) lower PBPC yield and higher percentage of mobilization failures for one (25.4 vs 5.8%) or two (39.4 vs 15.9%) transplants compared with VAD and a VAD-like induction regimen. The authors have pointed that thalidomide and CY with no previously reported negative impact on stem cell mobilization can have substantial impact when used in combination (Auner et al., 2011).

5.2 Lenalidomide

Lenalidomide in combination with dexamethasone (Len/dex) have been associated with better outcomes and improved survival rates in patients with PCM (Rajkumar et al., 2005, Dimopuolos et al., 2007, Wang et al., 2008). However, lenalidomide can cause myelosuppression and concerns have been raised that its use may negatively impact the ability to mobilize stem cells in patients who received lenalidomide as part of their induction therapies (Kumar et al., 2007; Mazumder et al., 2008; Paripati et al., 2008; Popat et al., 2009). Kumar have indicated that among patients mobilized with G-CSF alone there was a significant decrease in total CD34+ cells collected, average daily collection, day 1 collection and increased number of apheresis in patients treated with lenalidomide compared to patients treated with other regimens(Kumar et al., 2007). One retrospective analysis demonstrated higher mobilization failure rates with filgrastim among lenalidomide- treated patients compared with patients who had not received lenalidomide (25% vs 4%, $p<0.001$). Failure rate was very high in patients who received >3 cycles of lenalidomide. Majority of the lenalidomide-treated patients(77%) could be rescued with chemotherapy plus filgrastim(Popat et al., 2009). A multicenter prospective study of 346 patients with newly diagnosed PCM, has demonstrated that 21% of the patientswho received 4 cycles of len/dex as induction regimen, could not achieve the target 4×10^6 CD34+ cells/kg after CY plus G-CSF mobilization whereas only 9% of patients failed after a second mobilization attempt with the same mobilization protocol. Lenalidomide as a part of the induction regimen did not adversely affect the PBPC mobilization and a second mobilization procedure with CY plus G-CSF may be an appropriate strategy to rescue poor mobilizers(Cavallo et al., 2011). In different studies where patients were mobilized after len/dex induction therapy, mobilization with CY plus G-CSF yielded clearly higher (range 6.3 to 14.2×10^6/kg) number of stem cells with respect to mobilization with G-CSF alone (range 3.1 to 7.9×10^6/kg) (Kumar et al., 2007; Mark et al., 2008; Mazumder et al., 2008; Paripati et al., 2008; Popat et al., 2009). Incorporation of lenalidomide into induction therapy for PCM did not have clinically significant impact on PBPC mobilization when CY plus G-CSF was used as mobilization protocol. Sufficient stem cells for tandem auto-HCT were collected from all patients mobilized with CY plus G-CSF versus only 33% of patients mobilized with G-CSF alone. Some studies demonstarted lower stem cell yield with increasing duration of lenalidomide therapy but other studies could not demonstrate such correlation (Mark et al., 2008; Mazumder et al., 2008; Nazha et al., 2011). Since addition of CY + G-CSF does not increase the responses to myeloma therapy, exposing patients to the risks of chemomobilization for sole mobilization purposes should be avoided. Plerixafor is a promising alternative to chemomobilization in patients with PCM who received prior therapy with lenalidomide. Retrospective data analysis for 60 patients who received plerixafor plus G-CSF for front-line mobilization in a phase 3 clinical trial or for remobilization in a compassionate use program demonstrated that CD34+ cells can be successfully and predictably mobilized and collected in majority of patients with PCM who have been previously treated with lenalidomide (Micallef et al., 2010) (Table 6). The IMWG have published the consensus report focusing on the approach to stem cell mobilization in era of novel agents in PCM (Kumar et al., 2009)(Table 7).

	Frontline P + G-CSF	Remobilization P + G-CSF	Total
Minimal ≥ 2 x 10^6 CD34+ cells/kg	100%	80%	86.7%
Optimal ≥ 5 x 10^6 CD34+ cells/kg	95%	47.5%	63.3%

Table 6. Mobilization response to Plerixafor plus GCSF in lenalidomide-treated patients

5.3 Bortezomib

Bortezomib is effective in patients with relapsed or refractory disease as well as in untreated patients No definitive impact of initial therapy with bortezomib on stem cell harvest could be demonstrated (Benson et al., 2010; Corso et al., 2010; Horousseau et al., 2010; Jagannath et al., 2005). In the IFM2005/01 trial comparing bortezomib/dexamethasone to VAD, there was a trend towards lower CD34+ numbers among those receiving bortezomib. However, a single mobilization with G-CSF was adequate and allowed the harvest of sufficient number of CD34+ cells for a single transplant in 97% and for a tandem transplant 77% of the patients treated upfront with bortezomib/dexamethasone. Compared with VAD, a higher number of patients in bortezomib/dexamethasone arm required a second mobilization attempt to reach the target 5 x 10^6 CD34+ cells/kg for tandem transplantation (Horousseau et al., 2010; Moreau et al., 2010). HOVON65/GMMG-HD4 randomized phase 3 trial comparing bortezomib, adriamycin, dexamethasone (PAD) versus VAD, no impact of bortezomib was seen on ability to collect stem cells (Goldschmidt et al., 2008).

Studies combining bortezomib with lenalidomide or thalidomide also did not reveal any adverse effect of bortezomib on stem cell mobilization (Richardson et al., 2010; Bensinger et al., 2010; Kaufman et al., 2010). Simultaneous use of bortezomib in combination with thalidomide and chemotherapy (DT-PACE; cisplatin, doxorubicin, CY, etoposide and dexamethasone) was also effective, safe and allowed for adequate stem cell collection (Badros et al., 2006). Addition of alkylating agents to initial therapy especially in combination, may increase the risk of mobilization failures but no comparative data is available. Phase 2 studies combining CY with lenalidomide and CY with thalidomide reported mobilization failures while combination of CY with bortezomib did not reveal any failure (Reeder et al., 2009).

Condition	Recommended approach
Initial therapy with thalidomide or bortezomib plus dexamethasone Patients who received <4 cycles of lenalidomide plus dexamethasone and younger than 65 years	G-CSF alone
Patients who received ≥4 cycles of lenalidomide plus dexamethasone	CY + G-CSF
Patients who received ≥4 cycles of lenalidomide plus dexamethasone and older than 65 years	Reduced dose CY + G-CSF G-CSF alone with the addition of plerixafor before second apheresis if first apheresis yields <2 x 10^6 CD34+ cells/kg
Patients who received other myelosuppressive drugs in combination with lenalidomide	CY + G-CSF
Failed mobilization with G-CSF alone in lenalidomide-treated patients	CY + G-CSF G-CSF + Plerixafor G-CSF + GM-CSF

Table 7. Approach to stem cell mobilization in era of novel agents in PCM : IMWG consensus perspectives

6. Conclusions

As the novel anti-myeloma drugs (thalidomide, lenalidomide, bortezomib) in combination with dexamethasone or other agents have replaced the traditional VAD or single agent dexamethasone as first line therapy for myeloma, there has been concern about their impact on PBPC mobilization from the bone marrow. Studies could not demonstrate any deleretious effect of bortezomib on stem cell mobilization. There has been contraversy regarding thalidomide's impact especially when combined with other cytotoxic agents such as CY. However, the thal/dex combination has proved to allow for adequate PBPC yield for tandem transplantation. On the other hand, prolonged exposure to lenalidomide definitely affects the stem cell yield. Early PBPC mobilization with (<4 cycles) is recommended after lenalidomide-containing regimens. If this condition can not be satisfied, mobilization with CY+ G-CSF or addition of plerixafor to G-CSF should be considered. Although the integration of the novel anti-myeloma agents in the upfront treatment of PCM has started questioning the place of the high dose therapy supported with AHCT as first line approach, it is still the gold standard approach in elligible patients with PCM. This requires the mobilization and collection of adequate number of PBPCs following an initial induction threatment. Traditionally, G-CSF alone or after chemotherapy (mostly CY) have been the most commonly used protocols. Generally, CY plus G-CSF is used in the second mobilization attempt after failing G-CSF. However, this approach does not improve the overall outcome of the myeloma patients. So, it is unnecessary to expose the patients to toxic effects of chemotherapy for sole mobilization purposes. And the combined cytotoxic chemotherapies are better reserved for relapsed or refractory cases. Current studies focus on the novel investigational agents as adjuncts to G-CSF to improve the PBPC yields. Plerixafor, which selectively and reversibly antagonizes CXCR4 and disrupts its interaction with SDF-1, has the ability of rapid mobilization of PBPCs from BM and gained approval as an adjunct to G-CSF for poor mobilizers. At the present, it is challenging to search for the best approach using the available drugs with appropriate timing to provide sufficient CD34+ yield after initial mobilization attempt and in a cost-effective manner avoiding further mobilization attempts and exposure to chemotherapy.

7. References

Annunziata M, Celentano M, Pocali B, D'Amico MR, Palmieri S, Viola A, Copia C,Falco C, Del Vecchio L & Ferrara F.(2006). Vinorelbine plus intermediate dose cyclophosphamide is an effective and safe regimen for the mobilization of peripheral blood stem cells in patients with multiple myeloma. *Ann Hematol.*, 85(6):394-9.

Ataergin S, Arpaci F, Turan M, Solchaga L, Cetin T, Ozturk M, Ozet A, Komurcu S & Ozturk B.(2008). Reduced dose of lenograstim is as efficacious as standard dose of filgrastim for peripheral blood stem cell mobilization and transplantation: a randomized study in patients undergoing autologous peripheral stem cell transplantation. *Am J Hematol.*, 83(8):644-8.

Attal M, Harousseau JL, Stoppa AM, Sotto JJ, Fuzibet JG, Rossi JF, Casassus P,Maisonneuve H, Facon T, Ifrah N, Payen C,& Bataille R.(1996). A prospective, randomized trial of autologous bone marrow transplantation and chemotherapy in multiple myeloma. Intergroupe Français du Myélome. *N Engl J Med.*, 11;335(2):91-7.

Attal M, Harousseau JL, Facon T, Guilhot F, Doyen C, Fuzibet JG, Monconduit M,Hulin C, Caillot D, Bouabdallah R, Voillat L, Sotto JJ, Grosbois B & Bataille R;InterGroupe Francophone du Myélome.(2003). Single versus double autologous stem-cell transplantation for multiple myeloma. *N Engl J Med.*, 25;349(26):2495-502.

Auner HW, Mazzarella L, Cook L, Szydlo R, Saltarelli F, Pavlu J, Bua M, Giles C, Apperley JF & Rahemtulla A.(2011). High rate of stem cell mobilization failure after thalidomide and oral cyclophosphamide induction therapy for multiple myeloma. *Bone Marrow Transplant.*, 46(3):364-7.

Badros A, Goloubeva O, Fenton R, Rapoport AP, Akpek G, Harris C, Ruehle K,Westphal S & Meisenberg B.(2006). Phase I trial of first-line bortezomib/thalidomide plus chemotherapy for induction and stem cell mobilization in patients with multiple myeloma. *Clin Lymphoma Myeloma.*, 7(3):210-6.

Bakanay SM, Demirer T.(2011)Novel agents and approaches fors tem cell mobilization in normal donors and patients. *Bone Marrow Transplant.* (Epub ahead of print).

Barlogie B, Kyle RA, Anderson KC, Greipp PR, Lazarus HM, Hurd DD, McCoy J, Moore DF Jr, Dakhil SR, Lanier KS, Chapman RA, Cromer JN, Salmon SE, Durie B & Crowley JC.(2006). Standard chemotherapy compared with high-dose chemoradiotherapy for multiple myeloma: final results of phase III US Intergroup Trial S9321. *J Clin Oncol.*, 20;24(6):929-36.

Basak GW, Jaksic O, Koristek Z, Mikala G, Basic-Kinda S, Mayer J, Masszi T, Giebel S, Labar B & Wiktor-Jedrzejczak W; Central and Eastern European Leukaemia Group (CELG).(2011). Haematopoietic stem cell mobilization with plerixafor and G-CSF in patients with multiple myeloma transplanted with autologous stem cells. *Eur J Haematol.*, 86(6):488-95.

Basak GW, Knopinska-Posluszny W, Matuszak M, Kisiel E, Hawrylecka D, Szmigielska-Kaplon A, Urbaniak-Kujda D, Dybko J, Zielinska P, Dabrowska-Iwanicka A, Werkun J, Rzepecki P, Wroblewska W & Wiktor-Jedrzejczak W.(2011). Hematopoietic stem cell mobilization with the reversible CXCR4 receptor inhibitor plerixafor (AMD3100)-Polish compassionate use experience. *Ann Hematol.*,90(5):557-68.

Bensinger W, Appelbaum F, Rowley S, Storb R, Sanders J, Lilleby K, Gooley T,Demirer T, Schiffman K & Weaver C.(1995). Factors that influence collection and engraftment of autologous peripheral-blood stem cells. *J Clin Oncol,* 13(10):2547-55.

Bensinger W, DiPersio JF & McCarty JM.(2009). Improving stem cell mobilization strategies: future directions. *Bone Marrow Transplant,* 43(3):181-95.

Bensinger WI, Jagannath S, Vescio R, Camacho E, Wolf J, Irwin D, Capo G, McKinley M, Potts P, Vesole DH, Mazumder A, Crowley J, Becker P, Hilger J & Durie BG.(2010). Phase 2 study of two sequential three-drug combinations containing bortezomib,cyclophosphamide and dexamethasone, followed by bortezomib, thalidomide and dexamethasone as frontline therapy for multiple myeloma. *Br J Haematol,*148(4):562-8.

Benson DM Jr, Panzner K, Hamadani M, Hofmeister CC, Bakan CE, Smith MK, Elder P, Krugh D, O'Donnell L & Devine SM.(2010). Effects of induction with novel agents versus conventional chemotherapy on mobilization and autologous stem cell transplant outcomes in multiple myeloma. *Leuk Lymphoma.,* 51(2):243-51.

Breitkreutz I, Lokhorst HM, Raab MS, Holt B, Cremer FW, Herrmann D, Glasmacher A,Schmidt-Wolf IG, Blau IW, Martin H, Salwender H, Haenel A, Sonneveld P & Goldschmidt H. (2007). Thalidomide in newly diagnosed multiple myeloma: influence of thalidomide treatment on peripheral blood stem cell collection yield. *Leukemia.*, 21(6):1294-9.

Bruns I, Steidl U, Kronenwett R, Fenk R, Graef T, Rohr UP, Neumann F, Fischer J,Scheid C, Hübel K, Haas R & Kobbe G.(2006). A single dose of 6 or 12 mg of pegfilgrastim for peripheral blood progenitor cell mobilization results in similar yields of CD34+ progenitors in patients with multiple myeloma. *Transfusion,* 46:180-5.

Calandra G, McCarty J, McGuirk J, Tricot G, Crocker SA, Badel K, Grove B, Dye A & Bridger G.(2008). AMD3100 plus G-CSF can successfully mobilize CD34+ cells from non-Hodgkin's lymphoma, Hodgkin's disease and multiple myeloma patients previously failing mobilization with chemotherapy and/or cytokine treatment: compassionate use data. *Bone Marrow Transplant.,* 41: 331-8.

Cashen AF, Lazarus HM &Devine SM. (2007). Mobilizing stem cells from normal donors: is it possible to improve upon G-CSF ? *Bone Marrow Transplant,* 39: 577-88.

Cavallo F, Bringhen S, Milone G, Ben-Yehuda D, Nagler A, Calabrese E, Cascavilla N, Montefusco V, Lupo B, Liberati AM, Crippa C, Rossini F, Passera R, Patriarca F, Cafro AM, Omedè P, Carella AM, Peccatori J, Catalano L, Caravita T, Musto P,Petrucci MT, Boccadoro M & Palumbo A. Stem cell mobilization in patients with newly diagnosed multiple myeloma after lenalidomide induction therapy. *Leukemia.* 2011 Jun 3. [Epub ahead of print]

Cavo M, Zamagni E, Tosi P, Tacchetti P, Cellini C, Cangini D, de Vivo A, Testoni N, Nicci C, Terragna C, Grafone T, Perrone G, Ceccolini M, Tura S & Baccarani M;Bologna 2002 study.(2005). Superiority of thalidomide and dexamethasone over vincristine-doxorubicindexamethasone (VAD) as primary therapy in preparation for autologous transplantation for multiple myeloma. *Blood*,1;106(1):35-9.

Child JA, Morgan GJ, Davies FE, Owen RG, Bell SE, Hawkins K, Brown J, Drayson MT & Selby PJ; Medical Research Council Adult Leukaemia Working Party.(2003).High-dose chemotherapy with hematopoietic stem-cell rescue for multiple myeloma. *N Engl J Med*, 8;348(19):1875-83.

Corso A, Arcaini L, Caberlon S, Zappasodi P, Mangiacavalli S, Lorenzi A, Rusconi C, Troletti D, Maiocchi MA, Pascutto C, Morra E & Lazzarino M. (2002). A combination of dexamethasone, cyclophosphamide, etoposide, and cisplatin is less toxic and more effective than high-dose cyclophosphamide for peripheral stem cell mobilization in multiple myeloma. Haematologica, 87(10):1041-5.

Corso A, Mangiacavalli S, Nosari A, Castagnola C, Zappasodi P, Cafro AM, Astori C, Bonfichi M, Varettoni M, Rusconi C, Troletti D, Pascutto C, Morra E & Lazzarino M; HOST Group.(2005). Efficacy, toxicity and feasibility of a shorter schedule of DCEP regimen for stem cell mobilization in multiple myeloma. *Bone Marrow Transplant*, 36(11):951-4.

Corso A, Barbarano L, Mangiacavalli S, Spriano M, Alessandrino EP, Cafro AM,Pascutto C, Varettoni M, Bernasconi P, Grillo G, Carella AM, Montalbetti L,Lazzarino M & Morra E.(2010). Bortezomib plus dexamethasone can improve stem cell collection and overcome the need for additional chemotherapy before autologous transplant in patients with myeloma. *Leuk Lymphoma*, 51(2):236-42.

Costa LJ, Alexander ET, Hogan KR, Schaub C, Fouts TV & Stuart RK.(2011). Development and validation of a decision-making algorithm to guide the use of plerixafor for autologous hematopoietic stem cell mobilization. *Bone Marrow Transplant*, 46: 64-9.

Costa LJ, Miller AN, Alexander ET, Hogan KR, Shabbir M, Schaub C & Stuart RK.(2011).Growth factor and patient-adapted use of plerixafor is superior to CY and growth factor for autologous hematopoietic stem cells mobilization. *Bone Marrow Transplant*, 46:523-8.

Demirer T, Buckner CD, Gooley T, Appelbaum FR, Rowley S, Chauncey T, Lilleby K, Storb R & Bensinger WI. (1996). Factors influencing collection of peripheral blood stem cells in patients with multiple myeloma. *Bone Marrow Transplant,* 17(6):937-41.

Dimopoulos M, Spencer A, Attal M, Prince HM, Harousseau JL, Dmoszynska A, San Miguel J, Hellmann A, Facon T, Foà R, Corso A, Masliak Z, Olesnyckyj M, Yu Z,Patin J, Zeldis JB & Knight RD; Multiple Myeloma (010) Study Investigators. (2007). Lenalidomide plus dexamethasone for relapsed or refractory multiple myeloma. *N Engl J Med*, 22;357(21):2123-32.

Dingli D, Nowakowski GS, Dispenzieri A, Lacy MQ, Hayman S, Litzow MR, Gastineau DA & Gertz MA.(2006). Cyclophosphamide mobilization does not improve outcome in patients receiving stem cell transplantation for multiple myeloma. *Clin Lymphoma Myeloma*, 6:384-8.

DiPersio JF, Micallef IN, Stiff PJ, Bolwell BJ, Maziarz RT, Jacobsen E, Nademanee A, McCarty J, Bridger G & Calandra G ; 3101 Investigators.(2009).Phase III prospective randomized double-blind placebo-controlled trial of plerixafor plus granulocyte colony-stimulating factor compared with placebo plus granulocyte colony-stimulating factor for autologous stem-cell mobilization and transplantation for patients with non-Hodgkin's lymphoma. *J Clin Oncol*, 27: 4767-73.

DiPersio JF, Stadtmauer EA, Nademanee A, Micallef IN, Stiff PJ, Kaufman JL, Maziarz RT., Hosing C, Fruehauf S., Horwitz M., Cooper D.,Bridger G.,& Gary Calandra, for the 3102 Investigators.(2009). Plerixafor and G-CSF versus placebo and G-CSF to mobilize hematopoietic stem cells for autologous stem cell transplantation in patients with multiple myeloma. *Blood,* 113: 5720-6.

Douglas KW, Parker AN, Hayden PJ, Rahemtulla A, D'Addio A, Lemoli RM, Rao K, Maris M, Pagliuca A, Uberti J, Scheid C, Noppeney R, Cook G, Bokhari SW, Worel N, Mikala G, Masszi T, Taylor R & Treisman J. Plerixafor for PBPC mobilisation in myeloma patients with advanced renal failure: safety and efficacy data in a series of 21 patients from Europe and the USA. *Bone Marrow Transplant* 2011 Feb 28 (Epub ahead of print).

Duarte RF, Shaw BE, Marín P, Kottaridis P, Ortiz M, Morante C, Delgado J, Gayoso J, Goterriz R, Martínez-Chamorro C, Mateos-Mazón JJ, Ramírez C, de la Rubia J,Achtereekte H, Gandhi PJ, Douglas KW & Russell NH.(2011). Plerixafor plus granulocyte CSF can mobilize hematopoietic stem cells from multiple myeloma and lymphoma patients failing previous mobilization attempts: EU compassionate use data. *Bone Marrow Transplant,* 46(1):52-8.

Dugan MJ, Maziarz RT, Bensinger WI, Nademanee A, Liesveld J, Badel K, Dehner C, Gibney C, Bridger G & Calandra G.(2010). Safety and preliminary efficacy of plerixafor (Mozobil) in combination with chemotherapy and G-CSF: an open-label, multicenter, exploratory trial in patients with multiple myeloma and non-Hodgkin's lymphoma undergoing stem cell mobilization. *Bone Marrow Transplant,* 45: 39-47.

Duong HK, Bolwell BJ, Rybicki L, Koo A, Hsi ED, Figueroa P, Dean R, Pohlman B,Kalaycio M, Andresen S, Sobecks R & Copelan E. (2011).Predicting hematopoietic stem cell mobilization failure in patients with multiple myeloma: A simple method using day 1 CD34+ cell yield. *J Clin Apher,* 26:111-5.

Fenk R, Hieronimus N, Steidl U, Bruns I, Graef T, Zohren F, Ruf L, Haas R & Kobbe G.(2006). Sustained G-CSF plasma levels following administration of pegfilgrastim fasten neutrophil reconstitution after high-dose chemotherapy and autologous blood stem cell transplantation in patients with multiple myeloma. *Exp Hematol,* 34: 1296-302.

Fermand JP, Katsahian S, Divine M, Leblond V, Dreyfus F, Macro M, Arnulf B, Royer B, Mariette X, Pertuiset E, Belanger C, Janvier M, Chevret S, Brouet JC & Ravaud P; Group Myelome-Autogreffe.(2005). High-dose therapy and autologous blood stem-cell transplantation compared with conventional treatment in myeloma patients aged 55 to 65 years: long-term results of a randomized control trial from the Group Myelome-Autogreffe. *J Clin Oncol,* 20;23(36):9227-33.

Fitoussi O, Perreau V, Boiron JM, Bouzigon E, Cony-Makhoul P, Pigneux A, Agape P,Nicolini F, Dazey B, Reiffers J, Salmi R & Marit G.(2001). A comparison of toxicity following two different doses of cyclophosphamide for mobilization of peripheral blood progenitor cells in 116 multiple myeloma patients. *Bone Marrow Transplant,* 27(8):837-42.

Flomenberg N, Devine SM, Dipersio JF, Liesveld JL, McCarty JM, Rowley SD, Vesole DH, Badel K & Calandra G.(2005). The use of AMD3100 plus G-CSF for autologous hematopoietic progenitor cell mobilization is superior to G-CSF alone. *Blood,* 106: 1867-74.

Fruehauf S, Klaus J, Huesing J, Veldwijk MR, Buss EC, Topaly J, Seeger T, Zeller LW, Moehler T, Ho AD & Goldschmidt H.(2007). Efficient mobilization of peripheral blood stem cells following CAD chemotherapy and a single dose of pegylated G-CSF in patients with multiple myeloma. *Bone Marrow Transplant,* 39: 743-50.

Fruehauf S, Ehninger G, Hübel K, Topaly J, Goldschmidt H, Ho AD, Müller S, Moos M, Badel K & Calandra G.(2010). Mobilization of peripheral blood stem cells for autologous transplant in non-Hodgkin's lymphoma and multiple myeloma patients by plerixafor and G-CSF and detection of tumor cell mobilization by PCR in multiple myeloma patients. *Bone Marrow Transplant,* 45: 269-75.

Gerlach LO, Skerlj RT, Bridger GJ & Schwartz TW.(2001). Molecular interactions of cyclam and bicyclam non-peptide antagonists with the CXCR4 chemokine receptor. *J Biol Chem,* 276: 14153-60.

Gertz MA, Kumar SK, Lacy MQ, Dispenzieri A, Hayman SR, Buadi FK, Dingli D, Gastineau DA, Winters JL & Litzow MR.(2009). Comparison of high-dose CY and growth factor with growth factor alone for mobilization of stem cells for transplantation in patients with multiple myeloma. *Bone Marrow Transplant,* 43(8):619-25.

Gertz MA, Wolf RC, Micallef IN & Gastineau DA.(2010). Clinical impact and resource utilization after stem cell mobilization failure in patients with multiple myeloma and lymphoma. *Bone Marrow Transplant,* 45(9):1396-403.

Gertz MA. (2010).Current status of stem cell mobilization. *Br J Haematol,* 150: 647-62.

Giralt S, Stadtmauer EA, Harousseau JL, Palumbo A, Bensinger W, Comenzo RL, Kumar S, Munshi NC, Dispenzieri A, Kyle R, Merlini G, San Miguel J, Ludwig H, Hajek R, Jagannath S, Blade J, Lonial S, Dimopoulos MA, Einsele H, Barlogie B, Anderson KC, Gertz M, Attal M, Tosi P, Sonneveld P, Boccadoro M, Morgan G, Sezer O, Mateos MV, Cavo M, Joshua D, Turesson I, Chen W, Shimizu K, Powles R, Richardson PG,Niesvizky R, Rajkumar SV & Durie BG; IMWG.(2009). International myeloma working group (IMWG) consensus statement and guidelines regarding the current status of stem cell collection and high-dose therapy for multiple myeloma and the role of plerixafor (AMD 3100). *Leukemia,*23(10):1904-12.

Gojo I, Guo C, Sarkodee-Adoo C, Meisenberg B, Fassas A, Rapoport AP, Cottler-Fox M, Heyman M, Takebe N & Tricot G.(2004). High-dose cyclophosphamide with or without etoposide for mobilization of peripheral blood progenitor cells in patients with multiple myeloma: efficacy and toxicity. *Bone Marrow Transplant,* 34(1):69-76.

Goldschmidt H, Hegenbart U, Haas R & Hunstein W.(1996). Mobilization of peripheral blood progenitor cells with high-dose cyclophosphamide (4 or 7 g/m2) and granulocyte colony-stimulating factor in patients with multiple myeloma. *Bone Marrow Transplant,* 17(5):691-7.

Goldschmidt H, Lokhorst HM, Bertsch U, et al. Successful harvesting of peripheral hematopoietic stem cells after induction treatment with bortezomib,adriamycin, dexamethasone (PAD) in patients with newly diagnosed multiple myeloma (MM) [abstract]. *Blood (ASH Annual Meeting Abstracts).*2008;112:3470.

Gupta S, Zhou P, Hassoun H, Kewalramani T, Reich L, Costello S, Drake L, Klimek V, Dhodapkar M, Teruya-Feldstein J, Hedvat C, Kalakonda N, Fleisher M, Filippa D,Qin J, Nimer SD & Comenzo RL.(2005). Hematopoietic stem cell mobilization with intravenous melphalan and G-CSF in patients with chemoresponsive multiple myeloma: report of a phase II trial. *Bone Marrow Transplant,* 35(5):441-7.

Harousseau JL.(2008). Induction therapy in multiple myeloma. *Hematology Am Soc Hematol Educ Program*, 306-12.

Hart C, Blank C, Krause SW, Andreesen R & Hennemann B.(2007). Ifosfamide, epirubicin, and etoposide (IEV) mobilize peripheral blood stem cells more efficiently than cyclophosphamide/etoposide. *Ann Hematol*, 86(8):575-81.

Hendrix CW, Flexner C, MacFarland RT, Giandomenico C, Fuchs EJ, Redpath E, Bridger G & Henson GW.(2000). Pharmacokinetics and safety of AMD-3100, a novel antagonist of the CXCR-4 chemokine receptor, in human volunteers. *Antimicrob Agents Chemother*, 44: 1667-73.

Hiwase DK, Bollard G, Hiwase S, Bailey M, Muirhead J & Schwarer AP.(2007). Intermediate-dose CY and G-CSF more efficiently mobilize adequate numbers of PBSC for tandem autologous PBSC transplantation compared with low-dose CY in patients with multiple myeloma. *Cytotherapy*, 9(6):539-47.

Hosing C, Qazilbash MH, Kebriaei P, Giralt S, Davis MS, Popat U, Anderlini P, Shpall EJ, McMannis J, Körbling M & Champlin RE.(2006). Fixed-dose single agent pegfilgrastim for peripheral blood rogenitor cell mobilisation in patients with multiple myeloma. *Br J Haematol*,133: 533-7.

Hunter MG, Druhan LJ, Massullo PR &Avalos BR. (2003). Proteolytic cleavage of granulocyte colony-stimulating factor and its receptor by neutrophil elastase induces growth inhibition and decreased cell surface expression of the granulocyte colony-stimulating factor receptor. *Am J Hematol*, 74: 149-55.

Jagannath S, Durie BG, Wolf J, Camacho E, Irwin D, Lutzky J, McKinley M, Gabayan E, Mazumder A, Schenkein D & Crowley J.(2005). Bortezomib therapy alone and in combination with dexamethasone for previously untreated symptomatic multiple myeloma. *Br J Haematol*, 129(6):776-83.

Jantunen E, Putkonen M, Nousiainen T, Pelliniemi TT, Mahlamäki E & Remes K.(2003). Low-dose or intermediate-dose cyclophosphamide plus granulocyte colony-stimulating factor for progenitor cell mobilisation in patients with multiple myeloma. *Bone Marrow Transplant*, 31(5):347-51.

Jantunen E, Kuittinen T, Mahlamäki E, Pyörälä M, Mäntymaa P & Nousiainen T. (2011). Efficacy of pre-emptively used plerixafor in patients mobilizing poorly after chemomobilization: a single centre experience. *Eur J Haematol*, 86(4):299-304.

Kaufman JL, Nooka A, Vrana M, Gleason C, Heffner LT & Lonial S.(2010). Bortezomib, thalidomide, and dexamethasone as induction therapy for patients with symptomatic multiple myeloma: a retrospective study. *Cancer*, 1;116(13):3143-51.

Kopf B, De Giorgi U, Vertogen B, Monti G, Molinari A, Turci D, Dazzi C, Leoni M, Tienghi A, Cariello A, Argnani M, Frassineti L, Scarpi E, Rosti G & Marangolo M.(2006). A randomized study comparing filgrastim versus lenograstim versus molgramostim plus chemotherapy for peripheral blood progenitor cell mobilization. *Bone Marrow Transplant*, 38:407-12.

Koreth J, Cutler CS, Djulbegovic B, Behl R, Schlossman RL, Munshi NC, Richardson PG, Anderson KC, Soiffer RJ & Alyea EP 3rd.(2007). High-dose therapy with single autologous transplantation versus chemotherapy for newly diagnosed multiple myeloma: A systematic review and meta-analysis of randomized controlled trials. *Biol Blood Marrow Transplant*, 13(2):183-96.

Kumar S, Dispenzieri A, Lacy MQ, Hayman SR, Buadi FK, Gastineau DA, Litzow MR, Fonseca R, Roy V, Rajkumar SV& Gertz MA.(2007). Impact of lenalidomide therapy on stem cell mobilization and engraftment post-peripheral blood stem cell transplantation in patients with newly diagnosed myeloma. *Leukemia,* 21: 2035-42.

Kumar S, Giralt S, Stadtmauer EA, Harousseau JL, Palumbo A, Bensinger W, Comenzo RL, Lentzsch S, Munshi N, Niesvizky R, San Miguel J, Ludwig H, Bergsagel L, Blade J, Lonial S, Anderson KC, Tosi P, Sonneveld P, Sezer O, Vesole D, Cavo M, Einsele H, Richardson PG, Durie BG & Rajkumar SV; International Myeloma Working Group.(2009). Mobilization in myeloma revisited: IMWG consensus perspectives on stem cell collection following initial therapy with thalidomide-, lenalidomide-, or bortezomib-containing regimens. *Blood,* 27;114(9):1729-35.

Lazzarino M, Corso A, Barbarano L, Alessandrino EP, Cairoli R, Pinotti G, Ucci G,Uziel L, Rodeghiero F, Fava S, Ferrari D, Fiumanò M, Frigerio G, Isa L, Luraschi A, Montanara S, Morandi S, Perego D, Santagostino A, Savarè M, Vismara A & Morra E.(2001). DCEP (dexamethasone, cyclophosphamide, etoposide, and cisplatin) is an effective regimen for peripheral blood stem cell collection in multiple myeloma. *Bone Marrow Transplant,* 28(9):835-9.

Lefrère F, Bernard M, Audat F, Cavazzana-Calvo M, Belanger C, Hermine O, Arnulf B, Buzyn A & Varet B.(1999). Comparison of lenograstim vs filgrastim administration following chemotherapy for peripheral blood stem cell (PBSC) collection: a retrospective study of 126 patients. *Leuk Lymphoma,* 35(5-6):501-5.

Lefrère F, Zohar S, Ghez D, Delarue R, Audat F, Suarez F, Hermine O, Damaj G, Maillard N, Ribeil JA, Azagury M, Misbahi R, Jondeau K, Cavazzana-Calvo M, Dal Cortivo L & Varet B.(2006). The VAD chemotherapy regimen plus a G-CSF dose of 10 microg/kg is as effective and less toxic than high-dose cyclophosphamide plus a G-CSF dose of 5 microg/kg for progenitor cell mobilization: results from a monocentric study of 82 patients. *Bone Marrow Transplant,* 37(8):725-9.

Leung AY & Kwong YL.(2010). Haematopoietic stem cell transplantation: current concepts and novel therapeutic strategies. *Br Med Bull,* 93:85-103.

Ljungman P, Bregni M, Brune M, Cornelissen J, de Witte T, Dini G, Einsele H,Gaspar HB, Gratwohl A, Passweg J, Peters C, Rocha V, Saccardi R, Schouten H,Sureda A, Tichelli A, Velardi A & Niederwieser D; European Group for Blood and Marrow Transplantation.(2010). Allogeneic and autologous transplantation for haematological diseases, solid tumours and immune disorders: current practice in Europe 2009. *Bone Marrow Transplant,* 45(2):219-34.

MacFarland R, Hard ML, Scarborough R, Badel K & Calandra G.(2010). A pharmacokinetic study of plerixafor in subjects with varying degrees of renal impairment. *Biol Blood Marrow Transplant* 2010; 16: 95-101.

Mark T, Stern J, Furst JR, Jayabalan D, Zafar F, LaRow A, Pearse RN, Harpel J,Shore T, Schuster MW, Leonard JP, Christos PJ, Coleman M & Niesvizky R.(2008). Stem cell mobilization with cyclophosphamide overcomes the suppressive effect of lenalidomide therapy on stem cell collection in multiple myeloma. *Biol Blood Marrow Transplant* 2008; 14: 795-8.

Mazumder A, Kaufman J, Niesvizky R, Lonial S, Vesole D & Jagannath S.(2008). Effect of lenalidomide therapy on mobilization of peripheral blood stem cells in previously untreated multiple myeloma patients. *Leukemia,* 22(6):1280-1.

Micallef IN, Ho AD, Klein LM, Marulkar S, Gandhi PJ & McSweeney PA.(2011). Plerixafor (Mozobil) for stem cell mobilization in patients with multiple myeloma previously treated with lenalidomide. *Bone Marrow Transplant,* 46(3):350-5.

Molineux G, Kinstler O, Briddell B, Hartley C, McElroy P, Kerzic P, Sutherland W, Stoney G, Kern B, Fletcher FA, Cohen A, Korach E, Ulich T, McNiece I, Lockbaum P,Miller-Messana MA, Gardner S, Hunt T & Schwab G.(1999). A new form of Filgrastim with sustained duration in vivo and enhanced ability to mobilize PBPC in both mice and humans. *Exp Hematol*, 27: 1724-34.

Moreau P, Hulin C, Marit G, Caillot D, Facon T, Lenain P, Berthou C, Pégourié B, Stoppa AM, Casassus P, Michallet M, Benboubker L, Maisonneuve H, Doyen C, Leyvraz S, Mathiot C, Avet-Loiseau H, Attal M & Harousseau JL; IFM group.(2010). Stem cell collection in patients with de novo multiple myeloma treated with the combination of bortezomib and dexamethasone before autologous stem cell transplantation according to IFM 2005-01 trial. *Leukemia*, 24(6):1233-5.

Mozobil(Plerixafor)[Product information]. Genzyme Co.,Cambridge, MA 2008.

Nakasone H, Kanda Y, Ueda T, Matsumoto K, Shimizu N, Minami J, Sakai R, Hagihara M, Yokota A, Oshima K, Tsukada Y, Tachibana T, Nakaseko C, Fujisawa S, Yano S,Fujita H, Takahashi S, Kanamori H & Okamoto S; Kanto Study Group of Cell Therapy.(2009). Retrospective comparison of mobilization methods for autologous stem cell transplantation in multiple myeloma. *Am J Hematol*, 84(12):809-14.

Nazha A, Cook R, Vogl DT, Mangan PA, Gardler M, Hummel K, Cunningham K, Luger SM,Porter DL, Schuster S, O'Doherty U, Siegel D & Stadtmauer EA.(2011). Stem cell collection in patients with multiple myeloma: impact of induction therapy and mobilization regimen.*Bone Marrow Transplant*, 46(1):59-63.

Neulasta(pegfilgrastim) [package insert]. Amgen Inc.: Thousand Oaks, CA, 2007.

Ozcelik T, Topcuoglu P, Beksac M, Ozcan M, Arat M, Biyikli Z, Bakanay SM, Ilhan O, Gurman G, Arslan O &Demirer T.(2009). Mobilization of PBPCs with chemotherapy and recombinant human G-CSF: a randomized evaluation of early vs late administration of recombinant human G-CSF. *Bone Marrow Transplant*, 44:779-83.

Palumbo A, Bringhen S, Petrucci MT, Musto P, Rossini F, Nunzi M, Lauta VM,Bergonzi C, Barbui A, Caravita T, Capaldi A, Pregno P, Guglielmelli T, Grasso M, Callea V, Bertola A, Cavallo F, Falco P, Rus C, Massaia M, Mandelli F, Carella AM, Pogliani E, Liberati AM, Dammacco F, Ciccone G & Boccadoro M.(2004). Intermediate-dose melphalan improves survival of myeloma patients aged 50 to 70: results of a randomized controlled trial. *Blood*, 15;104(10):3052-7.

Paripati H, Stewart AK, Cabou S, Dueck A, Zepeda VJ, Pirooz N, Ehlenbeck C, Reeder C, Slack J, Leis JF, Boesiger J, Torloni AS, Fonseca R & Bergsagel PL.(2008). Compromised stem cell mobilization following induction therapy with lenalidomide in myeloma. *Leukemia*, 22(6):1282-4.

Petrucci MT, Avvisati G, La Verde G, De Fabritiis P, Ribersani M, Palumbo G, De Felice L, Rusignuolo A, Simone F, Meloni G & Mandelli F.(2003). Intermediate-dose cyclophosphamide and granulocyte colony-stimulating factor is a valid alternative to high-dose cyclophosphamide for mobilizing peripheral blood CD34+ cells in patients with multiple myeloma. *Acta Haematol*, 109(4):184-8.

Pinto V, Castelli A, Gaidano G & Conconi A.(2010). Safe and effective use of plerixafor plus G-CSF in dialysis-dependent renal failure. *Am J Hematol*, 85:461-2.

Popat U, Saliba R, Thandi R, Hosing C, Qazilbash M, Anderlini P, Shpall E,McMannis J, Körbling M, Alousi A, Andersson B, Nieto Y, Kebriaei P, Khouri I, de Lima M, Weber D, Thomas S, Wang M, Jones R, Champlin R & Giralt S.(2009). Impairment of filgrastim-induced stem cell mobilization after prior lenalidomide in patients with multiple myeloma. *Biol Blood Marrow Transplant,* 15: 718-23.

Pusic I, Jiang SY, Landua S, Uy GL, Rettig MP, Cashen AF, Westervelt P, Vij R,Abboud CN, Stockerl-Goldstein KE, Sempek DS, Smith AL & DiPersio JF.(2008). Impact of mobilization and remobilization strategies on achieving sufficient stem cell yields for autologous transplantation. *Biol Blood Marrow Transplant,* 14(9):1045-56.

Rajkumar SV, Hayman SR, Lacy MQ, Dispenzieri A, Geyer SM, Kabat B, Zeldenrust SR,Kumar S, Greipp PR, Fonseca R, Lust JA, Russell SJ, Kyle RA, Witzig TE & Gertz MA.(2005). Combination therapy with lenalidomide plus dexamethasone (Rev/Dex) for newly diagnosed myeloma. *Blood,* 15;106(13):4050-3.

Rajkumar SV, Blood E, Vesole D, Fonseca R & Greipp PR; Eastern Cooperative Oncology Group.(2006). Phase III clinical trial of thalidomide plus dexamethasone compared with dexamethasone alone in newly diagnosed multiple myeloma: a clinical trial coordinated by the Eastern Cooperative Oncology Group. *J Clin Oncol,* 20;24(3):431-6.

Reeder CB, Reece DE, Kukreti V, Chen C, Trudel S, Hentz J, Noble B, Pirooz NA,Spong JE, Piza JG, Zepeda VH, Mikhael JR, Leis JF, Bergsagel PL, Fonseca R & Stewart AK.(2009). Cyclophosphamide, bortezomib and dexamethasone induction for newly diagnosed multiple myeloma: high response rates in a phase II clinical trial. *Leukemia,* 23(7):1337-41.

Richardson PG, Weller E, Lonial S, Jakubowiak AJ, Jagannath S, Raje NS, Avigan DE, Xie W, Ghobrial IM, Schlossman RL, Mazumder A, Munshi NC, Vesole DH, Joyce R,Kaufman JL, Doss D, Warren DL, Lunde LE, Kaster S, Delaney C, Hideshima T,Mitsiades CS, Knight R, Esseltine DL & Anderson KC.(2010). Lenalidomide, bortezomib, and dexamethasone combination therapy in patients with newly diagnosed multiple myeloma. *Blood,* 5;116(5):679-86.

Roncon S, Barbosa IL, Campilho F, Lopes SM, Campos A & Carvalhais A.(2011). Mobilization and collection of peripheral blood stem cells in multiple myeloma patients older than 65 years. *Transplant Proc,* 43(1):244-6.

Shaughnessy P, Islas-Ohlmayer M, Murphy J, Hougham M, Macpherson J, Winkler K, Silva M, Steinberg M, Matous J, Selvey S, Maris M & McSweeney PA.(2011). Cost and Clinical Analysis of Autologous Hematopoietic Stem Cell Mobilization with G-CSF and Plerixafor compared to G-CSF and Cyclophosphamide. *Biol Blood Marrow Transplant,* 17:729-36.

Steidl U, Fenk R, Bruns I, Neumann F, Kondakci M, Hoyer B, Gräf T, Rohr UP, Bork S, Kronenwett R, Haas R & Kobbe G.(2005). Successful transplantation of peripheral blood stem cells mobilized by chemotherapy and a single dose of pegylated G-CSF in patients with multiple myeloma. *Bone Marrow Transplant,* 35: 33-6.

Stewart DA, Smith C, MacFarland R & Calandra G. (2009).Pharmacokinetics and pharmacodynamics of plerixafor in patients with non-Hodgkin lymphoma and multiple myeloma. *Biol Blood Marrow Transplant,* 15: 39-46.

Stiff P, Micallef I, McCarthy P, Magalhaes-Silverman M, Weisdorf D, Territo M, Badel K. & Calandra G. Treatment with plerixafor in non-Hodgkin's lymphoma and multiple myeloma patients to increase the number of peripheral blood stem cells when given a mobilizing regimen of G-CSF: implications for the heavily pretreated patient. *Biol Blood Marrow Transplant,* 2009; 15: 249-56.

Straka C, Hebart H, Adler-Reichel S, Werding N, Emmerich B & Einsele H.(2003). Blood stem cell collections after mobilization with combination chemotherapy containing ifosfamide followed by G-CSF in multiple myeloma. *Oncology*, 65 Suppl 2:94-8.

Sutherland DR, Anderson L, Keeney M, Nayar R & Chin-Yee I. (1996). The ISHAGE guidelines for CD34+ cell determination by flow cytometry. International Society of Hematotherapy and Graft Engineering. J Hematother, 5: 213-26.

Tempescul A, Ianotto JC, Hardy E, Quivoron F, Petrov L & Berthou C.(2010). Peripheral blood stem cell collection in elderly patients. *Ann Hematol*, 89(3):317-21.

To LB, Shepperd KM, Haylock DN, Dyson PG, Charles P, Thorp DL, Dale BM, Dart GW, Roberts MM & Sage RE.(1990). Single high doses of cyclophosphamide enable the collection of high numbers of hemopoietic stem cells from the peripheral blood. *Exp Hematol*, 18(5):442-7.

Tricot G, Barlogie B, Zangari M, van Rhee F, Hoering A, Szymonifka J & Cottler-Fox M. (2008).Mobilization of peripheral blood stem cells in myeloma with either pegfilgrastim or filgrastim following chemotherapy. *Haematologica*, 93: 1739-42.

Tricot G, Cottler-Fox MH & Calandra G.(2010). Safety and efficacy assessment of plerixafor in patients with multiple myeloma proven or predicted to be poor mobilizers, including assessment of tumor cell mobilization. *Bone Marrow Transplant*, 45(1):63-8.

Wang M, Dimopoulos MA, Chen C, Cibeira MT, Attal M, Spencer A, Rajkumar SV, Yu Z,Olesnyckyj M, Zeldis JB, Knight RD & Weber DM.(2008). Lenalidomide plus dexamethasone is more effective than dexamethasone alone in patients with relapsed or refractory multiple myeloma regardless of prior thalidomide exposure. *Blood*, 1;112(12):4445-51.

Willis F, Woll P, Theti D, Jamali H, Bacon P, Baker N & Pettengell R.(2009). Pegfilgrastim for peripheral CD34+ mobilization in patients with solid tumours. *Bone Marrow Transplant* , 43: 927-34.

Wood WA, Whitley J, Moore D, Sharf A, Irons R, Rao K, Serody J, Coghill J, Gabriel D & Shea T.(2011). Chemomobilization with Etoposide is Highly Effective in Patients with Multiple Myeloma and Overcomes the Effects of Age and Prior Therapy. *Biol Blood Marrow Transplant*, 17(1):141-6.

Wuchter P, Ran D, Bruckner T, Schmitt T, Witzens-Harig M, Neben K, Goldschmidt H & Ho AD.(2010). Poor mobilization of hematopoietic stem cells-definitions, incidence, risk factors, and impact on outcome of autologous transplantation. *Biol Blood Marrow Transplant*,16(4):490-9.

Zappasodi P, Nosari AM, Astori C, Ciapanna D, Bonfichi M, Varettoni M,Mangiacavalli S, Morra E, Lazzarino M & Corso A.(2008). DCEP chemotherapy followed by a single, fixed dose of pegylated filgrastim allows adequate stem cell mobilization in multiple myeloma patients. *Transfusion*,48(5):857-60.

14

The Current Role of Stem Cell Transplantation in Multiple Myeloma

Ajay Gupta
Medical Oncology, Max Cancer Centre, Saket, New Delhi, India

1. Introduction

Multiple myeloma accounts for 10% of hematological cancers and 1% of all cancers. It is currently the most common indication for ASCT in North America and Europe. ASCT remains the standard of care in eligible patients aged below 65-70 years (though age is not a criterion in the United States) performed either upfront or at relapse. It is mostly performed upfront after induction therapy. The attainment of complete response (CR) is held to be a surrogate for improved survival and is the aim of the ASCT. CR is characterized by undetectable serum and urine monoclonal proteins (by immnofixation), absence of plasmacytosis (<5% plasma cells in marrow), disappearance of plasmacytomas and stable or improving bone disease. Stringent CR (sCR) is a new criterion which refers to normalization of the free light chain ratios (FLC) as well as the absence of monoclonal plasma cells in the marrow. Very good partial response (VGPR) refers to the absence of monoclonal proteins by electrophoresis but not by immunofixation or more than 90% reduction in level of serum M component proteins as well as urinary M proteins less than 100 mg/24 hours.[1]

With conventional chemotherapy comprising melphalan and prednisolone, CR was attained in less than 5% patients. However the median OS in patients achieving CR was 5.1 years as compared to 3.3 years for other responders.[2] ASCT has helped improve CR and VGPR rates over and above CC and is usually performed after induction therapy as consolidation.

Introduction of agents like bortezomib, lenalidomide, thalidomide, liposomal doxorubicin has resulted in Higher rates of CR and very good partial response (VGPR).

Ongoing debates regarding redefining the inclusion criteria/timing and expected benefits of ASCT as compared to maintenance with these drugs however await further trials.

2. ASCT in myeloma

Prospective randomized trials have been conducted to evaluate the efficacy of ASCT in terms of attainment of CR, response rate (RR), improvements in progression free survival (PFS) and overall survival (OS) as well as transplant-related mortality (TRM). [3],[4],[5],[6],[7],[8]

CR rates, median PFS, median OS and TRM have ranged from 17 to 44.5%, 25 to 42 months, 47.8 to 67 months and 3 to 7%, respectively. [3],[4],[5],[6],[7],[8]

However, only two of the trials, the French Intergroup Study (IFM) [3] and the British (MRC VII trial,) [4] demonstrated a survival advantage with ASCT. The French trial demonstrated median OS of 57 months vs. 37 months and the British trial demonstrated a median OS of 54.1 months vs. 42.3 months of ASCT over conventional chemotherapy (CC).

However other trials had some deficiencies. The Spanish study (PETHEMA) demonstrated improved CR rates (30% vs. 11%) with ASCT as compared to CC but no improvement in OS (61 vs. 66 months). This has been ascribed to the fact that only responding patients were taken up for transplant. Refractory patients who were not taken up for the study could also have derived benefit from ASCT. [5]

Two of the trials were designed specifically to look at the effect of upfront vs. delayed transplant (in the case of relapse or refractory disease) upon the survival rates. There was no difference in OS though the French trial reported higher CR rates and better PFS in favor of early transplant. [6],[7]

In another large US intergroup trial comparing CC with ASCT no difference could be demonstrated partly because of the cross over allowed for transplant at relapse in patients on the CC arm as also the fact that the combination of total body irradiation and melphalan dose of 140 mg/m 2 rather than the standard 200 mg/m 2 resulted in a disappointing CR rate of 17%. [8]

The trials incorporating melphalan and TBI had lower CR rates (17-22%) [3],[8] as compared to those in which melphalan 200 mg/m2 was used resulting in CR rates of 30-44%. [4],[5],[6],[7] Thus melphalan 200 mg/m 2 is now the conditioning regimen of choice. These days, most centers claim a TRM of 1% or less, thus rendering ASCT an acceptably safe treatment modality.

CR has been demonstrated to be the most important factor influencing long term survival. In the French IFM study, patients achieving a CR/VGPR had significantly higher 5 year OS rates of 72% as compared to 39% among patients who had a PR. [3] In a retrospective analysis of 721 newly diagnosed patients who underwent ASCT it was found that patients achieving CR had a median survival of 9-14 years compared to 5.9 years for patients who achieved PR. [9]

3. Improving efficacy of ASCT

3.1 Induction therapy and ASCT

The most common treatment strategy involves use of induction chemotherapy followed by HDT- ASCT (in eligible patients).

Initial regimens (vincristine, adriamycin, dexamethasone /dexamethasone /thalidomide, dexamethasone)

Initially the most popular regimens used were single agent pulsed dexamethasone or vincristine, adriamycin and dexamethasone (VAD). Response rates (RR) of 40-43% (CR rates ranging from 0 to 3%) have been reported with dexamethasone. [10],[11],[12] With VAD RR ranging from 52 to 67% and CR rates ranging from 3 to 9% have been described. [13],[14]

Following VAD the next common induction regimen was the oral regimen of thalidomide and dexamethasone (TD). RR ranging from 76 to 80% and CR rates ranging from 7 to 25% have been observed. [12],[13],[14],[15]

After ASCT, CR rates ranging from 30 to 48.2% (post VAD induction) have been described. [13],[14],[16] However studies using thalidomide/dexamethasone and single agent dexamethasone have demonstrated essentially similar results. [10],[11],[12],[13],[14],[15],[16]

In a study it was found that at 6 months post-transplant, the benefit of ThalDex over VAD was not seen and the VGPR or better rates were comparable (44.4% in the ThalDex arm and 41.7% in the VAD arm). [14] Thus ASCT seems to cover for the seeming inefficiencies of these induction regimens.

4. Newer combinations

Bortezomib and dexamethasone

The doublet of bortezomib and dexamethasone (VD) has been associated with RR ranging from 67 to 88% (VGPR or better rates ranging from 23 to 47%) and CR/nCR rates ranging from 13 to 21%. Post-ASCT, RR in the range of 90%, CR/nCR rates of up to 35% and VGPR or better rates up to 62% have been described. [17],[18],[19],[20]

Lenalidomide and dexamethasone

Lenalidomide and dexamethasone (LD) use was associated with RR of 91% and 18% CR rates. In patients who underwent ASCT the 2 year OS and PFS was 92% and 83% respectively as compared to 90% and 59% for those who did not undergo ASCT. However the yield of stem cells diminished upon prolonged use of this combination and hence it has been suggested that an early stem cell harvest might be necessary in the case of patients planned for delayed ASCT. [21]

Bortezomib-based combinations with other drugs

Bortezomib, doxorubicin and dexamethasone (PAD) was evaluated as induction using bortezomib 1.3 mg/m 2 (PAD1, N=21) or 1.0 mg/m 2 (PAD2, N=20). Complete/very good partial response rates with PAD1/PAD2 were 62%/42% post-induction and 81%/53% post-transplant. PFS (29 vs. 24 months), OS (2 years: 95% vs. 73%) were statistically similar but favored PAD1 versus PAD2. [22] Thus standard dose bortezomib was associated with better response rates as compared to the lower dose in which however the toxicity was lesser. This result was also suggested in earlier reports. With low dose bortezomib, CR rates of 11% were seen which improved to 37% post-ASCT. [23] RR of 95% and CR rates of 24% was seen with standard dose bortezomib and post-ASCT CR rates improved to 57% (81% had VGPR or better responses). [24]

Liposomal doxorubicin-based regimens

Bortezomib, liposomal doxorubicin and dexamethasone have been used with RR 93% (63% VGPR or better) and CR rates of 43%. Following ASCT CR rates improved to 65% (75% of the responses were VGPR or better). [25]

In regimens excluding dexamethasone (Bortezomib, Liposomal Doxorubicin alone) RR of 79% and CR rates of 28% have been observed. [26]

The three drug regimen of dexamethasone, vincristine, liposomal doxorubicin (DVd) yielded response rates of 66%. [27] 4 drug regimens comprising of dexamethasone, vincristine, liposomal doxorubicin and thalidomide (DVd+T) have been used with RR 74-83% and CR rates varying from 10-36%. [28],[29]

Bortezomib and thalidomide/ lenalidomide combinations

The three drug combination (VTD) of bortezomib, thalidomide and dexamethasone has resulted in 87% RR and up to 36% CR/nCR rates. After ASCT, CR/nCR rates improved to 57%. VGPR or better rates were seen in 77% cases. In this GIMEMA trial the high CR rates achieved after induction with VTD were not influenced by the presence of deletion 13 or t(4;14) thus suggesting their role in overcoming high risk cytogenetics. [30]

Use of VDT PACE (cisplatin, doxorubicin, dexamethasone, etoposide) resulted in OR 89% and CR rates of 22%. After ASCT CR/nCR rates improved to 75%. [31]

The combination of lenalidomide, bortezomib, dexame-thasone yielded CR rates of 20% and RR of 87%. [32] Thus ASCT improves upon the response rates of the induction regimens including those incorporating newer agents.

4.1 Tandem transplants

Tandem transplants have been used to improve the results of ASCT. 69% CR rates were reported with tandem ASCT in a very select group of patients. [33] Barlogie reported a 41% CR rate with such a strategy (total therapy). [34] Attal et al compared single vs. tandem ASCT in 399 patients and found that though the CR rates were equivalent (42 vs. 50%), the 7 year EFS and OS were significantly improved (10% vs. 20% EFS, 21% vs. 42% OS), [35] while the Bologna [36] trial has not shown a significant benefit for tandem transplantation.

Tandem transplants are useful in patients having PR or stable disease in response to the first transplant and are not usually recommended in those who have had a CR or VGPR.

Additionally it has been suggested that the negative impact of having both cytogenetic abnormalities: deletion 13 and t(4;14), which were associated with very low VGPR rates with TD, were offset by tandem transplantation. The VGPR rates were 12% in this subgroup of patients as compared to VGPR rates of 41-50% in patients with either of these abnormalities when given an induction regimen comprising of TD. The 3 year PFS and OS were nearly identical after tandem ASCT (70% vs. 77% and 92% vs. 88%, respectively). [37]

4.2 Other agents in tandem ASCT

The total therapy II trial included thalidomide into the induction, consolidation, tandem ASCT and maintenance strategy. After transplantation the CR rate in the thalidomide arm was 62% vs. no thalidomide 43% and though the EFS improved (48% vs. 38%) there was no difference in OS because of the more aggressive nature of the disease at relapse in those who were on thalidomide. [38],[39]

The total therapy III trial has incorporated VDT-PACE into induction, consolidation, tandem ASCT and maintenance strategy and have reported 83% CR/nCR rates for patients 24 months into the program. [40]

With better CR/VGPR rates after a single ASCT seen upon incorporation of the newer induction regimens, the requirement of a tandem transplant is expected to reduce.

Use of drug combinations: Bortezomib and melphalan in the conditioning regimen

In a preliminary study, a combination of bortezomib and melphalan was used in the conditioning regimen in 35 poor risk patients (including those who did not achieve VGPR after a first transplant). Three months after ASCT, 63% VGPR including 31% CR was observed suggesting that the combination had the potential to better the responses seen with melphalan alone but this would require confirmation from other studies: especially from those in which bortezomib was used as the induction regimen. [41]

5. Renal failure and transplantation

The Arkansas group studied autologous SCT in 81 patients with renal failure (including 38 patients on dialysis). Melphalan 140 mg/ m 2 appeared as effective as melphalan 200 mg/ m 2 as a conditioning regimen and was less toxic. 13 (24%) of the 54 patients evaluable for renal function improvement became dialysis free at a median of 4 months after transplant. 5 year EFS and OS of 59 patients on dialysis at the time of ASCT were 24% and 36%. [42],[43]

The PETHEMA (Spanish) group reported studied 14 patients and reported a TRM of 29% and a 3 year OS of 49%. [44]

In another study involving 46 patients with myeloma and renal impairment (21% dialysis dependent), 15(32%) showed improvement of CrCl of at least 25% above baseline. TRM of 4% and 3 year PFS and OS of 36% and 64% were reported. [45]

6. Allogenic stem cell transplantation

Allogenic SCT has the potential to induce molecular remissions and is at least theoretically the only possible curative treatment modality. [46],[47] The high incidence of infections and GVHD has limited its utility.

Initial studies suggested a CR rate of 44%. The overall actuarial survival rate was 32% at 4 years and 28% at 7 years. The overall relapse-free survival rate of patients in CR after BMT was 34% at 6 years. [48]

Most studies have reported TRM's ranging from 37-55% while only the EBMT study (1994-1998) reported a TRM of 30%. [49] Data suggest that only 10-20% patients are long term survivors: many of them in molecular remission. [49],[50],[51],[52]

Neither use of peripheral blood stem cells or T cell depletion has resulted in a decrease in TRM. [53],[54]

In the Dutch-Belgian Hemato-Oncology Cooperative Group, T cell-depleted allogeneic transplantation in 53 patients resulted in a medial survival of only 25 months. [55]

A similar treatment strategy employed at Dana Farber in 66 patients resulted in a nonrelapse TRM of 35%, with a PFS at 4 years of 23%. [47]

The toxicities of the procedure limit it's use to the minority of patients who are less than 55 years of age and have a HLA matched donor. Even then, the high TRM results in short term survival benefits in favor of the auologous transplant as compared to the allogenic transplant thus making this treatment strategy unviable at most centers. [56]

7. Reduced intensity allogenic transplantation

This treatment strategy was implemented in order to reduce the TRM while retaining the graft versus myeloma effect. [57],[58],[59],[60],[61],[62],[63]

The conditioning regimens consisted of 1) Fludarabine /melphalan with / without in vivo T cell depletion with antithymocyte globulin (ATG) or alemtuzumab or 2) low dose TBI with/without fludarabine. [57],[58],[59],[60],[61],[62],[63]

This strategy has also been associated with substantial toxicity with a TRM of approximately 20%, acute GVHD rates of 30% and chronic GVHD rates of 50%. Low tumor burden at time of transplantation was associated with better survival. [57],[58],[59],[60],[61],[62],[63]

8. Tandem autologous and reduced intensity allogenic transplantation

The strategy of reducing tumor load with autologous transplant and following up with reduced intensity allogenic transplantation has also been studied. In one major study, TRM at 100 days was 11%, the incidence of acute and chronic GVHD were 38% and 40% respectively: the CR rate being 73%. [64]

Unrelated stem cell transplantation in multiple myeloma after a reduced-intensity conditioning with pretransplantation antithymocyte globulin has been studied and found to be effective with relatively low transplantation-related mortality: I year TRM of 26% and CR rate of 40%. [65]

RIST using TBI of 2 Gy as the conditioning regimen were associated with CR rates of 53-57%, chronic GVHD rates of 74% and an EFS of 36-37% with a PFS of 25-30% 6 years post transplant. [66],[67]

3 studies have compared tandem ASCT with tandem ASCT/ RIST. Tandem ASCT/RIST arms were associated with TRM ranging from 11-18%, 50% to 74% incidence of extensive chronic GVHD, one-third of the patients were on immunosuppressive drugs at 5 years, donor lymphocyte infusions were ineffective at relapse, and PFS and OS was similar to tandem ASCT except in the Italian study which found an increased CR rate and survival advantage with allogenic ASCT. [68],[69],[70] In view of these differing studies, the results of a major ongoing Bone Marrow Transplant Clinical Trial Network study are eagerly awaited.

In our opinion RIST should not be offered outside of a clinical trial in view of significant TRM and GVHD risks as compared to autologous SCT.

9. Conclusion

ASCT represents one of the most important therapeutic options in the treatment of eligible patients suffering from multiple myeloma.

Newer drugs like thalidomide, bortezomib and lenalidomide have resulted in a marked improvement in relapse rates.

Regimens like MPT (melphalan, prednisone and thalidomide), [71],[72],[73] MPV (melphalan, bortezomib and prednisone) [74] and MPR (melphalan, prednisone and lenalidomide) [75] have yielded impressive results with RR varying from 76% to 89% and CR rates varying from 15.6 to 30% in patients ineligible for transplantation.

The MPT regimen was in fact superior to the intermediate dose (melphalan 100 mg/m 2) ASCT. [73] However the survival benefit has to be assessed against high dose chemotherapy in order to claim equivalence or superiority to HDT-ASCT.

ASCT remains the standard of care in eligible patients. Better induction strategies will hopefully improve the results . There is a debate whether patients in CR/nCR or even VGPR after induction therapy should be subjected to upfront ASCT or placed on maintenance therapy. In such a situation ASCT could then serve as a treatment option at relapse. The role of allogenic transplantation also keeps evolving but is tempered by the spectre of increased procedure-related morbidity and mortality. Non myeloablative transplants done after initial ASCT offer some promise but at the expense of great morbidity and at present cannot be offered outside the purview of a clinical trial. .[76,77]

10. References

[1] Durie BG, Harousseau JL, Miguel JS, Bladé J, Barlogie B, Anderson K, et al. International uniform response criteria for multiple myeloma. Leukemia 2006;20:1467-73.

[2] Combination chemotherapy versus melphalan plus prednisone as treatment for multiple myeloma: An overview of 6633 patients from 27 randomized trials. Myeloma Trialists' Collaborative Group. J Clin Oncol 1998;16:3832-42.

[3] Attal M, Harousseau JL, Stoppa AM, Sotto JJ, Fuzibet JG, Rossi JF, et al. A prospective, randomized trial of autologous bone marrow transplantation and chemotherapy in multiple myeloma. N Engl J Med 1996;335:91-7

[4] Child JA, Morgan GJ, Davies FE, Owen RG, Bell SE, Hawkins K, et al. High-dose chemotherapy with hematopoietic stem-cell rescue for multiple myeloma. N Engl J Med 2003;348:1875-83.

[5] Bladé J, Rosiñol L, Sureda A, Ribera JM, Díaz-Mediavilla J, García-Laraña J, et al. High-dose therapy intensification compared with continued standard chemotherapy in multiple myeloma patients responding to the initial chemotherapy: Long-term results from a prospective randomized trial from the Spanish cooperative group PETHEMA. Blood 2005;106:3755-9.

[6] Fermand JP, Ravaud P, Chevret S, Divine M, Leblond V, Belanger C, et al. High-dose therapy and autologous peripheral blood stem cell transplantation in multiple myeloma: Up-front or rescue treatment? Results of a multicenter sequential randomized trial. Blood 1998;92:3131-6.

[7] Fermand JP, Katsahian S, Divine M, Leblond V, Dreyfus F, Macro M, et al. High-dose therapy and autologous blood stem-cell transplantation compared with conventional treatment in myeloma patients aged 55 to 65 years: Long-term results of a randomized control trial from the Group Myelome-Autogreffe. J Clin Oncol 2005;23:9227-33.

[8] Barlogie B, Kyle RA, Anderson KC, Greipp PR, Lazarus HM, Hurd DD, et al. Standard chemotherapy compared with high-dose chemoradiotherapy for multiple

myeloma: Final results of phase III US Intergroup Trial S9321. J Clin Oncol 2006;24:929-36.

[9] Wang M, Delasalle K, Thomas S. Complete remission represents the major surrogate marker of long term survival in multiple myeloma. Blood 2006;108:123a-4a.

[10] Alexanian R, Dimopoulos MA, Delasalle K, Barlogie B. Primary dexamethasone treatment of multiple myeloma. Blood 1992;80:887-90.

[11] Facon T, Mary JY, Pégourie B, Attal M, Renaud M, Sadoun A, et al. Dexamethasone-based regimens versus melphalan-prednisone for elderly multiple myeloma patients ineligible for high-dose therapy. Blood 2006;107:1292-8.

[12] Rajkumar SV, Blood E, Vesole D, Fonseca R, Greipp PR; Eastern Cooperative Oncology Group. Phase III clinical trial of thalidomide plus dexamethasone compared with dexam-ethasone alone in newly diagnosed multiple myeloma: A clinical trial coordinated by the Eastern Cooperative Oncology Group. J Clin Oncol 2006;24:431-6.

[13] Cavo M, Zamagni E, Tosi P, Tacchetti P, Cellini C, Cangini D, et al. Superiority of thalidomide and Dexamethsone over Vincristine-Doxorubicine-Dexamethasone (VAD) as primary therapy in preparation for autologous transplantation for multiple myeloma. Blood 2005;106:35-9

[14] Macro M, Divine M, Uzunban Y. Dexamethasone + Thalidomide compared to VAD as pre-transplant treatment in newly diagnosed multiple myeloma: A randomized trial. Blood Vol. 108. 2006.

[15] Lokhorst HM, Schmidt-Wolf I, Sonneveld P, van der Holt B, Martin H, Barge R, et al. Thalidomide in induction treatment increases the very good partial remission rate before and after high-dose therapy in previously untreated multiple myeloma. Haematologica 2008;93:124-7.

[16] Kumar SK, Dingli D, Dispenzieri A, Lacy MQ, Hayman SR, Buadi FK, et al. Impact of pretransplant therapy in patients with newly diagnosed myeloma undergoing autologous SCT. Bone Marrow Transplant 2008;41:1013-9.

[17] Harousseau JL, Attal M, Leleu X, Troncy J, Pegourie B, Stoppa AM, et al. Bortezomib plus dexamethasone as induction treatment prior to autologous transplantation in patients with newly diagnosed multiple myeloma: Results of an IFM phase II study. Haematologica 2006;91:1498-505.

[18] Jagannath S, Durie BG, Wolf JL. Long term follow up of patients treated with bortezomib alone and in combination wit dexamethasone as frontline therapy for multiple myeloma. Blood 2006;108:238a-9a.

[19] Rosiñol L, Oriol A, Mateos MV, Sureda A, García-Sánchez P, Gutiérrez N, et al. Phase II PETHEMA trial of alternating bortezomib and dexamethasone as induction regimen before autologous stem-cell transplantation in younger patients with multiple myeloma: efficacy and clinical implications of tumor response kinetics. J Clin Oncol 2007;25:4452-8.

[20] Harousseau JL, Marit G, Calliot D. VELCADE / dexamethasaone(Vel/Dex) versus VAD as induction treatment prior to autologous stem cell transplantation (ASCT) in newly diagnosed multiple myeloma: An interim analysis of the IFM 2005-01 randomized multicenter phase III trial. Blood 2006;108:21a.

[21] Rajkumar SV, Hayman SR, Lacy MQ, Dispenzieri A, Geyer SM, Kabat B, et al. Combination therapy with lenalidomide plus dexamethasone (Rev/Dex) for newly diagnosed myeloma. Blood 2005;106:4050-3.

[22] Popat R, Oakervee HE, Hallam S, Curry N, Odeh L, Foot N, et al. Bortezomib, doxorubicin and dexamethasone (PAD) front-line treatment of multiple myeloma: Updated results after long-term follow-up. Br J Haematol 2008;141:512-6.

[23] Oakervee HE, Popat R, Curry N, Smith P, Morris C, Drake M, et al. PAD combination therapy (PS-341/bortezomib, doxorubicin and dexamethasone) for previously untreated patients with multiple myeloma. Br J Haematol 2005;129:755-62.

[24] Popat R, Oakervee HE, Curry N. Reduced dose PAD combination therapy (PS-341/Bortezomib, adriamycin and dexamethasone) for previously untreated patients with multiple myeloma. Blood 2005;106:717a.

[25] Jakubowiak AJ, Al-Zoubi A, Kendall T. Combination therapy with bortezomib (VELCADE), Doxil, and dexamethasone (VDD) in newly diagnosed myeloma: Updated results of phase II clinical trial. Haematologica 2007;92:PO-721.

[26] Orlowski RZ, Peterson BL, Sanford B. Bortezomib and pegylated liposomal doxorubicin as induction therapy for adult patients with symptomatic multiple myeloma. Br J Haematol 2005;129:755-62.

[27] Zervas K, Mihou D, Katodritou I. VAD - doxil vs VAD doxil plus thalidomide as initial treatment in patients with multiple myeloma: a multicenter randomized trail of the Greek Myeloma Study Group. Blood 2006;108:238a.

[28] Hussein MA, Baz R, Srkalovic G, Agrawal N, Suppiah R, Hsi E, et al. Phase 2 study of pegylated liposomal doxorubicin, vincristine, decreased-frequency dexamethasone, and thalidomide in newly diagnosed and relapsed-refractory multiple myeloma. Mayo Clin Proc 2006;81:889-95.

[29] Zervas K, Dimopoulos MA, Hatzicharissi E, Anagnostopoulos A, Papaioannou M, Mitsouli Ch, et al. Primary treatment of multiple myeloma with thalidomide, vincristine, liposomal doxorubicin and dexamethasone (T-VAD doxil): A phase II multicenter study. Ann Oncol 2004;5:134-8.

[30] Cavo M, Patricia F, Tachetti P. Bortezomib (Velcade)-thalidomide-dexamethasone (VTD) vs thalidomide-dexamethasone (TD) in preparation for autologous stem cell transplantation (ASCT) in newly diagnosed multiple myeloma. Blood 2007;110:30a.

[31] Badros A, Goloubeva O, Fenton R, Rapoport AP, Akpek G, Harris C, et al. Phase I trial of first-line bortezomib/thalidomide plus chemotherapy for induction and stem cell mobilization in patients with multiple myeloma. Clin Lymphoma Myeloma 2006;7:210-6.

[32] Richardson PG, Jagannath S, Raje NS. Phase 1/2 study of upfront Rev/Vel/Dex in MM. Early results. Hematologica 2007;92:PO-715.

[33] Attal M, Harousseau JL. Randomized trial experience of the Intergroupe Francophone du Myélome. Semin Hematol 2001;38:226-30.

[34] Barlogie B, Jagannath S, Vesole DH, Naucke S, Cheson B, Mattox S, et al. Superiority of tandem autologous transplantation over standard therapy for previously untreated multiple myeloma. Blood 1997;89:789-93.

[35] Attal M, Harousseau JL, Facon T, Guilhot F, Doyen C, Fuzibet JG, et al. Single versus double autologous stem-cell transplantation for multiple myeloma. N Engl J Med 2003;349:2495-502.

[36] Cavo M, Tosi P, Zamagni E, Cellini C, Tacchetti P, Patriarca F, et al. Prospective, randomized study of single compared with double autologous stem-cell

transplantation for multiple myeloma: Bologna 96 clinical study. J Clin Oncol 2007;10:2434-41.

[37] Gertz MA, Lacy MQ, Dispenzieri A, Greipp PR, Litzow MR, Henderson KJ, et al. Clinical implications of t(11;14)(q13;q32), t(4;14)(p16.3;q32), and -17p13 in myeloma patients treated with high-dose therapy. Blood 2005;106:2837-40.

[38] Barlogie B, Tricot G, Anaissie E, Shaughnessy J, Rasmussen E, van Rhee F, et al. Thalidomide and hematopoietic-cell transplantation for multiple myeloma. N Engl J Med 2006;354:1021-30.

[39] Shaughnessy JD, Haessler J, Zeldis J. An update on the role of thalidomide (THAL) in Total Therapy 2 (TT2) for newly diagnosed patients with multiple myeloma (MM): Analysis of subgroups defined by standard prognostic factors (SPF) and gene expression profiling (GEP) - derived subgroups. Blood 2006;108:968a.

[40] Barlogie B, Anaissie E, van Rhee F, Haessler J, Hollmig K, Pineda-Roman M, et al. Incorporating bortezomib into upfront treatment for multiple myeloma: Early results of total therapy 3. Br J Hematol 2007;138:176-85.

[41] Attal M, Moreau P, Avet-Loiseau H, Harousseau JL. Stem cell transplantation in multiple myeloma. Hematology Am Soc Hematol Educ Program 2007. p. 311-6.

[42] Badros A, Barlogie B, Siegel E, Roberts J, Langmaid C, Zangari M, et al. Results of autologous stem cell transplant in multiple myeloma patients with renal failure. Br J Haematol 2001;114:822-9.

[43] Lee CK, Zangari M, Barlogie B, Fassas A, van Rhee F, Thertulien R, et al. Dialysis dependent renal failure in patients with myeloma can be reversed by high-dose myeloablative therapy and autotransplant. Bone Marrow Transplant 2004;33:823-8.

[44] San Miguel JF, Lahuerta JJ, García-Sanz R, Alegre A, Bladé J, Martinez R, et al. Are myeloma patients with renal failure candidates for autologous stem cell transplantation? Hematol J 2000;1:28-36.

[45] Parikh GC, Amjad AI, Saliba RM, Kazmi SM, Khan ZU, Lahoti A, et al. Autologous hematopoietic stem cell transplantation may reverse renal failure in patients with multiple myeloma. Biol Blood Marrow Transplant 2009;15:812-6.

[46] Tricot G, Vesole DH, Jagannath S, Hilton J, Munshi N, Barlogie B. Graft-versus-myeloma effect: proof of principle. Blood 1996;87:1196-8.

[47] Alyea E, Weller E, Schlossman R, Canning C, Mauch P, Ng A, et al. Outcome after autologous and allogeneic stem cell transplantation for patients with multiple myeloma: impact of graft-versus-myeloma effect. Bone Marrow Transplant 2003;32:1145-51.

[48] Gahrton G, Tura S, Ljungman P, Blade J, Brandt L, Cavo M, et al. Prognostic factors in allogeneic bone marrow transplantation for multiple myeloma. J Clin Oncol 1995;13:1312-22.

[49] Gahrton G, Svensson H, Cavo M, Bacigalupo A, Björkstrand B, Bladé J, et al. Progress in allogeneic bone marrow and peripheral blood stem cell transplantation for multiple myeloma: a comparison between transplants performed 1983-93 and 1994-98 at European Group for Blood and Marrow Transplantation centres. Br J Haematol 2001;113:209-16.

[50] Crawley C, Iacobelli S, Björkstrand B, Apperley JF, Niederwieser D, Gahrton G. Reduced-intensity conditioning for myeloma: lower nonrelapse mortality but

higher relapse rates compared with myeloablative conditioning. Blood 2007;109:3588-94.

[51] Gahrton G, Tura S, Ljungman P, Bladé J, Brandt L, Cavo M, et al. Prognostic factors in allogeneic bone marrow transplantation for multiple myeloma. J Clin Oncol 1995;13:1312-22.

[52] Bensinger WI, Buckner CD, Anasetti C, Clift R, Storb R, Barnett T, et al. Allogeneic marrow transplantation for multiple myeloma: an analysis of risk factors and outcome. Blood 1996;88:2787-93.

[53] Gahrton G, Iacobelli S, Bandini G, Björkstrand B, Corradini P, Crawley C, et al. Peripheral blood or bone marrow cells in reduced-intensity or myeloablative conditioning allogeneic HLA identical sibling donor transplantation for multiple myeloma. Haematologica 2007;92:1513-8.

[54] Bladé J, Rosiñol L, Cibeira MT, Rovira M, Carreras E. Hematopoietic stem cell transplantation for multiple myeloma beyond 2010. Blood 2010;115:3655-63.

[55] Lokhorst HM, Segeren CM, Verdonck LF, van der Holt B, Raymakers R, van Oers MH, et al. Partially T-cell depleted allogeneic stem-cell transplantation for first-line treatment of multiple myeloma: a prospective evaluation of patients treated in the phase III study Hovon 24 MM. J Clin Oncol 2003;21:1728-33.

[56] Harousseau JL. The allogeneic dilemma. Bone Marrow Transplant 2007;40:1123-8.

[57] Giralt S, Aleman A, Anagnostopoulos A, Weber D, Khouri I, Anderlini P, et al. Fludarabine/melphalan conditioning for allogeneic transplantation in patients with multiple myeloma. Bone Marrow Transplant 2002;30:367-73.

[58] Einsele H, Schafer HJ, Hebart H, Bader P, Meisner C, Plasswilm L, et al. Follow-up of patients with progressive multiple myeloma undergoing allograft after reduced-intensity conditioning. Br J Haematol 2003;121:411-8.

[59] Pérez-Simón JA, Martino R, Alegre A, Tomais JF, De Leon A, Caballero D, et al. Chronic but not acute graft-versus-host disease improves outcome in multiple myeloma patients after non-myeloablative allogeneic transplantation. Br J Haematol 2003;121:104-8.

[60] Lee CK, Badros A, Barlogie B, Morris C, Zangari M, Fassas A, et al. Prognostic factors in allogeneic transplantation for patients with high-risk multiple myeloma alter reduced intensity conditioning. Exp Hematol 2003;31:73-80.

[61] Peggs KS, MacKinnon S, Williams CD, D'Sa S, Thuraisundaram D, Kyriakou C, et al. Reduced-intensity transplantation with in vivo T-cell depletion and adjuvant dose-escalating donor lymphocyte infusions for chemotherapy-sensitive myeloma: limited efficacy of graft-versus-tumor activity. Biol Blood Marrow Transplant 2003;9:257-65.

[62] Crawley C, Lalancette M, Szydlo R, Gilleece M, Peggs K, Mackinnon S, et al. Outcomes for reduced-intensity allogeneic transplantation for multiple myeloma: an analysis of prognostic factors from the Chronic Leukemia Myeloma Working Party of the EBMT. Blood 2005;105:4532-9.

[63] Kröger N, Pérez-Simón JA, Myint H, Klingemann H, Shimoni A, Nagler A, et al. Relapse to prior autograft and chronic graft-versus-host disease are the strongest prognostic factors for outcome of melphalan/fludarabine-based dose-reduced allogeneic stem cell transplantation in patients with multiple myeloma. Biol Blood Marrow Transplant 2004;10:698-708.

[64] Kröger N, Schwerdtfeger R, Kiehl M, Sayer H, Helmut Renges H, Zabelina T, et al Autologous stem cell transplantation followed by a dose reduced allograft induces high complete remission rate in multiple myeloma. Blood 2002;100:755-60.

[65] Kröger N, Sayer H, Schweerdtfeger R, Kiehl M, Nagler A, Renges H, et al. Unrelated stem cell transplantation in multiple myeloma after reduced intensity conditioning with pre-transplantation antithymocyte globulin is highly effective with low transplantation-related mortality. Blood 2002;100:3919-24.

[66] Rotta M, Storer BE, Sahebi F, Shizuru JA, Bruno B, Lange T, et al. Long-term outcome of patients with multiple myeloma after autologous hematopoietic cell transplantation and nonmyeloablative allografting. Blood 2009;113:3383-91.

[67] Bruno B, Rotta M, Patriarca F, Mattei D, Allione B, Carnevale-Schianca F, et al. Nonmyeloablative allografting for newly diagnosed multiple myeloma: the experience of the Gruppo Italiano Trapianti di Midollo. Blood 2009;113:3375-82.

[68] Garban F, Attal M, Michallet M, Hulin C, Bourhis JH, Yakoub-Agha I, et al. Prospective comparison of autologous stem cell transplantation followed by dose-reduced allograft (IFM99-03 trial) with tandem autologous stem cell transplantation (IFM99-04 trial) in high risk de novo multiple myeloma. Blood 2006;107:3474-80.

[69] Bruno B, Rotta M, Patriarca F, Mordini N, Allione B, Carnevale-Schianca F, et al. A comparison of allografting with autograft for newly diagnosed myeloma. N Engl J Med 2007;356:1110-20.

[70] Rosiñol L, Pérez-Simón JA, Sureda A, de la Rubia J, de Arriba F, Lahuerta JJ, et al. A prospective PETHEMA study of tandem autologous transplantation versus autograft followed by reduced-intensity conditioning allogeneic transplantation in newly diagnosed multiple myeloma. Blood 2008;112:3591-93.

[71] Palumbo A, Bringhen S, Caravita T, Merla E, Capparella V, Callea V, et al. Oral melphalan and prednisone chemotherapy plus thalidomide compared with melphalan and prednisone alone in elderly patients with multiple myeloma: Randomised controlled trial. Lancet 2006;367:825-31.

[72] Palumbo A, Bringhen S, Liberati AM, Caravita T, Falcone A, Callea V, et al. Oral melphalan, prednisone, and thalidomide in elderly patients with multiple myeloma: Updated results of a randomized controlled trial. Blood 2008;112:3107-14.

[73] Facon T, Mary JY, Hulin C, Benboubker L, Attal M, Pegourie B, et al. Melphalan and prednisone plus thalidomide versus melphalan and prednisone alone or reduced-intensity autologous stem cell transplantation in elderly patients with multiple myeloma (IFM 99-06): A randomised trial. Lancet 2007;370:1209-18.

[74] San Miguel JF, Schlag R, Khuageva NK, Dimopoulos MA, Shpilberg O, Kropff M, et al. Bortezomib plus melphalan and prednisone for initial treatment of multiple myeloma. N Engl J Med 2008;359:906-17.

[75] Palumbo A, Falco P, Corradini P, Falcone A, Di Raimondo F, Giuliani N, et al. Melphalan, prednisone, and lenalidomide treatment for newly diagnosed myeloma: A report from the GIMEMA-Italian Multiple Myeloma Network. J Clin Oncol 2007;25:4459-65.

[76] Gupta A, Kumar L. Evolving role of high dose stem cell therapy in multiple myeloma. Indian J Med Paediatr Oncol 2011;32:17-24.

[77] Gupta A. Autologous Stem Cell Transplantation—An Important Step Toward Improving Survival in Multiple Myeloma. US Oncological Review, 2010;6:24–7

CPSIA information can be obtained
at www.ICGtesting.com
Printed in the USA
LVHW061532281222
736047LV00007B/160

9 789533 077680